SCIENCE *of*

UNDERSTAND THE ANATOMY AND PHYSIOLOGY TO TRANSFORM YOUR BODY

STRENGTH TRAINING

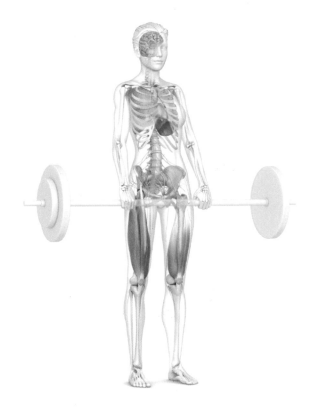

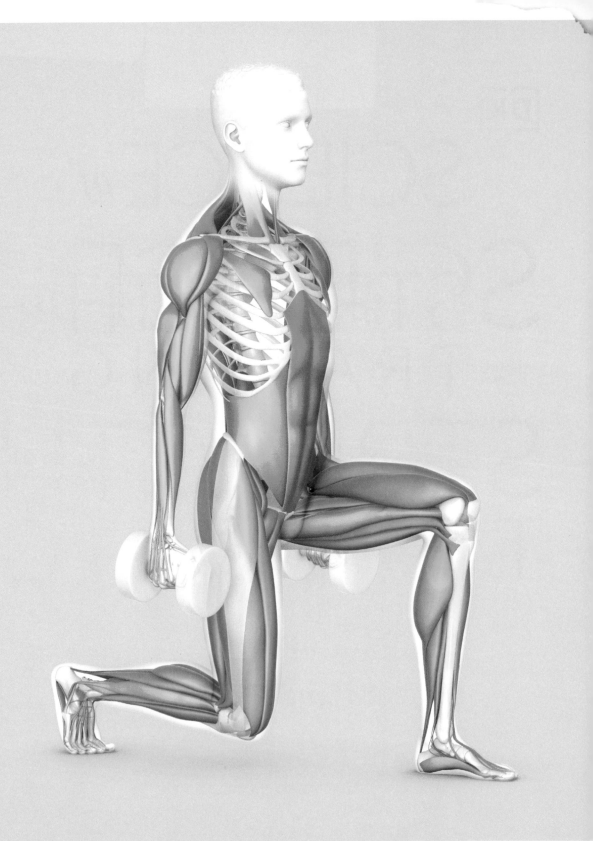

SCIENCE *of*

UNDERSTAND THE ANATOMY AND PHYSIOLOGY TO TRANSFORM YOUR BODY

STRENGTH TRAINING

Austin Current, CSCS, CISSN

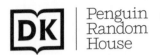

Senior Editor Nikki Sims
Senior Art Editor Clare Joyce
Editor Megan Lea
Project Art Editor Karen Constanti
Editorial Assistant Kiron Gill
Production Editor David Almond
US Editor Kayla Dugger
Production Controller Luca Bazzoli
Jacket Designer Amy Cox
Jacket Editor Lucy Philpott

Senior Editor Alastair Laing
Senior Art Editor Barbara Zuniga
Managing Editor Dawn Henderson
Managing Art Editor
Marianne Markham
Art Director Maxine Pedliham
Publishing Director Katie Cowan

Illustrations Arran Lewis

First American Edition, 2021
Published in the United States by
DK Publishing
1450 Broadway, Suite 801,
New York, NY 10018

A catalog record for this book
is available from the Library of Congress.
ISBN 978-0-7440-2695-5

Printed and bound in Latvia

For the curious
www.dk.com

CONTENTS

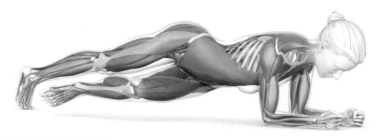

INTRODUCTION

When it comes to strength training, also known as resistance training, knowledge is power. Most often, the largest barrier for participation in strength training is the complexity of resistance programs or lack of knowledge in the gym. The aim of this book is to break down this barrier, teaching you both the science behind strength training, how to perform exercises properly (at the gym or at home), and offering clear and simple programs for beginners and those wanting to challenge themselves. Whatever your current level of knowledge or abilities, you'll find the information and tools you need to better learn, understand, and confidently perform strength training exercises—whether as a standalone activity or in combination with other forms of exercise.

THE BENEFITS OF STRENGTH TRAINING

The exercises in this book not only improve muscular strength and endurance, but also boost overall health. Incorporating strength training into your everyday life will bring with it a multitude of positive effects:

- **Lowers the risk of a number of diseases**, such as cardiovascular disease and type 2 diabetes
- **Promotes muscle growth and retention** and counters the age-related reductions in muscle mass and muscle strength and in bone density across a lifespan
- **Improves cognitive function, memory, and concentration**
- **Prevents age-related illness**, such as Alzheimer's disease and dementia
- **Lowers the risk and the severity of depression and anxiety**

HOW THE BOOK WORKS

The first section—human physiology—introduces you to the wonder that is skeletal muscle and the mechanisms that underpin strength training's demands on the body. It will help you understand how muscles work and grow and how resistance work stimulates muscles to develop size and strength, alongside its positive impacts on bones and connective tissue. It also explains how the body powers muscular work and shows you how to calculate your own daily fuel and macronutrient requirements. Last, but by no means least, comes an overview of the benefits to the brain and the crucial role it plays in attitude and mental health.

Much of the book is devoted to a comprehensive list of strength exercises to perform, along with many variations offered to complement your available training equipment, personal preferences, and level of challenge. The exercises are organized according to which muscle group they target. Each displays the

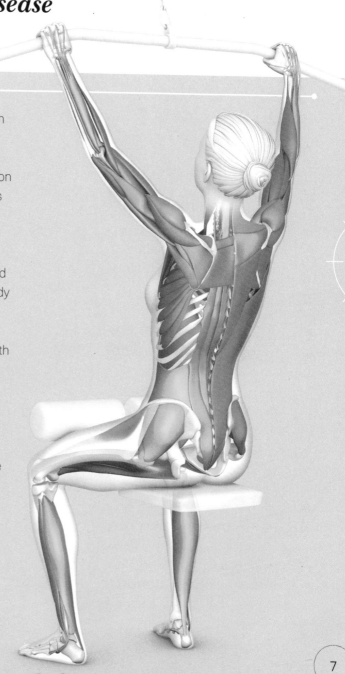

> ## *Consistent strength training improves **health** and **well-being** and **lowers the risk of disease** across a lifespan.*

muscles being used throughout the movement, with detailed instructions on how to achieve proper form and technique; and common mistakes are covered.

The section on preventing injury explores common injuries related to resistance work, with explanations of how to avoid them and how to return to training if you do suffer an injury. A consistent and structured routine, including a proper warm-up, prepares the body for work, and the various mobility exercises and stretches given will help you tune in to how your body is responding to the training.

The how to train section outlines everything you need to know about the variables of effective strength training, such as training volume and fatigue management. Whether you want to build muscle, strength, or endurance, you'll find an easy-to-follow program to suit, as well as alternatives for those wanting regular or more intense workouts. These programs form the base for your training and can be adjusted in the months and years to come.

Austin Current BSc, CSCS, CISSN
Fitness coach and educator

STRENGTH TRAINING FOR EVERYONE

We know now that everyone benefits from including strength training in their day-to-day lives. There is plenty of contradictory advice out there, but take a read through this debunking of common myths related to resistance work and discover what body type you are and if that matters.

MYTH   FACT

BODY TYPE OR GENETICS

*I have **bad** genes*

GENETICS MATTER BUT AREN'T EVERYTHING

Research has shown that being told you are bad at something, regardless of gene expression, can negatively impact your performance. As accurate genetic testing is out of reach for most, it's important to not limit yourself through labeling and to believe in yourself, which can produce a positive outcome.

*I haven't seen results. **It doesn't work***

IT DOES. INDIVIDUAL VARIATIONS MEAN A CHANGE OF PROGRAM IS NEEDED

Some people may respond more than others. Simply because you didn't respond to one specific program doesn't mean you will not have success with another. If you're not seeing results, it's time to revisit your current regime (see p.198).

AGE

*I am **too young** for strength training*

NO. WITH SUPERVISION, TRAINING CAN START AT 11 FOR GIRLS AND 13 FOR BOYS

A properly designed and supervised strength training program has been shown to be relatively safe, plus it comes with a host of other benefits from improved motor skills to enhanced well-being, as well as developing exercise habits early in life.

*I am **too old** for strength training*

NO. THE BENEFITS CAN COUNTERACT AGE-RELATED LOSSES

Strength training is the most effective standalone exercise strategy for counteracting age-related loss of muscle mass, strength, and power. Being stronger helps prevent the loss of physical function and independence common in older people.

MYTH

FACT

> *Strength training is* **only for men**

EVERYONE CAN BENEFIT

The manybenefits of resistance work (see also pp.6–7) are universal across genders. It's the most effective way of reshaping your body, adding muscle, and losing fat in areas you want to improve. Women benefit just as much as men do from strength training, whatever their improvement goals are.

> *Strength training causes* **women to get bulky**

EXCESSIVE MUSCLE IS LIMITED BY ESTROGEN

A woman's abilitiy to build excessive amounts of muscle tissue is limited by her natural hormones. Women have higher levels of estrogen and lower levels of testosterone, which can help in recovery and in retention of muscle tissue.

> *Men grow* **more muscle** *than women*

EVERYONE EXPERIENCES SIMILAR LEVELS OF MUSCLE GROWTH

Men and women have been shown to experience similar levels of muscle growth with strength training, but importantly, women start from a lower baseline. Men do experience more absolute gains due to their high levels of testosterone.

AM I LIMITED BY BODY SHAPE?

Your current body shape is not set for life; you can change and improve your physique through strength training. You may identify with one of the three body types (also known as somatotypes, see right) now, but you shouldn't let your current body shape dictate your training recommendations. Managing stress, sleep, and nutrition, as well as physical activity, will all impact your body shape.

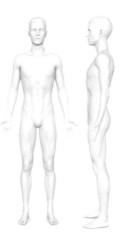

ECTOMORPH
Tall and leaner individuals who have a harder time building muscle but lose fat more easily.

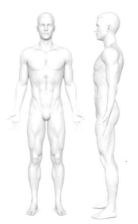

ENDOMORPH
Bulkier and larger individuals who have an easy time gaining muscle but a harder time losing body fat.

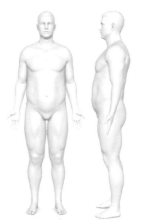

MESOMORPH
Lean and muscular individuals who have an easy time building muscle and do not have a challenge losing body fat.

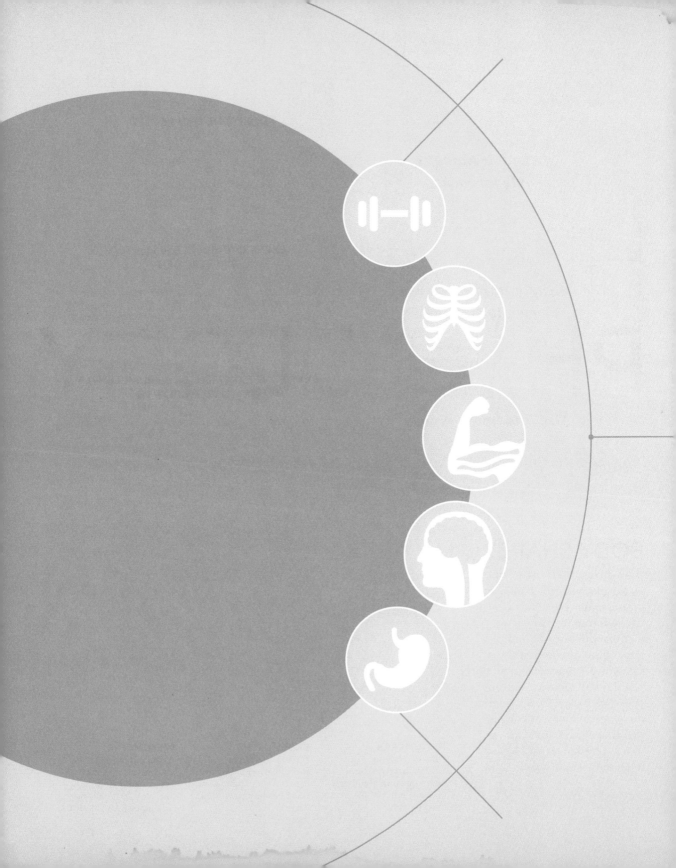

HUMAN
PHYSIOLOGY

As well as building strength and muscle, strength training also has positive impacts on bone density and connective tissue, on the risk of metabolic disorders and cardiovascular diseases, and on psychology and mental health. Grow your understanding of how strength training affects the body and the nutrition it takes to maximize health, performance, and recovery.

MUSCULAR
ANATOMY

There are over 600 muscles in your body—some deep inside your body, others more superficial. Skeletal muscles are attached to bones via tendons and facilitate movement.

SKELETAL MUSCLE

Muscle creates movement through coordinated contractions of skeletal muscle fibers. If you locate, study, and become familiar with the major muscle groups of your body, you can use this knowledge to visualize how the muscles function, as well as build greater mechanical tension during strength training exercises.

Pectorals
Pectoralis major
Pectoralis minor

Intercostal muscles

Brachialis

Abdominals
Rectus abdominis
External abdominal obliques
Internal abdominal obliques
(deep, not shown)
Transversus abdominis

Hip flexors
Iliopsoas (iliacus and psoas major)
Rectus femoris (see quadriceps)
Sartorius
Adductors (see below)

Adductors
Adductor longus
Adductor brevis
Adductor magnus
Pectineus
Gracilis

Quadriceps
Rectus femoris
Vastus medialis
Vastus lateralis
Vastus intermedius
(deep, not shown)

Ankle dorsiflexors
Tibialis anterior
Extensor digitorum longus
Extensor hallucis longus

SUPERFICIAL   **DEEP**

A zoomed-in view shows myofibrils lined up with one another

Elbow flexors
Biceps brachii
Brachialis (deep)
Brachioradialis

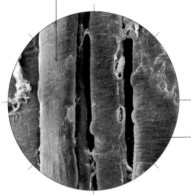

Visible stripes (striations) reflect the arrangement of muscle proteins (see p.15)

Skeletal muscle fibers
Striated skeletal muscle is responsible for producing force and creating movement during strength training. A single muscle comprises thousands of myofibrils arranged parallel to each other (see also pp.14–15).

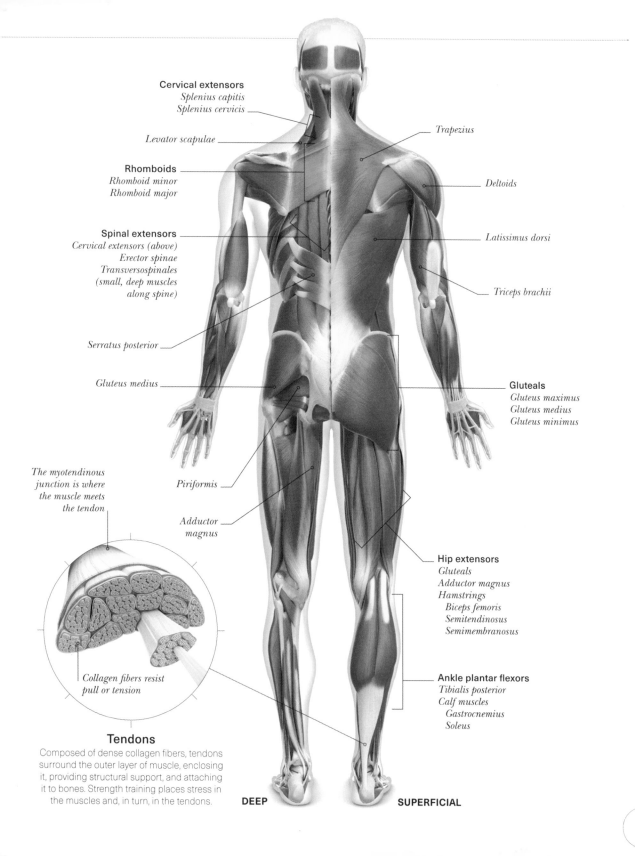

Cervical extensors
Splenius capitis
Splenius cervicis

Levator scapulae

Rhomboids
Rhomboid minor
Rhomboid major

Spinal extensors
Cervical extensors (above)
Erector spinae
Transversospinales
(small, deep muscles
along spine)

Serratus posterior

Gluteus medius

The myotendinous
junction is where
the muscle meets
the tendon

Piriformis

Adductor
magnus

Collagen fibers resist
pull or tension

Tendons
Composed of dense collagen fibers, tendons
surround the outer layer of muscle, enclosing
it, providing structural support, and attaching
it to bones. Strength training places stress in
the muscles and, in turn, in the tendons.

Trapezius

Deltoids

Latissimus dorsi

Triceps brachii

Gluteals
Gluteus maximus
Gluteus medius
Gluteus minimus

Hip extensors
Gluteals
Adductor magnus
Hamstrings
Biceps femoris
Semitendinosus
Semimembranosus

Ankle plantar flexors
Tibialis posterior
Calf muscles
Gastrocnemius
Soleus

DEEP   **SUPERFICIAL**

HOW MUSCLES WORK

Muscles are attached to bones via tendons, which can stretch to help deal with forces produced by movement. Muscles often work in antagonistic pairs to control the movement around a joint, such as the arm curl shown here. They can contract in many different ways.

TYPES OF CONTRACTION

In strength training, three types of contraction are referred to as isotonic—which is broken down into eccentric and concentric—and isometric. These names describe how a muscle is changing. For instance, isotonic involves a change in muscle length; eccentric contractions involve lengthening of a muscle, while concentric involve shortening. In an isometric movement, a muscle is activated but doesn't cause any movement, as there is no change in the muscle's length. (See also pp.20–21.)

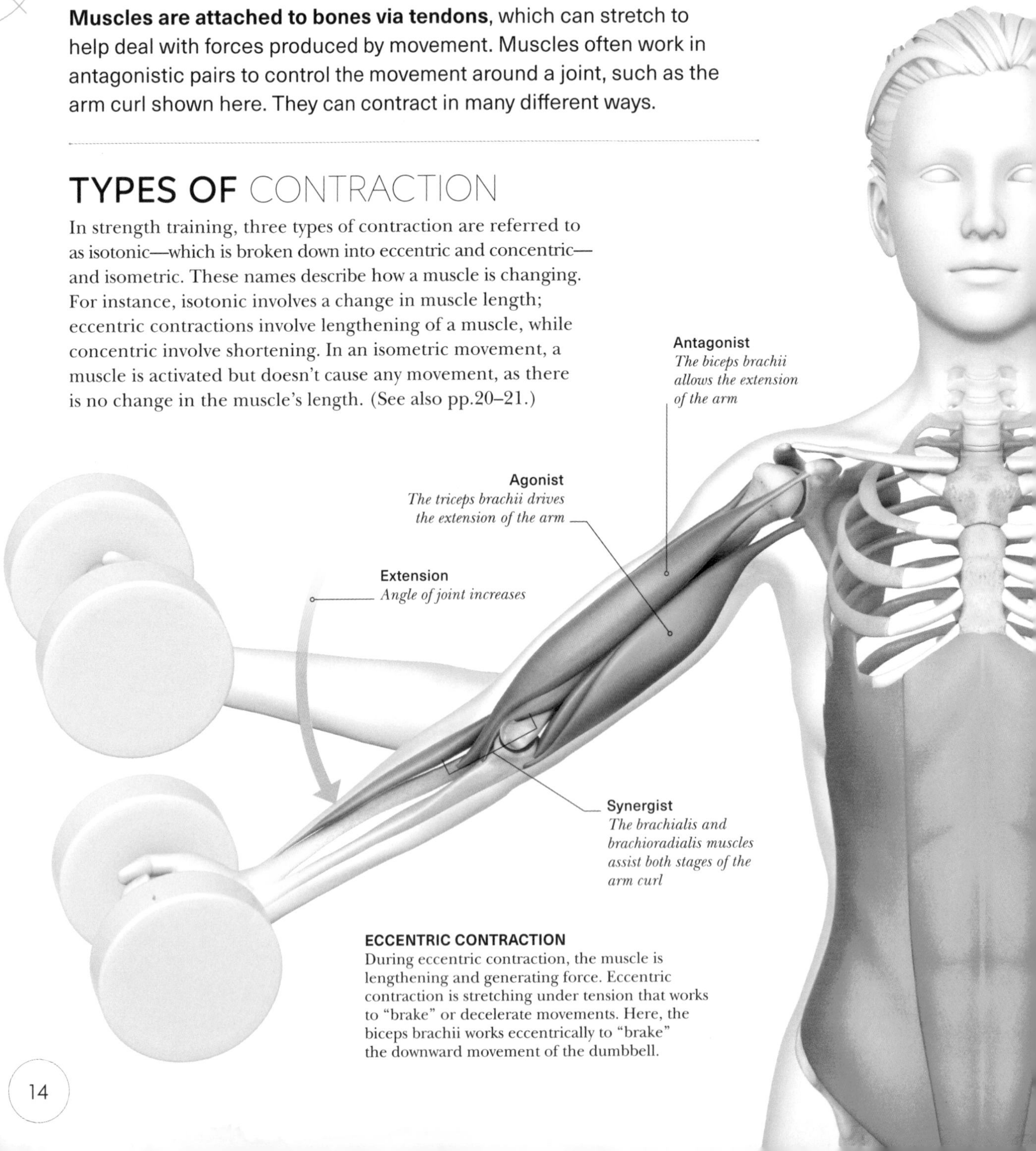

Antagonist
The biceps brachii allows the extension of the arm

Agonist
The triceps brachii drives the extension of the arm

Extension
Angle of joint increases

Synergist
The brachialis and brachioradialis muscles assist both stages of the arm curl

ECCENTRIC CONTRACTION
During eccentric contraction, the muscle is lengthening and generating force. Eccentric contraction is stretching under tension that works to "brake" or decelerate movements. Here, the biceps brachii works eccentrically to "brake" the downward movement of the dumbbell.

HOW MUSCLES
WORK TOGETHER

Muscles can only pull—they cannot push.
To that end, they often work in antagonistic
pairs. The prime mover, also known as the
agonist, works alongside the synergist to
create the joint motion. The antagonist,
the muscle that opposes the prime mover,
helps in controlling the movement on the
other side of the joint.

Refining movements

When you first start performing strength
training exercises, your nervous system tries
to activate both agonist and antagonist at the
same time, which results in "choppy" and
less coordinated movements. Over time and
with practice, your nervous system adapts
(see also p.37) and coactivation is reduced
in the antagonist muscle group, resulting in
a smoother and more efficient joint action,
as well as more potential force production.

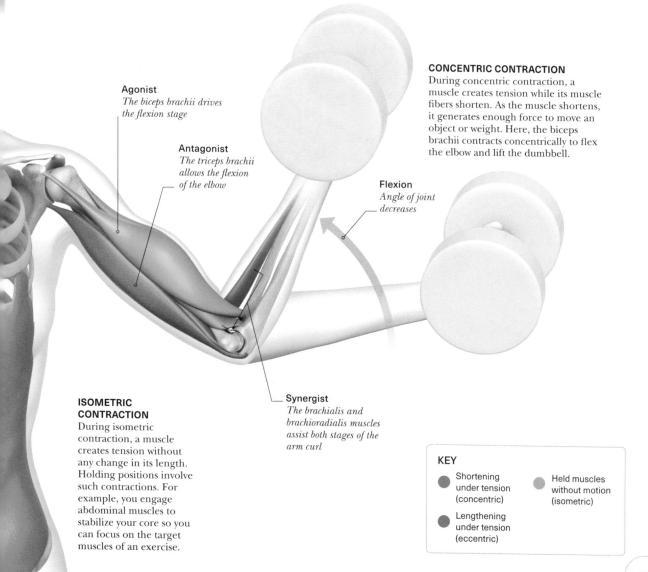

Agonist
*The biceps brachii drives
the flexion stage*

Antagonist
*The triceps brachii
allows the flexion
of the elbow*

Flexion
*Angle of joint
decreases*

CONCENTRIC CONTRACTION
During concentric contraction, a
muscle creates tension while its muscle
fibers shorten. As the muscle shortens,
it generates enough force to move an
object or weight. Here, the biceps
brachii contracts concentrically to flex
the elbow and lift the dumbbell.

**ISOMETRIC
CONTRACTION**
During isometric
contraction, a muscle
creates tension without
any change in its length.
Holding positions involve
such contractions. For
example, you engage
abdominal muscles to
stabilize your core so you
can focus on the target
muscles of an exercise.

Synergist
*The brachialis and
brachioradialis muscles
assist both stages of the
arm curl*

KEY

● Shortening
under tension
(concentric)

● Lengthening
under tension
(eccentric)

● Held muscles
without motion
(isometric)

UNRAVELING **A MUSCLE'S STRUCTURE**

Skeletal muscle comprises cylindrical bundles of muscle fibers known as fascicles. Each muscle fiber—also a muscle cell—is constructed from contractile protein filaments that produce muscle contraction. Each muscle also has a vascular network that transports oxygen and chemical substrates for energy production (see also pp.28–29) and removes waste generated by muscular contractions.

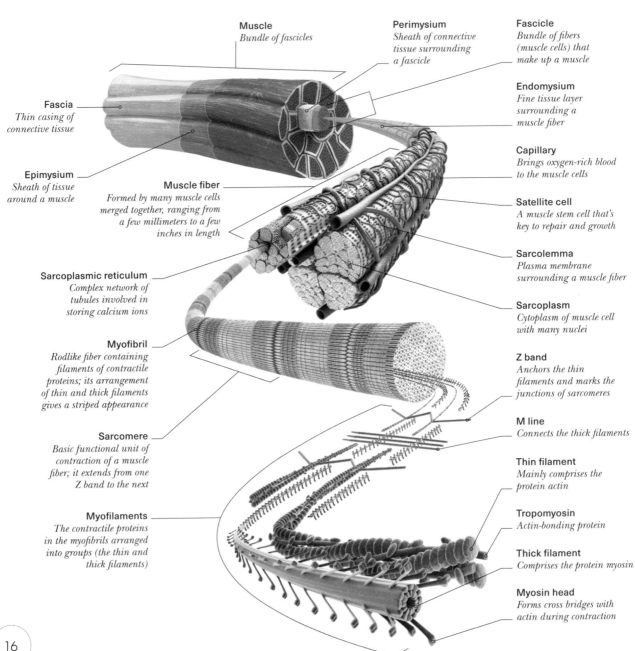

Muscle
Bundle of fascicles

Perimysium
Sheath of connective tissue surrounding a fascicle

Fascicle
Bundle of fibers (muscle cells) that make up a muscle

Fascia
Thin casing of connective tissue

Endomysium
Fine tissue layer surrounding a muscle fiber

Capillary
Brings oxygen-rich blood to the muscle cells

Epimysium
Sheath of tissue around a muscle

Muscle fiber
Formed by many muscle cells merged together, ranging from a few millimeters to a few inches in length

Satellite cell
A muscle stem cell that's key to repair and growth

Sarcolemma
Plasma membrane surrounding a muscle fiber

Sarcoplasmic reticulum
Complex network of tubules involved in storing calcium ions

Sarcoplasm
Cytoplasm of muscle cell with many nuclei

Myofibril
Rodlike fiber containing filaments of contractile proteins; its arrangement of thin and thick filaments gives a striped appearance

Z band
Anchors the thin filaments and marks the junctions of sarcomeres

M line
Connects the thick filaments

Sarcomere
Basic functional unit of contraction of a muscle fiber; it extends from one Z band to the next

Thin filament
Mainly comprises the protein actin

Tropomyosin
Actin-bonding protein

Myofilaments
The contractile proteins in the myofibrils arranged into groups (the thin and thick filaments)

Thick filament
Comprises the protein myosin

Myosin head
Forms cross bridges with actin during contraction

Slow- and fast-twitch muscle fibers

There are two main types of skeletal muscle fibers: slow-twitch (or type 1) and fast-twitch (type 2). Your nervous system automatically chooses the right type of fiber for the given exercise. The majority of skeletal muscles have a fairly even split of both types of fiber, allowing for the ability to perform a variety of tasks of different magnitudes and durations.

Fast-twitch fibers contract quickly but tire quickly; used for higher-intensity or explosive actions

Slow-twitch fibers contract more slowly and keep going for longer; used for endurance activities

FORCE

TIME (MSEC) 200

HOW SLOW- AND FAST-TWITCH MUSCLES COMPARE

Muscle contraction at the microscopic level

The shortening and lengthening of skeletal muscle is achieved by contractile protein filaments in the myofibril—actin and myosin. A nervous impulse triggers a cycle of events within the muscle fiber. The filaments of actin and myosin attach, bend, detach, and then reattach through a repeated sequence to pull the actin filaments toward the center of the sarcomere, creating tension within a muscle.

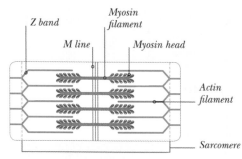

Z band
M line
Myosin filament
Myosin head
Actin filament
Sarcomere

RELAXED MUSCLE

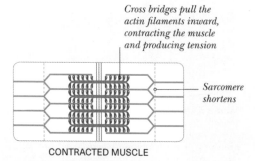

Cross bridges pull the actin filaments inward, contracting the muscle and producing tension

Sarcomere shortens

CONTRACTED MUSCLE

THE CYCLE OF CONTRACTION

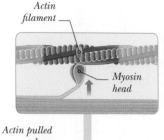

Actin filament
Myosin head

ATTACHMENT
The activated myosin head attaches to binding site on the actin filament, forming what's known as a cross bridge between the filaments.

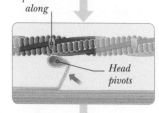

Actin pulled along
Head pivots

POWER STROKE
The myosin head pivots and bends, pulling the actin filament toward the M line and bringing the Z bands closer together.

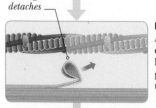

Cross bridge detaches

DETACHMENT
A molecule of ATP (chemical energy) binds to the myosin head, causing it to loosen its grip on the actin filament; the cross bridge detaches.

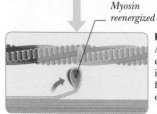

Myosin reenergized

REENERGIZING
ATP releases energy to convert the myosin head from its bent position to its upright form, ready for the next cycle of contraction to begin.

HOW MUSCLES GROW

Muscle cell growth—or muscle hypertrophy—can be generally defined as an increase in size of skeletal muscle tissue. Strength training stimulates muscle hypertrophy via various routes, and specialist cells maintain, repair, and grow new muscle.

STIMULI OF GROWTH

The current proposed understanding of what is occurring during the growth of skeletal muscle concerns three related stimuli: mechanical tension (the tension placed on a muscle fiber during strength training), metabolic stress (the accumulation of metabolic byproducts within the muscle fiber during training), and muscle damage (the microtears to the muscle fiber and disruption of the Z band).

The primary driver of muscle growth is mechanical tension. Fatigue, in part caused by the metabolic stress, raises mechanical tension, recruits more motor neurons to the muscle, and slows muscle fiber shortening. This combination of changes raises the number of muscles controlled, which accentuates the amount of mechanical tension produced. The resulting two-way relationship boosts tension further; metabolic stress is a byproduct of mechanical tension and also contributes to raising tension within a muscle.

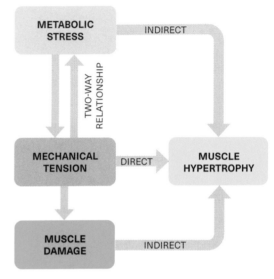

MECHANISMS OF HYPERTROPHY

HOW MUSCLES GET BIGGER

Skeletal muscle protein cycles through periods of synthesis and breakdown on a daily basis (see also p.34). Muscle growth occurs whenever the rate of muscle protein synthesis is greater than the rate of muscle protein breakdown. Muscle hypertrophy is thought to be a collection of adaptations to different components—the myofibrils, the sarcoplasmic fluid, and the connective tissue.

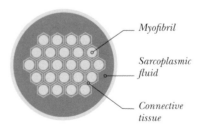

Myofibril

Sarcoplasmic fluid

Connective tissue

MUSCLE FIBER BEFORE GROWTH
The circle represents a muscle fiber in cross-section. Within there are many myofibrils, and surrounding them is sarcoplasmic fluid and a honeycomblike layer of connective tissue.

SATELLITE CELLS

Muscle satellite cells are a type of stem cell that plays a key role in the maintenance, repair (and growth), and remodeling of muscle fibers in response to exercise, especially strength training. Typically, they are dormant until needed. When stimulated, satellite cells can help form new muscle fibers, help an existing muscle fiber by donating their nuclei, or return to replenish the pool of satellite cells.

The decline of muscle mass with age

Muscle atrophy (the opposite of hypertrophy) is defined as the wasting or reduction in size of muscle tissue. Such a reduction in muscle is linked to poor quality of life and increased morbidity. After the age of 40, the body progressively loses muscle mass each year. However, consistent resistance training along with a good intake of protein (see pp.30–31) has been shown to reduce this progressive loss. The completion of physical activity, specifically strength training, can prevent and treat the conditions of sarcopenia (muscle loss) and dynapenia (loss of muscle strength and power).

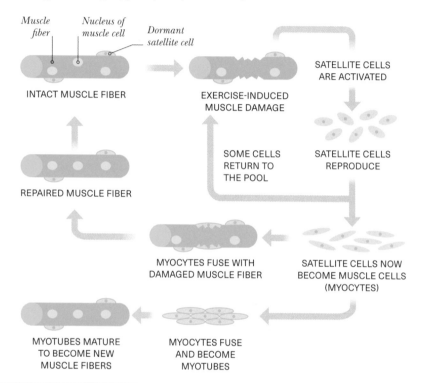

Muscle fiber *Nucleus of muscle cell* *Dormant satellite cell*

INTACT MUSCLE FIBER

EXERCISE-INDUCED MUSCLE DAMAGE

SATELLITE CELLS ARE ACTIVATED

SATELLITE CELLS REPRODUCE

SOME CELLS RETURN TO THE POOL

REPAIRED MUSCLE FIBER

MYOCYTES FUSE WITH DAMAGED MUSCLE FIBER

SATELLITE CELLS NOW BECOME MUSCLE CELLS (MYOCYTES)

MYOTUBES MATURE TO BECOME NEW MUSCLE FIBERS

MYOCYTES FUSE AND BECOME MYOTUBES

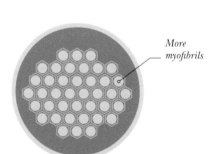

More myofibrils

MYOFIBRILLAR HYPERTROPHY
Myofibrillar protein makes up 60–70 percent of the protein in a muscle cell. Myofibrillar hypertrophy is the increase in number and/or size of myofibrils by the addition of sarcomeres.

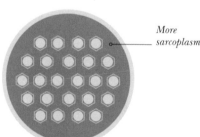

More sarcoplasm

SARCOPLASMIC HYPERTROPHY
A rise in the volume of the sarcoplasm (which includes mitochondria; sarcoplasmic reticulum; t-tubules; enzymes; and substrates, such as glycogen) also enlarges the muscle fiber.

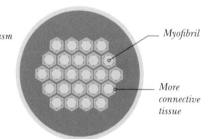

Myofibril

More connective tissue

CONNECTIVE TISSUE HYPERTROPHY
The extracellular matrix of the muscle fiber is a three-dimensional scaffolding of connective tissue. Increases in its mineral and protein content lead to muscles getting bigger.

HOW TRAINING PROMOTES MUSCLE GROWTH

The three stimuli of muscle hypertrophy all work quite differently. The primary driver is mechanical tension, with metabolic stress and muscle damage working on a less direct basis (see also p.18).

MECHANICAL TENSION

For muscle hypertrophy to occur, there must be a mechanical stimulus (or stress). This mechanical stimulus is referred to as mechanical tension or muscular tension. When you contract your muscles against resistance, you create mechanical tension via the force placed on your muscles. Once mechanoreceptors within the muscle detect such tension, a cascade of chemical reactions leading to muscle growth begins.

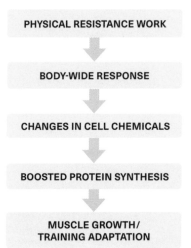

PHYSICAL RESISTANCE WORK

↓

BODY-WIDE RESPONSE

↓

CHANGES IN CELL CHEMICALS

↓

BOOSTED PROTEIN SYNTHESIS

↓

MUSCLE GROWTH/ TRAINING ADAPTATION

FROM WORK TO GROWTH
The physical stimulus of resistance work on mechanical tension, in turn, stimulates a range of chemical and biological responses that result in bigger and stronger muscles.

 The creation of tension in muscles

When actively contracting (see pp.14–15), muscles can generate mechanical, or muscular, tension while shortening, lengthening, or staying the same length. The tension depends on how big or small the overlap is between the actin and the myosin myofilaments within a sarcomere (see p.17).

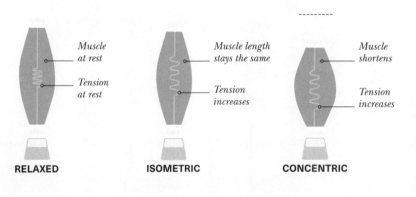

Muscle at rest

Tension at rest

RELAXED

Muscle length stays the same

Tension increases

ISOMETRIC

Muscle shortens

Tension increases

CONCENTRIC

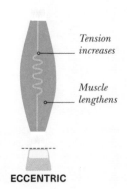

Tension increases

Muscle lengthens

ECCENTRIC

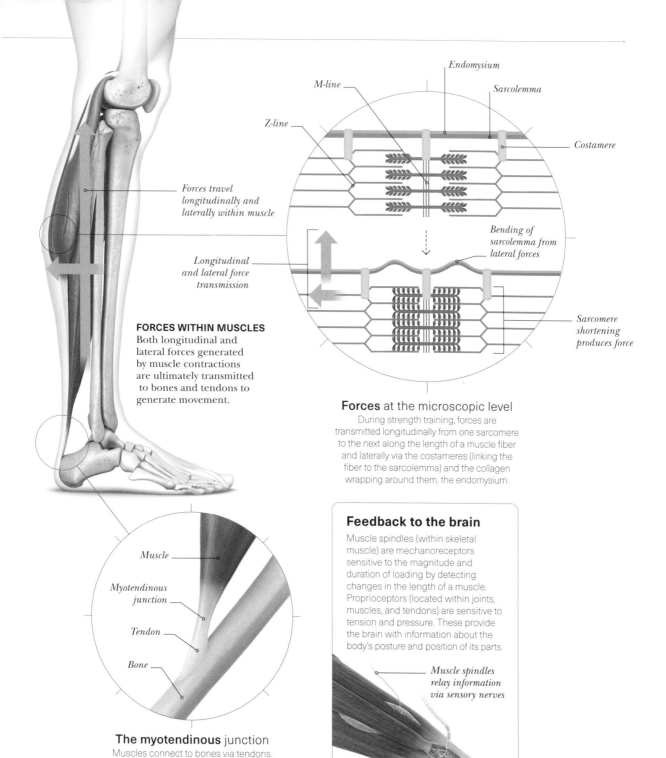

Endomysium

M-line

Sarcolemma

Z-line

Costamere

Forces travel
longitudinally and
laterally within muscle

Bending of
sarcolemma from
lateral forces

Longitudinal
and lateral force
transmission

Sarcomere
shortening
produces force

FORCES WITHIN MUSCLES
Both longitudinal and
lateral forces generated
by muscle contractions
are ultimately transmitted
to bones and tendons to
generate movement.

Forces at the microscopic level
During strength training, forces are
transmitted longitudinally from one sarcomere
to the next along the length of a muscle fiber
and laterally via the costameres (linking the
fiber to the sarcolemma) and the collagen
wrapping around them, the endomysium.

Muscle

Myotendinous
junction

Tendon

Bone

Feedback to the brain
Muscle spindles (within skeletal
muscle) are mechanoreceptors
sensitive to the magnitude and
duration of loading by detecting
changes in the length of a muscle.
Proprioceptors (located within joints,
muscles, and tendons) are sensitive to
tension and pressure. These provide
the brain with information about the
body's posture and position of its parts.

Muscle spindles
relay information
via sensory nerves

The myotendinous junction
Muscles connect to bones via tendons.
Where the tendon meets the muscle is
known as the myotendinous junction.
This area is a common site of injury
(see also p.178).

METABOLIC STRESS

This secondary driver of muscle hypertrophy is an exercise-induced accumulation of metabolites—the intermediate products of metabolic reactions catalyzed by enzymes within a cell; common metabolites are lactate (see also p.26), inorganic phosphate, and hydrogen. Low blood oxygen (hypoxia) can also promote the release of hormones and cytokines (signaling proteins) during contraction. The main theory explains that as muscular fatigue and metabolites build, it leads to higher levels of tension in fast-twitch fibers, stimulating them to grow.

Another by-product of metabolic stress that is thought to contribute to the amount of mechanical tension during muscle contraction is cell swelling (also called "the muscle pump"). Raised internal pressure within the muscle leads to more tension being produced—boosting the total amount of mechanical tension during contraction.

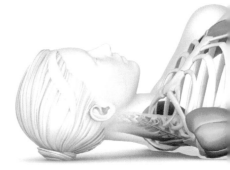

HAMSTRING BALL CURL
Within one exercise, different muscles are contracting isometrically, concentrically, and eccentrically. Controlling eccentric contractions is crucial to minimizing mechanistic damage to muscle cells.

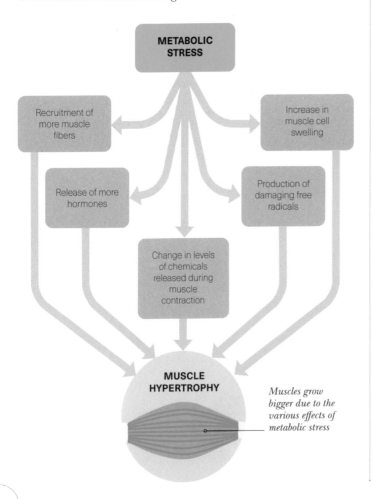

METABOLIC STRESS

Recruitment of more muscle fibers

Increase in muscle cell swelling

Release of more hormones

Production of damaging free radicals

Change in levels of chemicals released during muscle contraction

MUSCLE HYPERTROPHY

Muscles grow bigger due to the various effects of metabolic stress

MUSCLE DAMAGE

This contributor to muscle growth is specifically exercise-induced muscle damage. It exists on a continuum spanning from mild damage, which can be potentially helpful toward muscle growth, to severe damage, which can cause great disruption of tissues and negative effects across the body.

More damage is not better

A common mistake is that more exercise-induced muscle damage (and soreness) is better. Although muscle soreness is a sign you placed tension in the target muscles, large amounts of muscle damage limit your ability to improve over time. It was once thought that muscle damage was a positive because it impacts on building new muscle. But it's now known that the higher levels of muscle protein synthesis seen are mainly helping rebuild and repair the muscle after the damage of an intense training session rather than adding new contractile proteins.

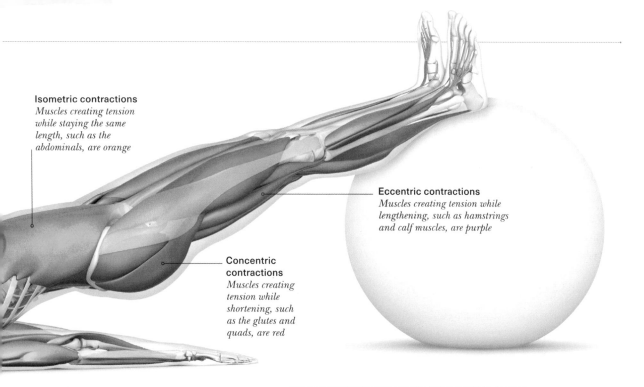

Isometric contractions
Muscles creating tension while staying the same length, such as the abdominals, are orange

Eccentric contractions
Muscles creating tension while lengthening, such as hamstrings and calf muscles, are purple

Concentric contractions
Muscles creating tension while shortening, such as the glutes and quads, are red

Damaging eccentric contractions

Muscle damage is caused most often with high training volumes (see p.198) and more exaggerated eccentric contractions, which can cause more mechanistic damages to a muscle cell compared to concentric or isometric contractions. The damage caused by eccentric contractions is due to the mechanical disruption of actin–myosin bonds rather than the ATP-dependent detachment (see p.17). During intense eccentric actions, sarcomeres are being stretched so much that they start to "pop"—think of the folds in the bendy section of a straw—one after the other along the muscle fiber length. The filaments fit back together afterward, but it results in muscle soreness.

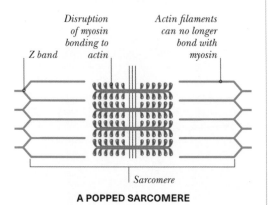

Disruption of myosin bonding to actin

Actin filaments can no longer bond with myosin

Z band

Sarcomere

A POPPED SARCOMERE

Recovery is vital to build muscle

The short period of muscle damage due to the intensity of a workout is followed by a longer recovery time, which is key for rebuilding damaged muscle fibers. If you train without enough chance for muscles to recover between sessions, you'll miss out on the opportunity to rebuild muscle, which will detrimentally affect your performance (see also p.177).

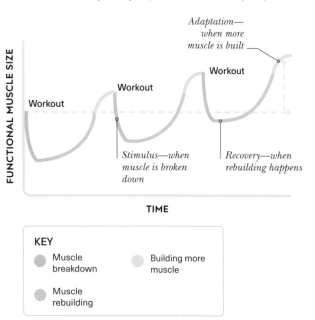

Adaptation—when more muscle is built

Workout

Workout

Workout

FUNCTIONAL MUSCLE SIZE

Stimulus—when muscle is broken down

Recovery—when rebuilding happens

TIME

KEY
- Muscle breakdown
- Muscle rebuilding
- Building more muscle

HOW TRAINING PROMOTES BONE STRENGTH

Bone is one of the most overlooked, sophisticated properties in the human body. It forms the functional framework for human movement (see pp.26–27) and is directly associated with injury incidence, quality of life, and mortality.

HOW **BONE** IS **MADE**

Bones increase in size and strength, via the action of osteoblasts, when placed under stress or mechanical load. When inactive or not challenged, bone is resorbed by the action of osteoclasts, resulting in the loss of strength, size, and overall density. The structure of bone is maintained by gravitational forces placed on your body, alongside the lateral forces associated with muscle contraction acting directly on the bone through connective tissue.

Periosteum
Fibrous membrane covering surface of bones (except in joints)

Bone marrow
Tissue filling the bone's cavity; source of blood cells

Blood vessels
Rich network of arteries and veins supplies the bone tissue

Spongy bone
Latticework of bone spikes (trabeculae), which are arranged along lines of stress

Osteon
Rod-shaped building block of compact bone

Femur
The long bone of the thigh

Compact bone
Gives bone its strength and is comprised of osteons

Epiphysis
Expanded head of bone that forms a joint surface

Cross-section of a long bone
A long bone (such as the femur) has a central core of bone marrow, a rich network of blood vessels to nourish the bone, and two types of bone—compact and spongy.

LOOK INSIDE A BONE
Bone is a living connective tissue made up of specialized cells and protein fibers. Its layers—compact bone around spongy bone—give it immense strength while being light.

Strengthening bones and muscles for life

Regular strength training has been shown to reduce the risk of both osteoporosis (weak and fragile bones) and sarcopenia (loss of muscle mass). In fact, these two diseases are a "hazardous duet" (osteosarcopenia), because they add to the susceptibility of falls and broken bones in older people.

HOW BONE AND MUSCLE CHANGES

Regular resistance training has been shown to positively impact bone mineral density and content, which reduces the risk of osteoporosis.

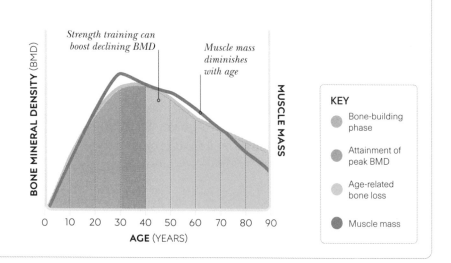

Strength training can boost declining BMD

Muscle mass diminishes with age

BONE MINERAL DENSITY (BMD)

MUSCLE MASS

AGE (YEARS)
0 10 20 30 40 50 60 70 80 90

KEY

- Bone-building phase
- Attainment of peak BMD
- Age-related bone loss
- Muscle mass

HOW **BONE** IS REMODELED

Your skeleton is in a constant state of flux, with osteoclasts breaking it down and osteoblasts making new bone. The force of a load—which can just be your bodyweight—confers different influences on this cyclical process depending on whether tension or compression forces dominate. If there is no external load on the skeleton, such as when sitting, osteoclast activity predominates. So a sedentary life is particularly bad for bones.

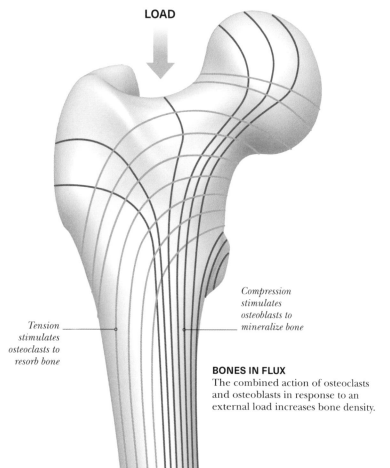

LOAD

Tension stimulates osteoclasts to resorb bone

Compression stimulates osteoblasts to mineralize bone

BONES IN FLUX
The combined action of osteoclasts and osteoblasts in response to an external load increases bone density.

THE **MECHANICS** OF **MOVEMENT**

The primary mechanical role of the skeleton is to provide rigid levers for muscles to act against. Strength training capitalizes on the opposing forces of muscles and external load to work hard to move both the body and the external resistance.

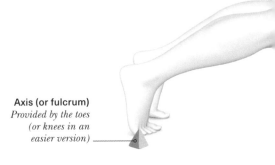

PUSH-UP
(SEE P.95)

Axis (or fulcrum)
Provided by the toes (or knees in an easier version)

HOW MUSCLES
MOVE THE BODY

Your body is basically a system of lever arrangements. Any lever set-up has a lever arm (bones), an axis (joints), force to move the load (provided by muscles, which pull on the bones), and the resistance offered by the weight of your body or by an external load.

A lever is useful to transform a small force into a much bigger one—what's known as mechanical advantage—so you can generate useful forces over short distances, which give speed with strength.

Whereabout on the lever arm the muscular force and resistance are applied in relation to a joint determines the leverage in lifting a weight. In the human body, there are three different lever systems differentiated into classes: first, second, and third.

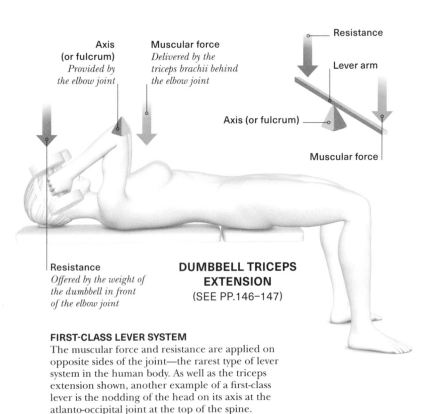

Axis
(or fulcrum)
Provided by the elbow joint

Muscular force
Delivered by the triceps brachii behind the elbow joint

Resistance

Lever arm

Axis (or fulcrum)

Muscular force

Resistance
Offered by the weight of the dumbbell in front of the elbow joint

DUMBBELL TRICEPS EXTENSION
(SEE PP.146–147)

FIRST-CLASS LEVER SYSTEM
The muscular force and resistance are applied on opposite sides of the joint—the rarest type of lever system in the human body. As well as the triceps extension shown, another example of a first-class lever is the nodding of the head on its axis at the atlanto-occipital joint at the top of the spine.

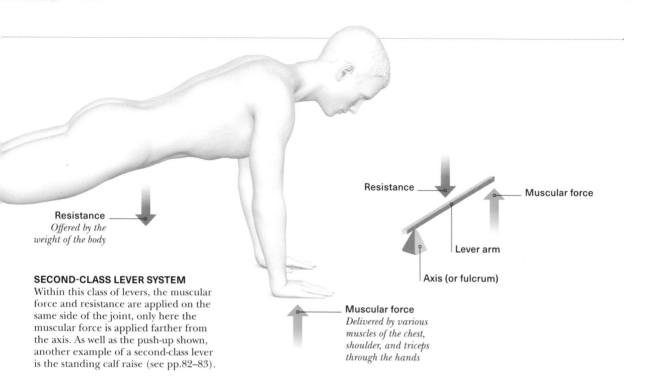

Resistance
Offered by the weight of the body

SECOND-CLASS LEVER SYSTEM
Within this class of levers, the muscular force and resistance are applied on the same side of the joint, only here the muscular force is applied farther from the axis. As well as the push-up shown, another example of a second-class lever is the standing calf raise (see pp.82–83).

Resistance

Muscular force

Lever arm

Axis (or fulcrum)

Muscular force
Delivered by various muscles of the chest, shoulder, and triceps through the hands

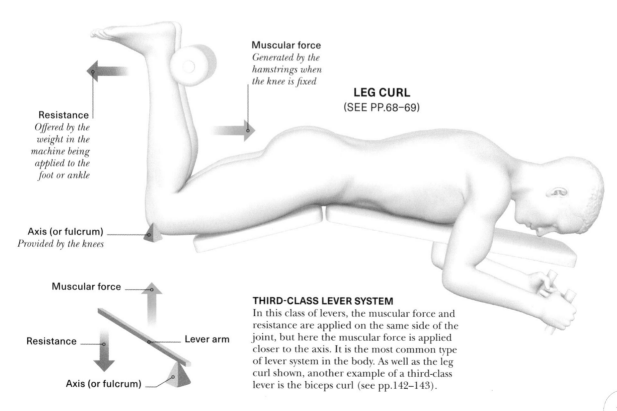

Muscular force
Generated by the hamstrings when the knee is fixed

LEG CURL
(SEE PP.68–69)

Resistance
Offered by the weight in the machine being applied to the foot or ankle

Axis (or fulcrum)
Provided by the knees

Muscular force

Resistance

Lever arm

Axis (or fulcrum)

THIRD-CLASS LEVER SYSTEM
In this class of levers, the muscular force and resistance are applied on the same side of the joint, but here the muscular force is applied closer to the axis. It is the most common type of lever system in the body. As well as the leg curl shown, another example of a third-class lever is the biceps curl (see pp.142–143).

27

POWERING
MUSCLE ACTION

Your body is a finely tuned machine that can respond to fast, explosive movements, such as a barbell back squat; as well as endurance activities, such as marathon running; plus everything in between. To do this, it relies on not one but three different systems of energy production.

ENERGY CONVERSION

The flow of energy in a biological system (bioenergetics) happens primarily by the conversion of chemical energy in stored glycogen and macronutrients, such as fats, protein, and carbohydrates (see pp.30–31), into biologically usable forms of energy.

Adenosine triphosphate, or ATP, is the body's principal molecule for storing and transferring energy in cells.

ATP—the cell's energy currency

Almost all cellular processes need ATP, including powering muscular activity. ATP is a nucleotide consisting of an adenine base attached to a ribose sugar, which is attached to three phosphate groups. The three phosphates are linked to one another by high-energy bonds. An ATP molecule releases energy when one phosphate group is removed and, in turn, becomes downgraded to the lower-energy molecule adenosine diphosphate (ADP). ADP and ATP cycle continuously between these two forms, as they provide a constant stream of energy for all the body's biological reactions.

Aerobic—oxidative metabolism

The body's oxidative system primarily produces energy for activities that are of longer duration and low intensity, such as runs over 1 mile (1,600 m), as well as helping the recovery of energy between moderate- and high-intensity activities—for instance, the rest periods during a strength training session. Adaptations to the oxidative system carry over to strength training via more muscle mitochondria (a cell's energy-producing units), increased myoglobin (the protein that helps extract oxygen from blood), and higher capillary density—all of which promote the exchange of oxygen into the muscle tissue.

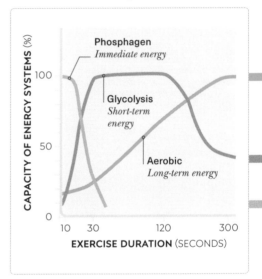

HOW THE BODY MAKES ENERGY

Energy processes can be broadly broken down into those that are anaerobic (not dependent on oxygen) and those that are aerobic (oxygen dependent). Anaerobic metabolism involves the phosphagen and glycolytic systems, while aerobic metabolism involves the oxidative system. It is important to note that all three systems are active at any given time. Which system is more dominant—and is being used to a greater magnitude—is relative to the intensity and the duration of the activity.

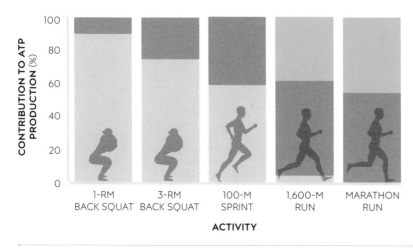

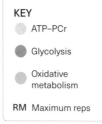

KEY

- ATP–PCr
- Glycolysis
- Oxidative metabolism
- **RM** Maximum reps

ENERGY FOR ACTIVITIES

The contribution the three energy systems supply to enable a range of activities varies. The ATP–PCr system powers strength training work, but other systems help replenish ATP between sets.

Anaerobic—glycolysis

The body's glycolytic system kicks in for activities of moderate duration and high intensity, such as higher volume resistance training and sprint endurance work. During high-intensity exercise, the process of glycolysis utilizes glucose in the blood but also creates lactate as it tries to match the energy (ATP) demands of muscles. When lactate accumulates in the bloodstream, it causes lactic acidosis with various unpleasant symptoms, such as muscle ache, burning muscles, fatigue, rapid breathing, stomach pain, and nausea. Luckily, the process is usually temporary and is reversible; lactate can be metabolized into pyruvate for reuse in other cellular energy pathways. Adaptations to the glycolytic energy route can happen via higher levels of glycolytic enzymes and more effective production of ATP during exercise, as well as a higher storage of glycogen within the muscle.

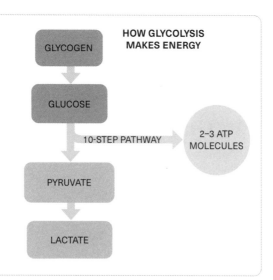

HOW GLYCOLYSIS MAKES ENERGY

GLYCOGEN → GLUCOSE → 10-STEP PATHWAY → 2–3 ATP MOLECULES

GLUCOSE → PYRUVATE → LACTATE

Anaerobic—phosphagen

The body's phosphagen system (sometimes called the ATP–PCr system, as it uses and remakes phosphocreatine (PCr) in the process) is primarily used for short, intense activities such as high-intensity resistance training (1–3 reps) and sprinting (100-m dash). This system is highly active at the beginning of any activity, regardless of intensity. Adaptations to this system from strength training are possible. The most substantial improvements in intramuscular storage result from a supplement of creatine monohydrate (see p.36).

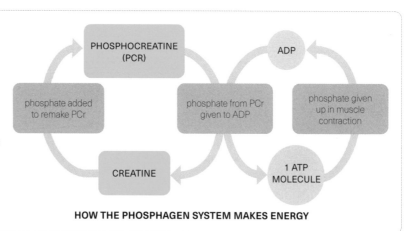

PHOSPHOCREATINE (PCR)

ADP

phosphate added to remake PCR

phosphate from PCr given to ADP

phosphate given up in muscle contraction

CREATINE

1 ATP MOLECULE

HOW THE PHOSPHAGEN SYSTEM MAKES ENERGY

FUELS FOR
STRENGTH TRAINING

The term "macronutrient" may not be familiar, but you've probably heard of the three types: carbohydrates, fats, and protein. The calories within these macronutrients are released for energy to be used in chemical reactions in the body, including powering muscles to work against resistance. There are also "micronutrients"—the vitamins and minerals crucial to a wide and varied range of body processes.

MACRONUTRIENTS

Each of the three macronutrients is made up of components that can be assembled and then broken down to facilitate energy production—a process called bioenergetics (see pp.28–29). Carbohydrates exist as glucose but are also stored in the form of glycogen (in muscles and in the liver). Proteins are made from amino acids. Fats exist as triacylglycerols and free fatty acids.

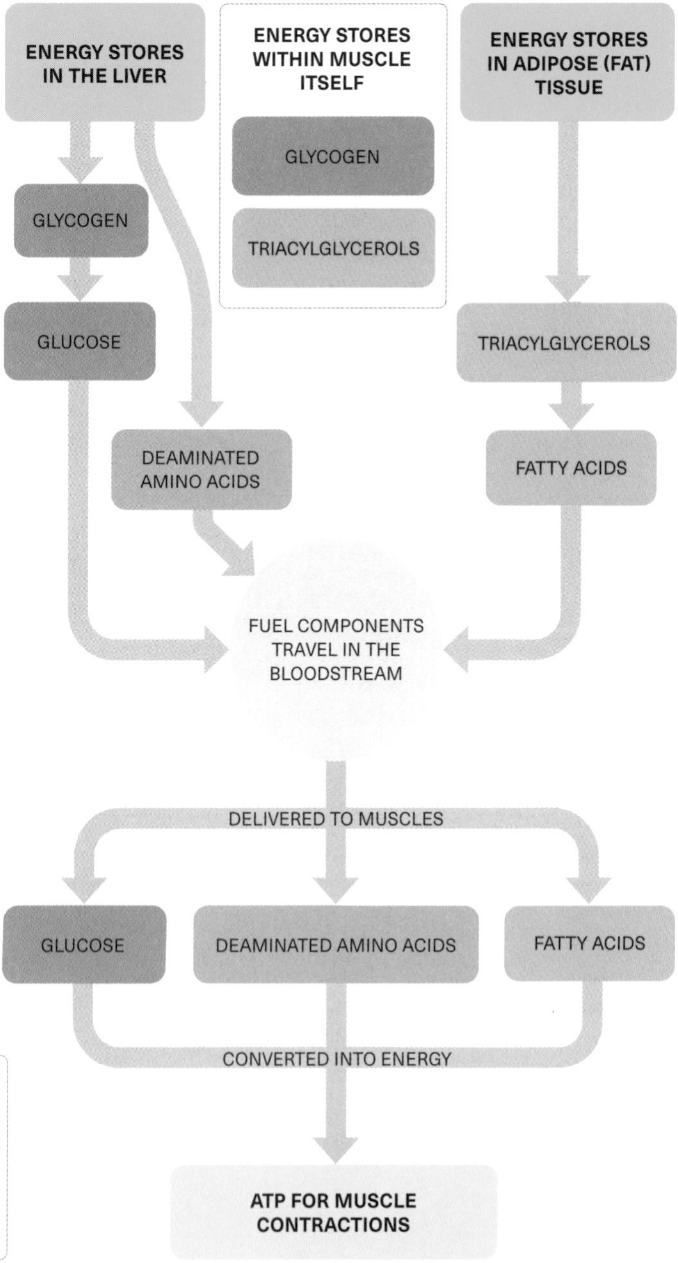

MACRONUTRIENT FUEL SOURCES

Whether the fuel comes in the form of carbohydrates, proteins, or fats, the body breaks it down and delivers components to the muscles in the blood. Muscle cells use these fuels to make energy—ATP (see pp.28–29). In addition to glycogen and triacylglycerols, muscles have stores of ATP and amino acids.

KEY

- ● Carbohydrates
- ● Protein
- ● Fats

ENERGY STORES IN THE LIVER

GLYCOGEN

GLUCOSE

ENERGY STORES WITHIN MUSCLE ITSELF

GLYCOGEN

TRIACYLGLYCEROLS

ENERGY STORES IN ADIPOSE (FAT) TISSUE

TRIACYLGLYCEROLS

FATTY ACIDS

DEAMINATED AMINO ACIDS

FUEL COMPONENTS TRAVEL IN THE BLOODSTREAM

DELIVERED TO MUSCLES

GLUCOSE

DEAMINATED AMINO ACIDS

FATTY ACIDS

CONVERTED INTO ENERGY

ATP FOR MUSCLE CONTRACTIONS

Carbohydrates

In strength training, the predominant source of fuels comes from carbohydrates, stored in the form of glycogen and converted into energy through anaerobic metabolism (see pp.28–29). Eating carbs is key to replenish glycogen stores between training sessions to ensure adequate recovery and subsequent performance. Although your body can manufacture glucose from protein and fat, carbohydrates should make up the largest percentage of your daily energy requirements—especially if you are strength training. Carbs are responsible for as much as 80 percent of ATP production during strength training.

Protein

Dietary protein is essential to life and the maintenance of health, especially when considering its importance in building and maintaining muscle; the growth and repair of tissues and cells; and structural roles in connective tissue, bones, and organs. Unlike carbs and fats, the body does not have reserves of protein to use when availability is low, which is why it is crucial to eat enough protein every day. Twenty amino acids are used in human bodily functions; these can be further broken down as essential and nonessential. Essential amino acids have to be consumed in our diet, while the body can synthesize nonessential acids from other protein sources.

Fat

Fat, also known as lipid, is an essential nutrient that plays a vital role in many body functions, including the protective cushioning of internal organs and nerve signal transmission, assisting the absorption of vitamins, and helping facilitate the production of cell membranes and hormones. In the body, fat is stored in adipose tissue. Adequate fat intake has been shown to have an impact on testosterone levels, playing an important role in building muscle and regulating metabolism. Dietitians recommend that the majority of your fat intake comes from high-quality essential fatty acids, especially polyunsaturated fatty acids.

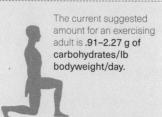

Carbohydrates provide 4 kcal of energy per g

The current suggested amount for an exercising adult is .91–2.27 g of carbohydrates/lb bodyweight/day.

A 154-LB (70-KG) ADULT REQUIRES 140–350 G* OF CARBS A DAY

*depending on energy demands and body composition

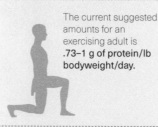

Protein provides 4 kcal of energy per g

The current suggested amounts for an exercising adult is .73–1 g of protein/lb bodyweight/day.

A 154-LB (70-KG) ADULT REQUIRES 112–154 G* OF PROTEIN A DAY

*depending on energy demands and body composition

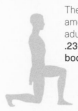

Fat provides 9 kcal of energy per g

The current suggested amount for an exercising adult is .23–.46 g of fat/lb bodyweight/day.

A 154-LB (70-KG) ADULT REQUIRES 35–70 G* OF FAT A DAY

*depending on energy demands and body composition

Micronutrient magic wands

Micronutrients are the vitamins and minerals required by the body in "micro," or small, amounts compared to macronutrients. The World Health Organization has labeled micronutrients the "magic wands" that help our body produce enzymes and hormones needed for growth and development. Vitamins and minerals play an important role, helping us best prepare for the physiological demands of everyday life and reducing the risk of age-related decline. The more active you are, the greater the need for you to consume a wide variety of micronutrient-rich foods such as fruits and vegetables. Research from 2018 shows it's best to consume micronutrients within foods rather than simply topping up levels via supplements.

DETERMINING YOUR ENERGY REQUIREMENTS

Your total daily energy balance refers to the relationship between the amount of energy you consume (in calories from macronutrients) and the amount that you use for activity. The amount of calories you take in has a direct impact on your ability to gain, lose, or maintain your bodyweight.

YOUR DAILY ENERGY BALANCE

Often simplified to "calories in versus calories out," energy balance is a little more complex than simply thinking about what you consume and the energy you use through exercise. Your body's total daily energy expenditure covers all kinds of activities, not just exercise (see below; percentages are for an average person). When you consume fewer calories than you expend, you're in a deficit energy balance; when you consume more calories than you expend, you're in a surplus energy balance.

Your daily calorie intake

In order to best understand how much energy it takes for you to maintain your current bodyweight or body fat levels, you have to do a little bit of math. Determining maintenance calories is typically done by taking your bodyweight and multiplying it by 10 (for weights in lb) or by 22 (for weights in kg). Select the activity level from the chart below that best describes you and use this to work out your daily calorie intake to maintain your bodyweight.

How active are you?

Sedentary (<8,000 steps a day) plus 3–6 days of strength training	Lightly active (8–10,000 steps a day) plus 3–6 days of strength training
1.3–1.6	**1.5–1.8**
Active (10–15,000 steps a day) plus 3–6 days of strength training	**Very active** (15,000+ steps a day) plus 3–6 days of strength training
1.7–2.0	**1.9–2.2**

10 kcal x weight in lb x activity multiplier

For a 202-lb person
10 x 202.8 = 2,028 kcal
who fits the sedentary level (1.3–1.6)
2,028 x 1.3–1.6
= 2,636–3,243 kcal per day

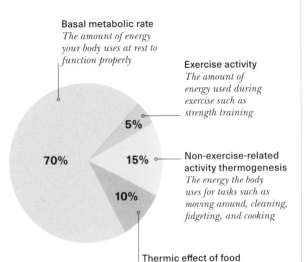

Basal metabolic rate
The amount of energy your body uses at rest to function properly

Exercise activity
The amount of energy used during exercise such as strength training

5%

70%

15%

10%

Non-exercise-related activity thermogenesis
The energy the body uses for tasks such as moving around, cleaning, fidgeting, and cooking

Thermic effect of food
The amount of energy the body uses to digest macronutrients

CALCULATE DAILY CALORIE TARGET

After finding your calorie range, choose a calorie mark you feel might best represent a maintenance level. Then calculate your macronutrient needs based on this (see below).

Take a **154-lb (70-kg) person** who is **lightly active** and strength training **3 days** per week.

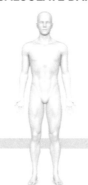

154 (lb) x 10 (kcal) x 1.5 (chosen activity multiplier) **= an estimated 2,310 kcal per day** to **maintain** your **bodyweight**.

To ensure this is your maintenance calories, you could **track your calories** for a **1–2-week period** and see how your bodyweight changes over that duration.

If your **bodyweight drops** over this period of time, try **adding 100 kcal** and see if this allows you to best maintain weight. Likewise, if your **bodyweight rises** over this **1–2-week period**, reduce intake by **100 kcal** and see if this helps maintain weight.

CALCULATE DAILY MACRONUTRIENT TARGETS

Protein

The current suggested amounts for protein intake for exercising adults is **.73–1 g protein/lb/day**

154 (lb) x .73 g protein/lb/day **= 112 g protein/day**

1

Fats

The current suggested amount for fat consumption is around **.23–.46 g fats/lb/day**

154 (lb) x .32 g fats/lb/day **= 49 g fats/day**

2

Carbohydrates

To calculate the carbs component, you add up how many calories would be collectively supplied by protein and fats and subtract that from your daily calorie target. What's left is your calories from carbohydrates*.

112 g x 4 kcal/g = 448 kcal from protein
49 g x 9 kcal/g = 441 kcal from fats
combined total = 889 kcal

For a daily energy intake of 2,310 kcal, you need to take away the **889 kcal** from **protein** and **fats** and then **divide by 4 kcal/g** to find your calories from carbs.

2,310 – 889 = 1,421 kcal

1,421 divided by **4 = 355 g** carbs

3

**FATS
19%**

**PROTEIN
20%**

**CARBOHYDRATES
61%**

*If you'd like to eat more of a particular macronutrient to better meet your nutritional preferences, then you can "steal" from one macronutrient intake as long as you stick within the suggested ranges.

Start with a calorie deficit—to lose weight

To adjust the figures to cut your calories in a balanced way, you'll need to first find your maintenance calorie level. Then **multiply the calories** by 10–15%—a good size deficit—and take that away. This uses a **15% deficit** on the above example.
2,310 kcal x 0.15 = ~346.5 kcal
2,310 – 346.5 = 1,963.5 kcal—the new calorie amount

Start with a calorie surplus—to gain weight

To adjust the figures to boost your calories in a balanced way, you'll need to multiply your maintenance calorie level by **10–15%**—a good size surplus—and add that to the daily goal. This uses a **15% surplus** on the above example.
2,310 kcal x 0.15 = ~346.5 kcal
2,310 + 346.5 = 2,656.5 kcal—the new calorie amount

EATING FOR STRENGTH TRAINING

A well-balanced meal can power your strength training routine, but it does involve some preparation and planning to include a good variety of vegetables, fruits, lean proteins, and healthy fats. Knowing when to eat, be it before or after a workout, can also make a big difference in your performance and your recovery.

CREATING A WELL-BALANCED MEAL

For muscles to work optimally, they need a constant supply of energy (see pp.30–31) and a source of the macro- and micronutrients needed for repair and recovery. So your meals should reflect that. Choose any vegetable with the exception of potatoes (classed as a starch) and opt for lean protein (such as chicken, fish, tofu, and yogurt), as well as healthy fats (in nuts, seeds, and oil-rich foods such as avocado and olive oil).

Protein, in particular

When combined with regularly strength training, daily protein intake has been linked in older adults to higher step count, positive impacts on living independently, and improved grip strength (a measure of muscle strength). And these benefits affect younger populations, too. There is evidence to suggest that boosting daily protein intake, such as with high-protein foods or protein powder (see p.36), can further minimize protein breakdown and promote muscle protein synthesis.

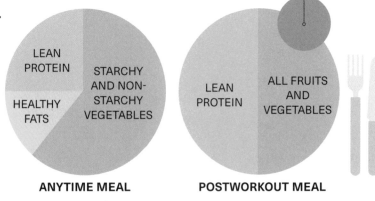

Extra starches
Potatoes, pasta, rice, or bread

ANYTIME MEAL

LEAN PROTEIN
HEALTHY FATS
STARCHY AND NON-STARCHY VEGETABLES

POSTWORKOUT MEAL

LEAN PROTEIN
ALL FRUITS AND VEGETABLES

THE RIGHT PROPORTIONS
These "plates" show you what you should be filling up on for most of your meals and how these proportions skew when eating after a strength training session.

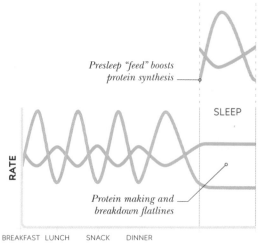

Presleep "feed" boosts protein synthesis

SLEEP

RATE

Protein making and breakdown flatlines

BREAKFAST   LUNCH   SNACK   DINNER

MUSCLE PROTEIN AND ITS DAILY FLUCTUATIONS

KEY
— Muscle protein synthesis
— Muscle protein breakdown

FEED MUSCLES WITH PROTEIN
Work with your body's cycles of protein synthesis and breakdown to create an opportunity to transform sleep into a time busy with protein manufacture instead of not much going on.

PRE- AND **POSTWORKOUT** NUTRITION

The nutrition surrounding your workout can be an important component of your overall performance and recovery. When choosing a snack before or after a training session, realize that carbohydrate sources differ in digestion rates and their ability to be used for energy. Glucose- and fructose-based sources are great for replenishing muscle and liver glycogen storage (supplying energy for the next workout).

WHAT TO EAT WHEN
The timing of nutrient intake, particularly the "anabolic window" postworkout, has been heavily debated. That said, the middle ground agrees that consuming high-quality protein postworkout (as a supplement or as a meal) has muscle-building benefits.

BEFORE WORKOUT

Snacks combining carbs and protein are key if you're training long after a meal or first thing in the morning in a fasted state. Such foods replenish glycogen stores and can stimulate protein synthesis. Avoid high-fiber foods though, as they take longer to digest.

DURING WORKOUT

There's no need to drink anything but water during a strength training session. Eating the right nutrients beforehand will fuel your workout, so there's no need to eat while you're training.

AFTER WORKOUT

Some experts recommend consuming protein as soon as your training session is over to maximize recovery, while others advise that a high-protein meal should be eaten within 1–3 hours. Such protein "feeding" stops protein breakdown and stimulates protein synthesis.

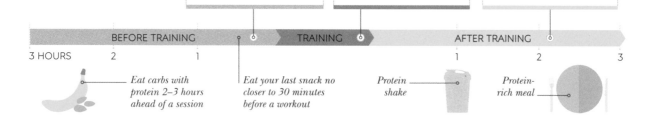

BEFORE TRAINING   TRAINING   AFTER TRAINING

3 HOURS   2   1   1   2   3

Eat carbs with protein 2–3 hours ahead of a session

Eat your last snack no closer to 30 minutes before a workout

Protein shake

Protein-rich meal

Your fluid balance

Because water makes up 55–60 percent of a human body, it is a crucial component of day-to-day consumption and one of the most important factors in survival. Water acts as a solvent, a catalyst for chemical reactions, a lubricant and shock absorber, and a source of important minerals, as well as enabling temperature control (sweating). The management of water in and out of the body is known as fluid balance. This delicate equilibrium is essential for performance, as well as health. It's vital that this is kept in check and does not turn into dehydration (from not drinking enough water) or hyperhydration (drinking too much water), as both come with health consequences.

HOW MUCH WATER TO DRINK A DAY
Current advice recommends ½ fl oz/lb (30–40 ml/kg) bodyweight. It's crucial to tailor your water intake depending on your weight, activity level, perspiration rate, and environmental factors on a daily basis.

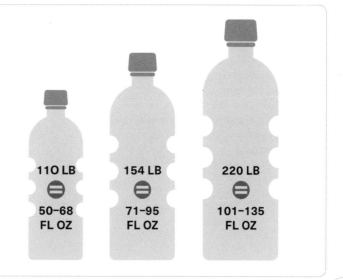

110 LB
50–68 FL OZ

154 LB
71–95 FL OZ

220 LB
101–135 FL OZ

ARE **SUPPLEMENTS** NECESSARY?

There are benefits to supplementation for overall health, performance, and recovery. That said, it's better to focus on eating a well-balanced diet than not to eat nutritious meals and rely on supplements to top you up. The supplements with the most comprehensive impact on health and performance are listed below left. As the research stands, there is no detriment to taking the "add-on" supplements, so view them as an extra or luxury item.

SUPPLEMENTS FOR HEALTH AND PERFORMANCE

PROVEN SUPPLEMENTS	"ADD-ON" SUPPLEMENTS
fish oil* vitamins D and K* creatine* whey protein* melatonin multivitamins caffeine calcium**	BCAAs—branched chain amino acids EAAs—essential amino acids citrulline malate

*These have been shown to have positive benefits across all ages.

** Calcium citrate is the best source of supplemental calcium.

 Protein powders—what's the deal?

If you're already getting enough high-quality protein, the likelihood is that you won't see much benefit from adding protein powder to your diet. But if you're regularly lifting weights, you may find that such powder can maximize muscle gain, and it's useful for those struggling to meet protein needs if following a vegan or vegetarian diet (see right). Protein powders are concentrated sources of protein; some are based on animal protein (whey and casein from milk, or egg), while others are based on plant protein (pea, hemp, soy, and rice). If you think a protein powder would help you reach your goals, discuss options with a trainer or dietitian.

TRAINING ON **VEGAN** OR **VEGETARIAN DIETS**

Strength training on a plant-based diet can be just as effective as on an animal-based diet. Although it can be more challenging, it utilizes the same principles of energy availability. Protein intake (specific to the amino acid leucine) is the most challenging of the macronutrients to maximize. Protein intake is invaluable to the maintenance and growth of muscle tissue and overall metabolic health, so learning how best to consume the required nutrients is important for anyone following a plant-based diet.

The case for leucine

Leucine is an essential amino acid, specifically one of the branched chain amino acids. It is important in the regulation of skeletal muscle, as it can stimulate muscle protein synthesis (see p.34). There is a certain leucine threshold (amount) per meal to stimulate this process to occur. Although leucine has been shown to switch on muscle protein synthesis, it cannot carry out and sustain this process without other essential amino acids. A complete protein source is required—from protein-rich foods or from a protein supplement. Research has shown that older adults need about double the amount of leucine per meal on average to reach the threshold to boost the synthesis of muscle protein.

Pay extra attention to all nutrients

While nutrition is important for the health of everyone, a poorly constructed plant-based diet can put you at risk of macronutrient deficiencies and micronutrient deficiencies for various vitamins and minerals. Look to these vegan-friendly food sources to provide the most commonly lacking nutrients in plant-based diets.

Protein Pulses, grains, legumes, tofu, quinoa, nuts, seeds, vegetables
Vitamin B12 Fortified foods, plant milks, nutritional yeast
Vitamin D Fortified foods, plant milks, nutritional yeast
Iron Legumes, grains, nuts, seeds, fortified foods, green vegetables

Zinc Beans, nuts, seeds, oats, wheat germ
Calcium Tofu, kale, broccoli, sprouts, cauliflower, bok choy, fortified plant milk
Iodine Seaweed, cranberries, potatoes, prunes, navy beans, iodized salt

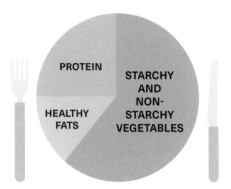

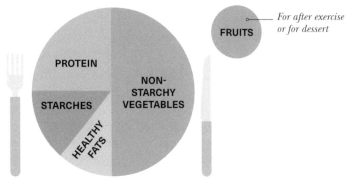

For after exercise or for dessert

ANYTIME ANIMAL-BASED MEAL
These are the proportions of nutrients recommended for eating a well-balanced diet while doing regular strength training.

ANYTIME PLANT-BASED MEALS
While the proportions of nutrients varies, the most vital nutrient is protein for those on a vegetarian or vegan diet.

Think "complete protein"

To build skeletal muscle, high-quality protein is of paramount importance. The quality of protein relates to its composition of the essential amino acids (those the body cannot make). A protein is defined as "complete" when it contains all nine essential amino acids in the amounts needed to support the growth and maintenance of lean muscle tissue. An "incomplete" protein is low in essential amino acids. All animal-based proteins (aside from gelatin) are complete proteins. Plant proteins, however, often lack enough essential amino acids and are by definition incomplete proteins. So anyone following a plant-based diet has to be more aware of protein quality and how to best pair two incomplete proteins to create a complete one.

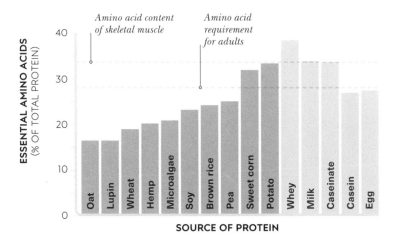

HOW PROTEINS COMPARE
Plant proteins mostly fall below the amino acid requirement, while animal proteins mostly surpass it.

KEY
- Plant-based protein
- Animal-based **protein**

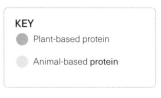

Veggie protein powders

Whey protein is the most common choice of protein supplements (see opposite) due to its high leucine content, rapid digestibility, and ability to stimulate protein synthesis. Those following a plant-based diet have different choices. Soy protein has been the most comparable alternative. But pea protein has more recently been proposed as the best alternative to whey protein supplements, as it has shown similar increases in muscular size and strength.

STRENGTH TRAINING AND YOUR BRAIN

The physical adaptations made early in response to strength training are predominantly in the nervous system. Experts believe that nervous-system-based responses account for the gains made in the first two to four weeks of strength training.

THE **CONTROL** OF **MUSCLES**

The nervous system comprises your brain and spinal cord and countless nerves taking messages from your brain to your body and back again. Motor nerves transmit signals about movement from the brain's motor cortex via the spinal cord, whereas sensory nerves relay information from the muscles to the brain and spinal cord.

Neural adaptations

Adaptation is a dynamic process whereby the body adjusts to a particular environment. Strength training helps develop motor pathways that enhance brain–body coordination. These "neural adaptations" describe how the brain recruits muscles to contract to produce a particular movement. Practice trains the brain to activate the right muscles for that motion; with time, the movement becomes more automatic. Adaptations in both nervous and muscular systems (which kick in later) result in improved technique, coordination, and efficiency of movement over time.

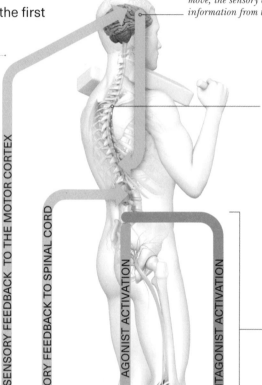

Brain
The motor cortex sends instructions to muscles to move; the sensory cortex receives information from the muscles

Spinal cord
A relay for messages coming from and going to the brain

SENSORY FEEDBACK TO THE MOTOR CORTEX

SENSORY FEEDBACK TO SPINAL CORD

AGONIST ACTIVATION

ANTAGONIST ACTIVATION

With practice, there is less coactivation of the antagonist muscle in a movement

Agonist muscles
The gastrocnemius and soleus drive the raise

Antagonist muscle
The tibialis anterior allows the raise

SMOOTHER MOVES
Your brain sends a signal to activate the agonist of an action. Initially, it also signals to the antagonist at the same time (coactivation). With repetition, the amount of coactivation diminishes and your technique improves.

STRENGTH TRAINING'S **BRAIN GAINS**

Regular strength training has been shown to increase levels of neurotrophins—a family of growth and survival factors that regulate the development and the maintenance of nerve cells or neurons. Two neurotrophins in particular—brain-derived neurotrophic factor (BDNF) and insulinlike growth factor 1 (IGF-1)—have both been shown to have positive effects on neurogenesis and neuroplasticity.

Neurogenesis

The creation of new neurons—neurogenesis—is just one of the positive ways that strength training and exercise impacts the brain. Scientists used to believe that you were born with a certain number of neurons—around 86 billion—and that you couldn't grow new ones. Research has since revealed that neurogenesis can happen and it does so in key areas of the brain, such as in the hippocampus, which is important in memory.

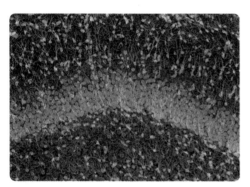

NEW BRAIN CELLS
In this microscopic image of the brain's hippocampus, neuron cell bodies are colored pink. Strength training promotes neurogenesis, the making of new neurons.

 Mind–muscle connection

When strength training, it's good to work without distractions so that you can pay attention to each and every exercise. You can also boost your workout gains by developing a mind–muscle connection. It's the act of consciously and deliberately thinking about moving the target muscle, because research shows that this can really boost muscle strength. Practicing such a conscious approach leads to the recruitment of more muscle fibers in a movement, which ultimately means better-quality muscle contractions and a more successful workout.

Neuroplasticity

Pathways within the brain become more permanent the more you use them; repetition strengthens and continues to build a neural network. This ability to form new connections and pathways—known as neuroplasticity—changes how brain circuits are wired. Learning a new skill, such as that needed in strength training, improves how existing neurons work and offers positive benefits across brain function.

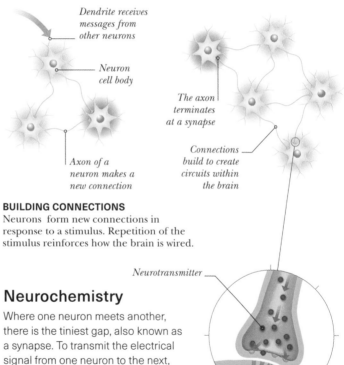

Dendrite receives messages from other neurons

Neuron cell body

Axon of a neuron makes a new connection

The axon terminates at a synapse

Connections build to create circuits within the brain

BUILDING CONNECTIONS
Neurons form new connections in response to a stimulus. Repetition of the stimulus reinforces how the brain is wired.

Neurotransmitter

Neurochemistry

Where one neuron meets another, there is the tiniest gap, also known as a synapse. To transmit the electrical signal from one neuron to the next, your brain uses a system of molecules called neurotransmitters. These chemicals diffuse across the gap and initiate the signal in the next connected neuron. Strength training exercise boosts levels of certain neurotransmitters, such as dopamine, as well as levels of endorphins, which lift mood and quell anxiety.

Synapse up close
Molecules of neurotransmitter prompted by the signal in one neuron flow across the synapse in about 1 millisecond, relaying the signal to the next connected neuron.

BRAIN-BASED BENEFITS

In addition to the physical health benefits (see pp.6–7), research is uncovering a host of positive impacts on mental health and the brain from doing regular strength training—reducing stress, boosting productivity, focusing the mind, and enhancing memory are just a few of them.

BOOSTS LONG-TERM MEMORY

Research shows that the participation in physical activity—most notably, aerobic exercise combined with strength training—helps increase the size of the hippocampus alongside raising levels of neurotrophins, leading to improvements in memory.

ENHANCES COGNITIVE FUNCTION

Strength training boosts levels of neurotrophins, such as brain-derived neurotrophic factor (BDNF), which positively influence neurogenesis and neuroplasticity, leading to improvements in learning and cognition.

IMPROVES CONCENTRATION

Strength training requires large amounts of focus and skill acquisition, which can help improve concentration. Such efforts can boost mental health status, leading to improvements in ability to concentrate on a singular task.

PROTECTS AGAINST DEPRESSION

A meta-review of studies consistently showed that exercise—specifically resistance training—has been found to decrease or help prevent depressive symptoms.

BOOSTS CREATIVITY

Strength training boosts levels of the neurotrophin BDNF, which encourages the growth of new neurons in the brain's hippocampus. These neurons build new connections, offering fresh and novel solutions.

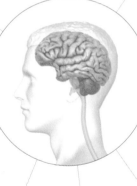

LIFTS MOOD

The endorphins that result from a strength training session perk you up. It has also been shown that they reduce the likelihood that exercisers experience bouts of sadness compared to those not weight training.

SPEEDS UP BRAIN FUNCTION

A recent meta-analysis of studies showed the positive effects of both aerobic exercise and resistance training on improving cognitive and executive function in older adults.

CREATES MUSCLE MEMORY

Returning to the gym after time away is made easier by your brain's memory of past movement patterns and tasks. Such memory helps improve the speed of recovery at the muscular level because less time is spent relearning the exercises.

STAVES OFF DEMENTIA

Strength training has been shown to raise levels of neurotrophins, which appear to lessen brain tissue loss and the lesions and plaques that are linked to conditions such as Alzheimer's disease.

ALLEVIATES STRESS AND ANXIETY

Training at the gym is often a social activity, which can ease stress. Plus, resistance training has been shown to significantly improve stress- and anxiety-related symptoms, both among healthy individuals and people with a physical or a mental illness.

PSYCHOLOGICAL WINS

Use psychological techniques to discover what drives you to do strength training and to establish sustainable habits based around achieving goals in the long term. Think of goals as a way of setting a direction, but your daily habits are the system for making progress.

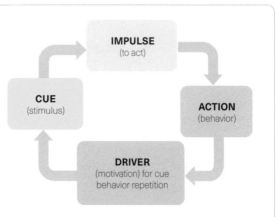

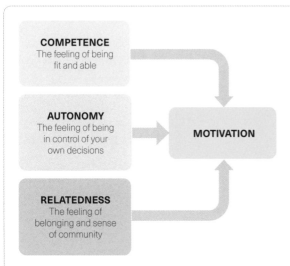

Establish sustainable habits

Creating long-lasting routines and habits ensures you set yourself up for success and perform tasks without having to think much about them. The more you repeat the cycle, the more you will strengthen the bond between the cue and the action. At first, this process can be difficult, but the more you execute this routine, the more automatic it will become. If you struggle to get started, keep in mind that it's important to begin with small steps and to find something you enjoy doing.

Find your motivation

Your basic psychological needs all feed into your motivation toward achieving a goal. But you also need to understand why you want to reach that goal. Motivation can be intrinsic (driven by basic needs; things that are satisfying; things that you're good at) and extrinsic (focused on appeasing others). While you work toward your goals, it has been shown that extrinsic motivations fade, while intrinsic motivations take over.

Set reliable goals

Once you've identified your motivations for creating change, it's important to understand how to set goals you can attain. Setting goals is known to be a positive contributor to achieving what you have set out to accomplish while lowering the potential to be overwhelmed or discouraged. When setting a goal, you need to be sure it is SMART (see below).

SMART goals work

The acronym SMART is useful to help you remember the characteristics of goal setting. For maximum success, a goal needs to be **S**pecific (identify what you would like to accomplish); **M**easurable (set a timeline and what you will track); **A**chievable (start slow and increase the intensity or commitment over time); **R**ealistic (consider the impact on your daily life); and **T**imely (start by setting an initial time frame for the goal).

THE RIGHT BALANCE

To hit the Goldilocks zone (not too hard, not too easy—just right), it's crucial to find the right level of challenge.

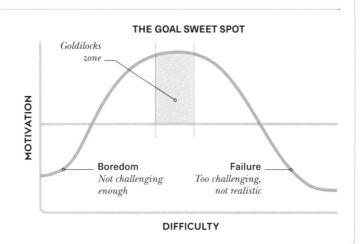

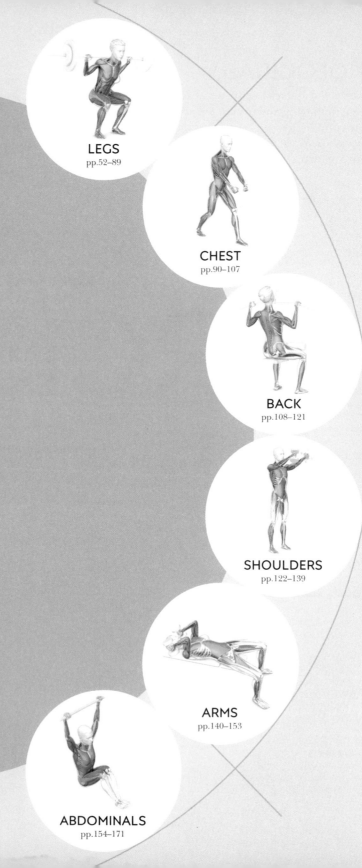

LEGS
pp.52–89

CHEST
pp.90–107

BACK
pp.108–121

SHOULDERS
pp.122–139

ARMS
pp.140–153

ABDOMINALS
pp.154–171

STRENGTH
EXERCISES

When it comes to strength training, the goal is to get the maximum benefit from every workout. This section comprises 31 main exercises, many with additional variations to do at home or with different equipment, that show you how best to execute each movement to maximize the benefits while limiting the risk of injury. You'll find the best exercises to challenge each major muscle group of the body.

INTRODUCTION TO THE **EXERCISES**

The exercises in this section show you how best to challenge a specific muscle group(s). But first, find out the basics of proper execution, how to master breathing, and how to exercise safely wherever you choose to train—at home or in the gym.

> **❗ Common mistakes**
>
> On most exercises, there is a box relating to commonly seen errors when performing the exercise. As well as these prompts, it's also crucial not to obsess over details (what's known as "paralysis by analysis"); not to move loads without thought of the muscles being worked (intention and focus are key for mind–muscle connection); and not to sacrifice execution or proper technique for a higher load on the bar or to adapt your form to make things easier (cheating reps).

MAINS AND VARIATIONS

The exercises are organized by muscle group, and further into "main" and "variation" exercises. Each main exercise has been chosen as an effective way to train specific muscle group(s), commonly using a multijoint compound exercise. Each variation helps complement the main exercise while adding new ways of challenging the muscle(s). The muscles used in each stage of a main exercise are illustrated anatomically, alongside the steps on how to best perform the movement. Exercises are also organized into goal-specific training programs (see pp.201–214), where you can take what you learn from each structured grouping and apply it to an organized workout at the gym or at home.

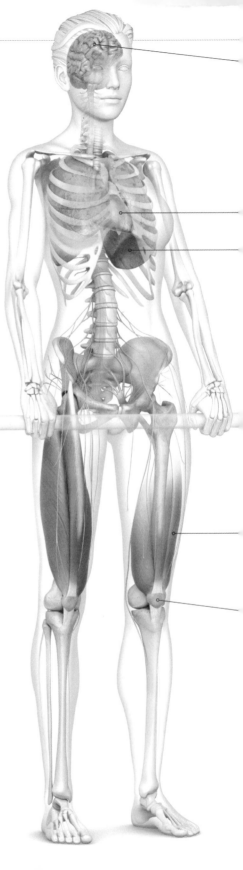
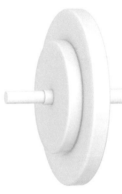

Brain and nervous system
A better connection between your nervous system and your muscles can lead to more strength and improved coordination

Cardiovascular system
Blood carrying oxygen and fuels is pumped to energize muscles and to remove waste products

Respiratory system
Breathing in sync with the right stages of a movement is key. You'll need to learn how to breathe while braced (see right)

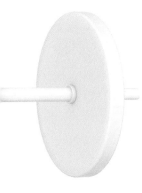

Muscular system
Placing more mechanical tension and stress on the desired muscle means more potential for muscle growth

Skeletal system
Muscles pull on bones to move the body in a series of levers. Correct set-up and execution means less tension placed on passive tissues and less injury

CORRECT EXERCISE EXECUTION
It takes a whole body to power muscles and to control and coordinate limbs within a movement. Proper execution of an exercise is vital to place tension on the target muscles, to build muscle, to gain strength and coordination, to avoid injury, and to maximize training stress (more work in less time).

THE IMPORTANCE OF **BREATHING**

The respiratory and circulatory systems work to respond to the demands of the exercise to fuel the muscles. To maximize a workout's efficiency, it's key to engage your abdominal muscles throughout. Breathing instructions are given for all exercises so that you know during which stage of an exercise to breathe in and to breathe out.

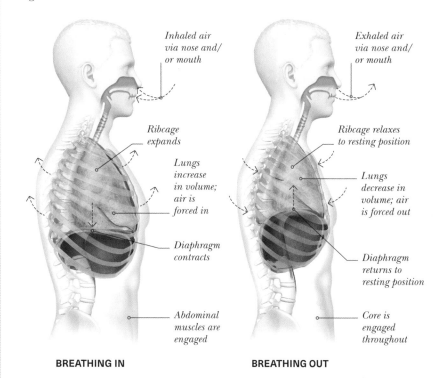

Inhaled air via nose and/ or mouth

Ribcage expands

Lungs increase in volume; air is forced in

Diaphragm contracts

Abdominal muscles are engaged

BREATHING IN

Exhaled air via nose and/ or mouth

Ribcage relaxes to resting position

Lungs decrease in volume; air is forced out

Diaphragm returns to resting position

Core is engaged throughout

BREATHING OUT

Exercise terminology
Knowing what terms mean is crucial to understanding instructions related to the exercises (see also pp.198–199 and the glossary, pp.215–216). The most important ones to learn from the start are explained here.

REPETITION (REP)
One completion of an exercise (concentric and eccentric, or vice versa). The number of reps is generally relative to the weight being lifted.

TRAINING VOLUME
The amount of exercise or work performed over a given period of time, whether that's the training session or a week of training.

SET
A series of repetitions (or reps) performed sequentially—such as "3 sets of 6–8 reps." You'll find the suggested number of reps and sets to perform for each exercise listed within a goal-specific training program (see pp.201–214).

TEMPO
The speed at which you perform an exercise. The tempo should be controlled at all times in both stages of the exercise.

WHERE TO TRAIN?

Unlike some types of exercise modalities, strength training provides flexibility to be done at the gym or from the comfort (and convenience) of your own home. Choosing the right environment to work out in can be important in avoiding somewhere you feel you do not belong, the feeling of intimidation, or the worry around proper hygiene by those around you. Whether you like to train solely in the gym, always at home, or a mix of the two, it's good to know that you can progress toward your goals no matter where you choose to strength train.

Caution

If you have a preexisting condition and any exercise in this section causes you pain, consult a qualified professional.

At home

If your home has space for you to train, then it offers you the most customizable option in terms of equipment and facilities. Working out at home allows you to control the environment (room temperature and music, for instance), omits the potential of feeling intimidated (if that's a concern), and puts you in sole charge of proper gym hygiene and potential spread of germs.

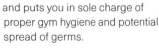

Pros

The potential upsides of training at home are:

- **More exercises are possible**—new innovations in multifunctional equipment, resistance bands, and free weights make training at home easier than ever

- **Choosing your own playlist**—motivate yourself through the music playing during workouts; the right music can motivate you to work harder

- **Working out anytime**—interested in a workout now? Then you can get set up and get right to it

Cons

The potential downsides of working out at home can be:

- **Feeling unmotivated**—it's easy not to feel the drive to push yourself during home-based workouts, plus you miss out on other social interactions

- **Affordability of equipment**—building up what you need to work out effectively can be expensive, though equipment has become more affordable

- **Potential limits on resistance (weight)**—free weights are available only up to a certain size, so you're limited to those you can buy and use

At the gym

The gym should be a warm, inviting, and motivating place to do a workout. That said, it's key to find a gym where you feel you belong and where you don't feel intimidated. If there isn't a gym nearby that you feel fits your preferences, training at home is a viable option.

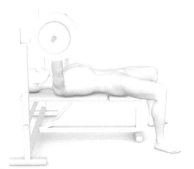

Pros

The potential upsides of gym-based training are:

- **The greatest value in terms of equipment and facilities**—a good gym has everything you need and more, including access to a personal trainer

- **A motivating environment**—training in a gym can encourage you to push yourself

- **A more social set-up**—you can form new relationships and be around others who are like-minded and have similar goals of improving their health and body composition

Cons

The potential downsides can be:

- **Lack of control of the environment**—working out with others has social advantages, but if the music is limited (or annoying) and the gym is too hot or too cold, this can throw off the experience

- **Feelings of intimidation**—it may be due to inexperience or the attitudes of others, but if you feel intimidated, find another gym instead

- **Gym hygiene**—you need to be happy with the cleanliness and measures taken to prevent germ transmission

At-home training equipment

Training at home has never been easier with the advent of more affordable multifunctional equipment. You may not want to buy all of the items listed below, but if you do, you'll be well on your way to be able to perform most of the exercises in the comfort of your own home.

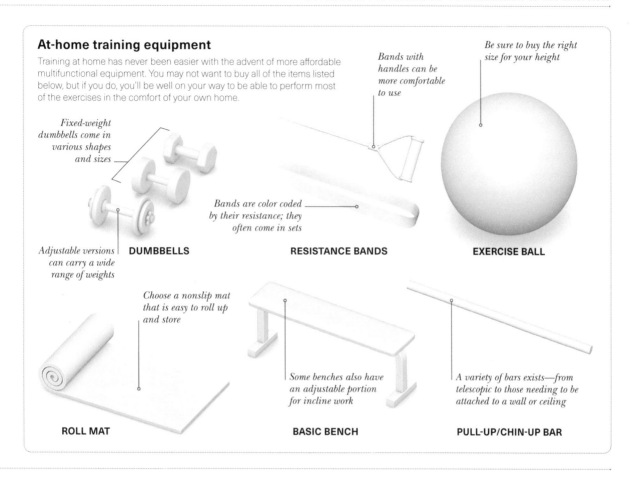

Bands with handles can be more comfortable to use

Be sure to buy the right size for your height

Fixed-weight dumbbells come in various shapes and sizes

Bands are color coded by their resistance; they often come in sets

Adjustable versions can carry a wide range of weights

DUMBBELLS

RESISTANCE BANDS

EXERCISE BALL

Choose a nonslip mat that is easy to roll up and store

Some benches also have an adjustable portion for incline work

A variety of bars exists—from telescopic to those needing to be attached to a wall or ceiling

ROLL MAT

BASIC BENCH

PULL-UP/CHIN-UP BAR

Good gym etiquette

When training in a public place, such as a gym, it's important to be respectful of others. Here are just a few things to be aware of that can keep a harmonious atmosphere and make others see that you are being considerate to them.

Rerack weights after use
Don't leave weights on the floor. Rerack barbells, move weights back to the stack, and wipe them down so they're ready for the next person.

Be aware of others using equipment
Find out who's waiting for a particular machine or piece of equipment. Do not take over someone's claimed machine.

Be socially aware
Respect boundaries, personal space, and eye contact. Get a sense for the feel of the gym and act appropriately.

Taking a photo or video
Ensure the gym's policy allows you to do so; when in doubt, ask management, as well as the permission of those around you.

Share equipment equally
Respect others and do not overstay your welcome at specific machines or stations, especially if the gym is busy.

Wear headphones if listening to music
Keep your music to yourself. Loud music from a speaker can interrupt and irritate those working out around you.

Extra-special measures
Cleaning equipment or weights after use was always part of a gym's protocol. But now, due to health concerns across the globe, gyms are required to take very serious measures to ensure the health and safety of their members and help prevent the spread of disease. Be sure to wipe down equipment before and after use, cover all coughs and sneezes, wash hands often (or use hand sanitizer), not share towels or drinks with others, and not go to the gym if you feel unwell.

CHOOSING **WEIGHTS**

When you first join a gym, you will be given instructions on how to safely use all the equipment. Understanding how to choose weights (load selection) to best fit your structure can impact the safety and efficacy of your lifting. Start each exercise with a light weight that you know you can lift easily and progress the weight based on assessment and the desired rep range.

Machines

You will likely see machines of two different styles: the "selectorize" machines are loaded with a pin system and the "plate-loaded" ones use weight plates on designated horns—the same plates used on a barbell. Machines that focus on large muscle groups (legs, chest, and back) typically have heavier weight stacks compared to machines that focus on smaller muscle groups (arms, shoulders, and calf). If you are unsure of what is "light enough," start by placing the selectorize pin in the first slot and perform one rep.

Free weights

Free weights include barbells and dumbbells. Barbells are commonly 45 lb (20 kg), 1 1/10 in (28.5 mm) in diameter, and 85 in (2.15 m) in length; shorter ones are sometimes available. When loading a barbell, slide the plates on and lock with a clip or collar. The weight of a dumbbell is identified by its label. Dumbbells are typically found in pairs (two of the same weight and size). Start with a weight you know you can lift for the designated rep range. If new to barbells, start with the bar only and increase weight in 5–10-lb (2.25–4.5-kg) increments.

WORKING ON **MACHINES**

Each machine will need to be adjusted to best fit your individual structure. It's a good idea if you are new to training with machines to have a session with a trainer to learn how each machine works and what settings are best for you. The most common adjustments are for the seat pad, back pad, and thigh pad, but also note any axis of rotations on the machine to best line up your legs. If something feels uncomfortable when you perform your first reps, adjust the available settings until the exercise feels comfortable.

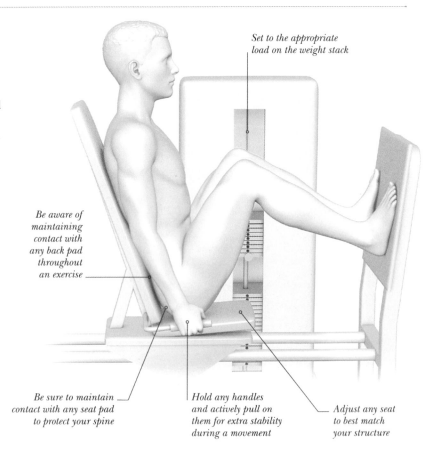

Set to the appropriate load on the weight stack

Be aware of maintaining contact with any back pad throughout an exercise

Be sure to maintain contact with any seat pad to protect your spine

Hold any handles and actively pull on them for extra stability during a movement

Adjust any seat to best match your structure

LIFTING **SAFELY**

Arguably the most important component of strength training is safety. Lifting weights safely takes constant thought and attention to what you are doing, whether you are training in the gym or working out at home. Such focus on execution of an exercise not only keeps you safe, but also ensures you're able to work out sustainably within your regular program. Grip is key—both in how you hold a weight (a barbell or dumbbell) and in how far apart your hands are when performing an exercise.

How to grip

Gripping the bar in a certain way is essential for securely holding the weight in whatever position is needed and for limiting any soreness in your hands. Common grips are supinated, neutral, and pronated (see below, and the wrist, p.50); semisupinated is halfway between a supinated and a neutral position.

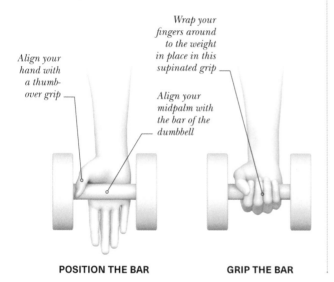

Align your hand with a thumb-over grip

Align your midpalm with the bar of the dumbbell

Wrap your fingers around to the weight in place in this supinated grip

POSITION THE BAR　　　**GRIP THE BAR**

Grip positions and types

Like other parts of the set-up, the width of the grip you use on a bar or a machine attachment (see pp.110–111), as well as your wrist's position, directly impacts which muscles have more leverage and can best contribute to the movement. So switching from a wide to a narrow or neutral grip for the same exercise targets slightly different muscles.

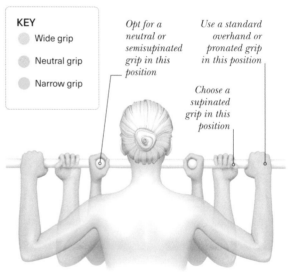

KEY
- Wide grip
- Neutral grip
- Narrow grip

Opt for a neutral or semisupinated grip in this position

Use a standard overhand or pronated grip in this position

Choose a supinated grip in this position

Log your workouts

Keeping notes on each workout helps you track and maintain progress. For example, you can see at a glance the weight used last week for an exercise and can increase accordingly, unless it was flagged as too challenging. Keeping a log—whether it's an actual book, a spreadsheet, or an app—is a good habit to get into. The table, shown here, gives you an idea of the details you need to track.

WORKOUT DATE

EXERCISE	REPS AND SETS	WEIGHT USED PER SET	REST	NOTES
LEG PRESS	4 sets of 10 reps	Set 1 XX lb/kg	60 seconds	Go up in weight next week by XX lb/kg
SHOULDER PRESS	4 sets of 10 reps	Set 1 XX lb/kg	60 seconds	Challenging; stay with same weight next time

TERMINOLOGY GUIDE

The body's joints facilitate an incredible and wide range of movements, and each movement is described using the illustrations on these pages. Throughout this book, instructions use terminology and directional terms that will help guide you in a specific stage of an exercise or the exercise as a whole, so it's a good idea to mark this page for easy reference.

Spine

As well as providing structural support for the upper body, the spine helps transfer loads between the lower and upper body. It can extend, flex, rotate, and flex to the side, as well as combinations of these.

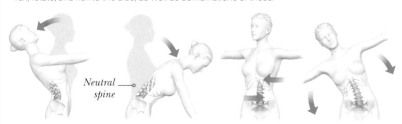

Neutral spine

EXTENSION
Bending at the waist to move the torso backward.

FLEXION
Bending at the waist to move the torso forward.

ROTATION
Turning the trunk to the right or left on the midline.

SIDE FLEXION
Bending the trunk to the right or left from the midline.

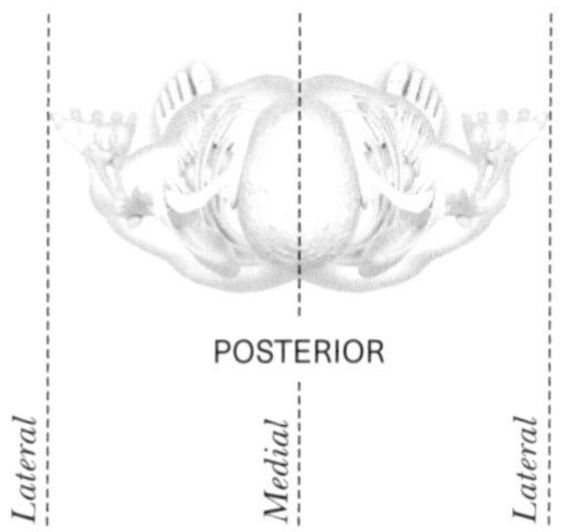

Orientations

ANTERIOR

POSTERIOR

Lateral
Medial
Lateral

SUPERIOR VIEW

ORIENTATIONS

Elbow

The elbow is involved in any exercise using hand-held resistance, as well as specific arm movements.

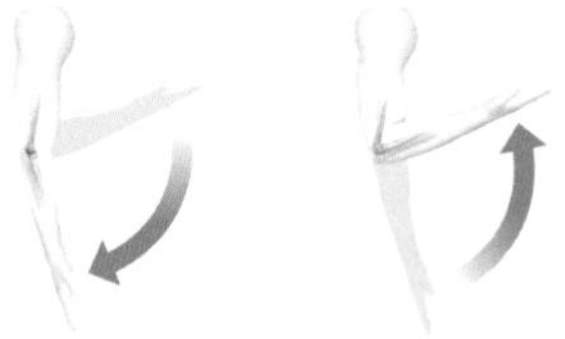

EXTENSION
Straightening the arm, increasing the joint angle.

FLEXION
Bending the arm, decreasing the joint angle.

Wrist

The wrist should remain neutral (in straight alignment with the forearm) unless otherwise directed.

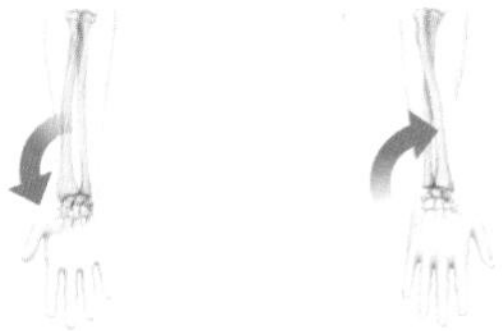

SUPINATION
Rotating the forearm so the palm faces up.

PRONATION
Rotating the forearm so the palm faces down.

Hip

The hip joint is capable of a wide range of motion in multiple planes, all involving a straight leg, as shown here.

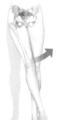
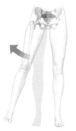
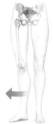
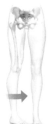
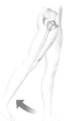
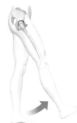

ADDUCTION
Moving the thigh inward toward the midline.

ABDUCTION
Moving the thigh away from the midline.

EXTERNAL ROTATION
Rotating the thigh outward.

INTERNAL ROTATION
Rotating the thigh inward.

EXTENSION
Extending the thigh backward, straightening the body at the hip.

FLEXION
Moving the thigh forward, bending the body at the hip.

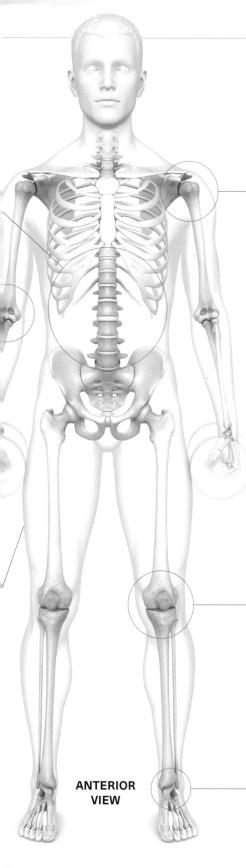

ANTERIOR VIEW

Shoulder

This complex joint has a wide range of movements in multiple planes. It can move the arm forward and backward and up and down at the side, as well as rotating at the shoulder joint itself.

FLEXION
Moving the arm forward at the shoulder.

EXTENSION
Moving the arm backward at the shoulder.

ADDUCTION
Moving the arm toward the body.

ABDUCTION
Moving the arm away from the body.

EXTERNAL ROTATION
Rotating the arm outward at the shoulder.

INTERNAL ROTATION
Rotating the arm inward at the shoulder.

Knee

The knee has to be able to sustain loads of up to 10 times the body's weight. Its main actions are flexing and extending, both of which are involved in lots of strength training exercises.

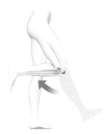
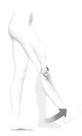

FLEXION
Bending at the knee, which decreases the joint angle.

EXTENSION
Straightening at the knee, which increases the joint angle.

Ankle

In strength training, the important movements of this joint involve its dorsiflexion and plantarflexion.

DORSIFLEXION
Bending at the ankle so that the toes point upward.

PLANTARFLEXION
Bending at the ankle so that the toes point downward.

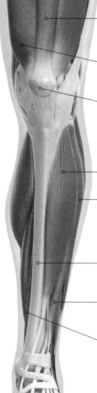

Gluteus medius
Fan-shaped muscle that extends the hip more laterally and rotates the leg

Gluteus maximus
One of the biggest muscles in the body; it extends the hip and rotates the leg

Adductor magnus
Known as an adductor of the hip but also acts as a powerful hip extensor

Vastus lateralis
Division of the quadriceps

Biceps femoris long head
The most lateral of the hamstrings, which extend the hip, flex the knee, and rotate the leg

Semitendinosus
A division of the hamstrings

Semimembranosus
A division of the hamstrings

Biceps femoris short head
A division of the hamstrings

Femur
The thighbone; the longest, strongest, and heaviest bone in the body

Gastrocnemius
Forms the major bulk of the calf; it has two heads and helps plantarflex the ankle and flex the knee

Soleus
Large, flat muscle lying beneath the gastrocnemius; its name comes from the Latin for sole or flatish

Achilles (calcaneal) tendon
This common tendon, shared between the gastrocnemius and soleus muscles, winds 90° on its path toward the heel

Fibula
A thin bone that sits on the outside of the lower leg

Calcaneus
The heel bone

POSTERIOR VIEW

Iliopsoas
Formed of two merged muscles (psoas and iliacus), it flexes the hip

Tensor fascia latae
Often abbreviated to TFL, it helps stabilize the femur, alongside the hip and knee joints

Pectineus
Flexes and adducts the hip

Adductor longus
Fan-shaped muscle that is one of the adductor muscles

Gracilis
Long, thin, superficial muscle that aids in flexion and adduction at the hip and knee

Sartorius
Flexes, abducts, and laterally rotates the hip, and flexes the knee

Rectus femoris
Division of the quadriceps; flexes the hip and extends the knee

Vastus medialis
Division of the quadriceps

Patella
Also called the kneecap, attached to the quadriceps tendon

Tibialis anterior
Dorsiflexes the ankle

Peroneus (fibularis) longus
Moves the foot and ankle in various directions; its tendon wraps under the foot

Tibia
The shinbone

Extensor digitorum longus
Extends lateral four digits and dorsiflexes the ankle

Flexor digitorum longus
Flexes the second to fifth toes and helps plantarflexion of the ankle

Extensor hallucis longus
Flexes the big toe and helps plantarflexion of the ankle

ANTERIOR VIEW

LEG EXERCISES

The main muscle groups responsible for movement of the lower body are: the quadriceps, the muscles that give the upper front leg its shape; the hamstrings, the equivalent muscle group at the back of the upper leg; the gluteal muscles, resting on the back of the pelvis; and the calves, at the back of the lower leg.

The main role of the quadriceps (or quads) is to extend the knee, with one division (rectus femoris) specifically also enabling hip flexion. Hamstrings, meanwhile, extend the hips and flex the knee. The glutes work to extend the hips, as well as aiding internal and external rotation of the leg at the hip. The calves mainly plantarflex the ankle and flex the knee.

Within lower-body training, multiple muscle groups combine to help coordinate movement around the hip, knee, and ankle joints.

- **When performing compound exercises** (which involve more than one joint), you will be using muscles across the lower body to perform the movement while controlling the forces around

each joint. Examples include back squats and deadlifts.

- **When performing isolation exercises** (which involve only one joint), you will be biasing one muscle group over others. You still use other muscles though—to stabilize the forces around the working joint. Examples are leg extensions and calf raises.

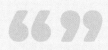

*Building muscle and **strength in your legs** can improve your performance across workouts.*

BARBELL
BACK SQUAT

This multijoint exercise—also known as a compound exercise—helps strengthen the quadriceps, adductors, and glutes; it also challenges the hamstrings, spinal erectors, and abdominals. Maintaining the correct form is key to protect the spine from injury.

THE BIG PICTURE

Proper coordination and mechanics are crucial here. Engaging the core increases stability and control and prevents lower-back strain. Start off with a low weight and only increase the load when you're comfortable with the move.

Beginners can start with 4 sets of 8–10 reps; discover other variations on pp.56–57 and other targeted sets in the training programs (see pp.201–214).

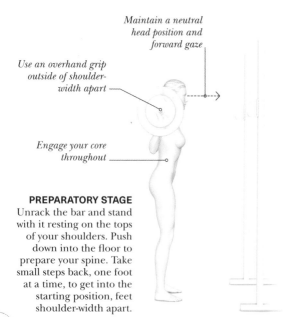

Maintain a neutral head position and forward gaze

Use an overhand grip outside of shoulder-width apart

Engage your core throughout

PREPARATORY STAGE
Unrack the bar and stand with it resting on the tops of your shoulders. Push down into the floor to prepare your spine. Take small steps back, one foot at a time, to get into the starting position, feet shoulder-width apart.

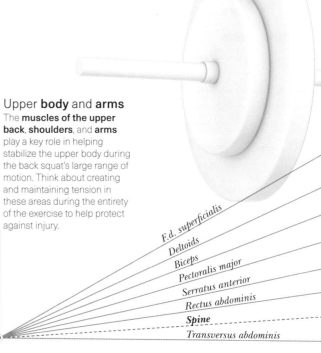

Upper **body** and **arms**
The **muscles of the upper back**, **shoulders**, and **arms** play a key role in helping stabilize the upper body during the back squat's large range of motion. Think about creating and maintaining tension in these areas during the entirety of the exercise to help protect against injury.

F.d. superficialis
Deltoids
Biceps
Pectoralis major
Serratus anterior
Rectus abdominis
Spine
Transversus abdominis

STAGE ONE
Breathe in and, with core engaged, push your hips back to begin the squat. Flex at your knees, keeping them in line with your feet as they move forward. Slow down as you approach the bottom position; your thighs should be roughly parallel to the floor.

Legs
The **quadriceps**, **glutes**, and **adductors** will be the main movers, while the **hamstrings** and **calf muscles** will help stabilize the pelvis and knee, respectively. This lowering-into-the-squat move is an eccentric action. This exercise can place large amounts of tension across many tissues of the lower body.

Psoas major
Gluteus maximus
Rectus femoris
Biceps femoris
Knee
Gastrocnemius
Soleus
Tibialis anterior
Peroneus longus
Ankle
Extensor digitorum longus

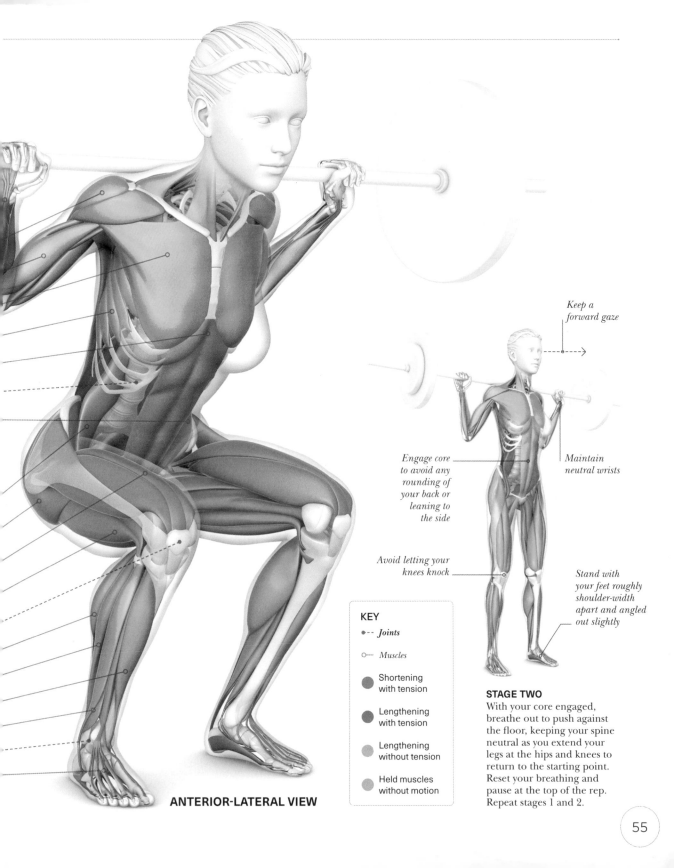

KEY

●--- *Joints*

○— *Muscles*

● Shortening
with tension

● Lengthening
with tension

● Lengthening
without tension

● Held muscles
without motion

ANTERIOR-LATERAL VIEW

*Keep a
forward gaze*

*Engage core
to avoid any
rounding of
your back or
leaning to
the side*

*Maintain
neutral wrists*

*Avoid letting your
knees knock*

*Stand with
your feet roughly
shoulder-width
apart and angled
out slightly*

STAGE TWO
With your core engaged,
breathe out to push against
the floor, keeping your spine
neutral as you extend your
legs at the hips and knees to
return to the starting point.
Reset your breathing and
pause at the top of the rep.
Repeat stages 1 and 2.

›› VARIATIONS

While all use a squatting movement that targets the glutes and quads along with the hamstrings, these variations to the barbell back squat use weights held in different ways to offer an easier version or one that challenges other muscles more. Master your squatting execution first with the dumbbell squats before tackling the barbell front squat.

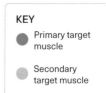

KEY

● Primary target muscle

● Secondary target muscle

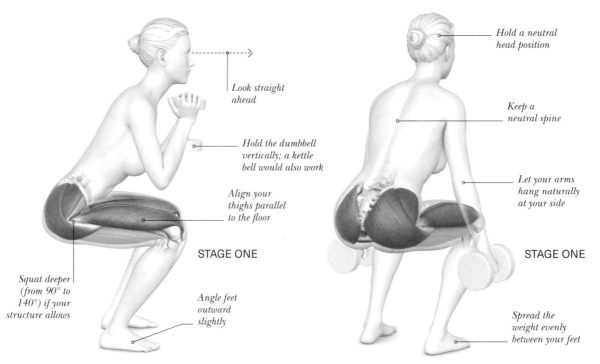

Look straight ahead

Hold the dumbbell vertically; a kettle bell would also work

Align your thighs parallel to the floor

STAGE ONE

Squat deeper (from 90° to 140°) if your structure allows

Angle feet outward slightly

Hold a neutral head position

Keep a neutral spine

Let your arms hang naturally at your side

STAGE ONE

Spread the weight evenly between your feet

DUMBBELL GOBLET SQUAT

Without the need for a barbell, this variation can be done at home. If you are new to squatting, start with this easier version. Holding a weight at the front skews the load to the upper back and allows the torso to be more upright.

PREPARATORY STAGE
Plant your feet shoulder-width apart. With both hands, hold the dumbbell in front of your chest, under your chin. Keep your forearms near vertical.

STAGE ONE
Breathe in and push your hips back, bending at the knee and squatting deeply. Keep your knees wide, tracking in line with your toes; don't let them knock in.

STAGE TWO
Drive out of the squat to return to the standing position, breathing out as you do so. Keep your abs engaged throughout. Repeat stages 1 and 2.

DUMBBELL SQUAT

Using a pair of dumbbells, this squatting movement offers another easier variation. Holding the weights at your sides and naturally carrying them into the squat offers more work for muscles of the forearms, arms, and upper back.

PREPARATORY STAGE
Stand tall with your feet roughly shoulder-width apart and parallel. Hold the dumbbells with straight arms at your sides. Look ahead and tense your torso.

STAGE ONE
With the core engaged, breathe in and flex at the hips and knees to squat, with the knees aligned over the feet. Look ahead and keep your arms hanging vertically.

STAGE TWO
Breathe out as you drive out of the squat to return to the standing position, keeping your abs engaged at all times. Repeat stages 1 and 2.

"" ""

*Squatting is a **multi-joint exercise** that challenges muscles around the knee, hip, and torso; improved **mobility** and **balance** and **stronger muscles** benefit day-to-day life.*

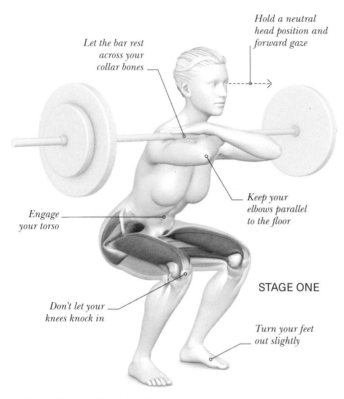

Hold a neutral head position and forward gaze

Let the bar rest across your collar bones

Keep your elbows parallel to the floor

Engage your torso

Don't let your knees knock in

Turn your feet out slightly

STAGE ONE

BARBELL **FRONT SQUAT**

If you find the barbell back squat aggravates your lower back or you have a shoulder injury, this variation might suit you instead. This version challenges the muscles of the upper back more due to the load shifting from back to front.

PREPARATORY STAGE
Stand tall with your feet roughly shoulder-width apart. Lift the barbell and allow it to settle at the top of your shoulders in line with your collar bones.

STAGE ONE
Breathe in, engage your core, and "sit" into a deep squat, keeping your torso as upright as possible. Hold a forward gaze and keep the barbell still.

STAGE TWO
Breathe out as you push through your feet and stand up, extending your legs at the hip and knee with your core engaged. Repeat stages 1 and 2.

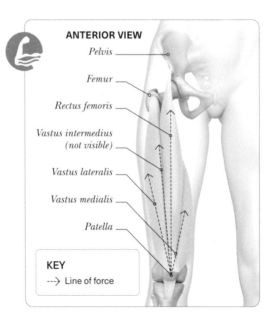

ANTERIOR VIEW

Pelvis

Femur

Rectus femoris

Vastus intermedius (not visible)

Vastus lateralis

Vastus medialis

Patella

KEY

--> Line of force

Force lines in the quadriceps
The quadriceps is not one muscle, but several divisions of muscle working together; these divisions have varying lines of force, or pull, depending on when they are most needed throughout a range of motion of an action. For example, in a squat exercise, different divisions of the quadriceps come into play more at particular points of the squatting movement. Overall, then, the divisions of the quadriceps work in synchronicity.

LEG PRESS

This straightforward movement works a wide range of leg muscles. The machine-based leg press helps strengthen the quadriceps, adductors, and glutes while also challenging the hamstrings. This compound movement mimics the back squat (see pp.54–55) but without the need to load the spine, so it's particularly good for protecting against injury or helping work around preexisting injuries.

KEY
- •-- *Joints*
- ○— *Muscles*
- ● Shortening with tension
- ● Lengthening with tension
- ● Lengthening without tension
- ● Held muscles without motion

THE BIG PICTURE

The leg press offers a full leg workout. Set the weights, sit back on the pad, and adjust the foot platform position. For maximum effectiveness, you need to bend only at the hips and knees. Grip the handles on the machine to offer stability to your torso and pull yourself down into the seat.

Beginners can start with 4 sets of 8–10 reps; discover other targeted sets in the training programs (see pp.201–214).

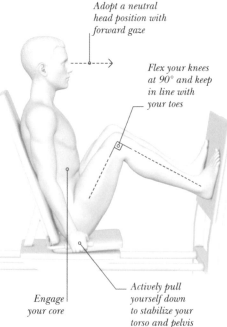

Adopt a neutral head position with forward gaze

Flex your knees at 90° and keep in line with your toes

Engage your core

Actively pull yourself down to stabilize your torso and pelvis

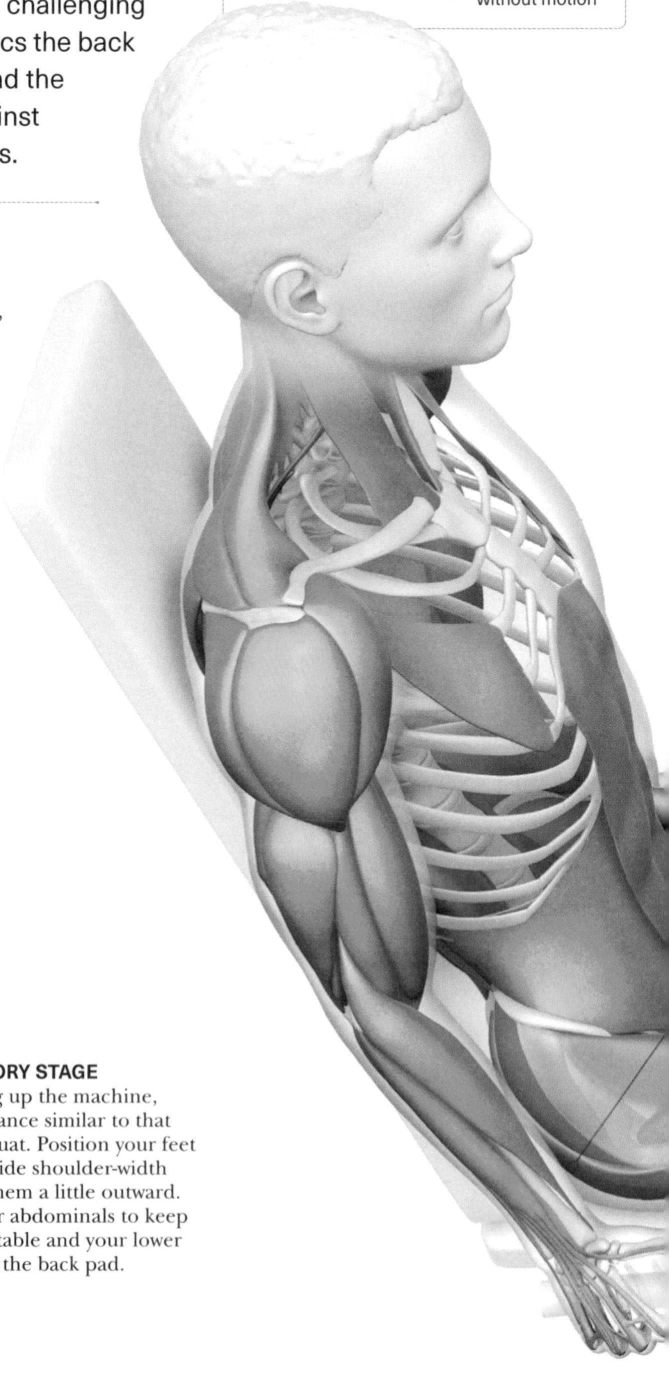

PREPARATORY STAGE
After setting up the machine, get into a stance similar to that of a back squat. Position your feet slightly outside shoulder-width and angle them a little outward. Engage your abdominals to keep your torso stable and your lower back flat on the back pad.

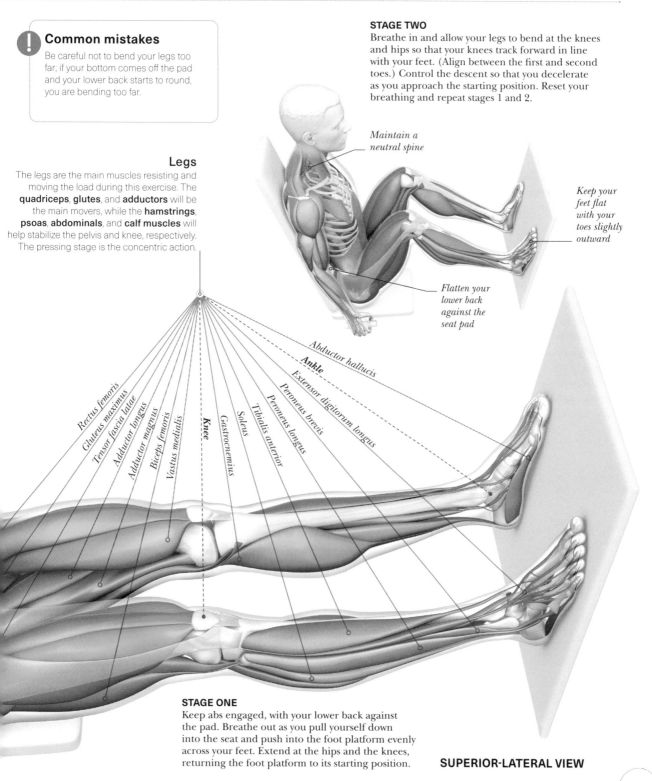

Common mistakes

Be careful not to bend your legs too far; if your bottom comes off the pad and your lower back starts to round, you are bending too far.

STAGE TWO
Breathe in and allow your legs to bend at the knees and hips so that your knees track forward in line with your feet. (Align between the first and second toes.) Control the descent so that you decelerate as you approach the starting position. Reset your breathing and repeat stages 1 and 2.

Maintain a neutral spine

Legs

The legs are the main muscles resisting and moving the load during this exercise. The **quadriceps**, **glutes**, and **adductors** will be the main movers, while the **hamstrings**, **psoas**, **abdominals**, and **calf muscles** will help stabilize the pelvis and knee, respectively. The pressing stage is the concentric action.

Keep your feet flat with your toes slightly outward

Flatten your lower back against the seat pad

Abductor hallucis

Rectus femoris

Gluteus maximus

Tensor fascia latae

Adductor longus

Adductor magnus

Biceps femoris

Vastus medialis

Knee

Gastrocnemius

Soleus

Tibialis anterior

Peroneus longus

Peroneus brevis

Extensor digitorum longus

Ankle

STAGE ONE
Keep abs engaged, with your lower back against the pad. Breathe out as you pull yourself down into the seat and push into the foot platform evenly across your feet. Extend at the hips and the knees, returning the foot platform to its starting position.

SUPERIOR-LATERAL VIEW

HACK SQUAT

This squat strengthens the quadriceps, adductors, and glutes, and also challenges the hamstrings. This machine-based exercise has a predefined movement pattern, so it works the big leg muscles while minimizing injury risk or working around preexisting injuries.

THE **BIG PICTURE**

This compound or multijoint squatting move is often built into workouts to complement other lower-body strength movements. Keep your core engaged to avoid straining your lower back and be sure to train within your available (active) range of motion. Before you start, set the weights and check your movement up and down on the machine.

Beginners can start with 4 sets of 8–10 reps; discover other targeted sets in the training programs (see pp.201–214).

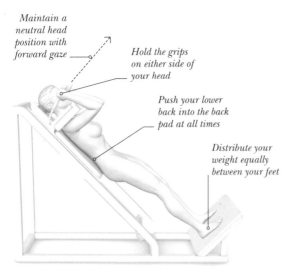

Maintain a neutral head position with forward gaze

Hold the grips on either side of your head

Push your lower back into the back pad at all times

Distribute your weight equally between your feet

PREPARATORY STAGE
Position yourself onto the machine and get into the standing starting position. Your stance on the foot platform will closely mimic that in the back squat (see pp.54–55)—your feet should be slightly outside shoulder-width with feet angled slightly outward.

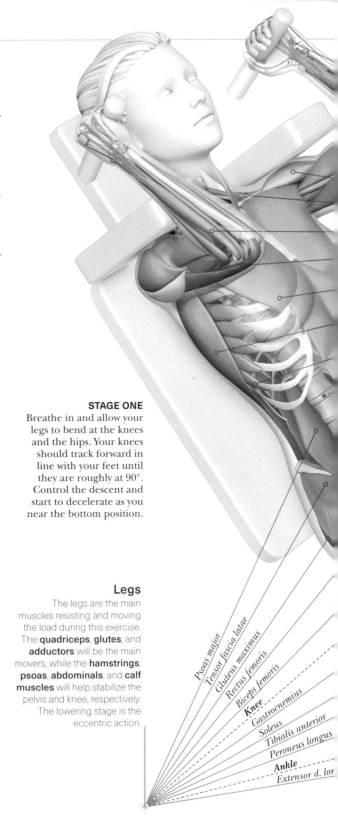

STAGE ONE
Breathe in and allow your legs to bend at the knees and the hips. Your knees should track forward in line with your feet until they are roughly at 90°. Control the descent and start to decelerate as you near the bottom position.

Legs
The legs are the main muscles resisting and moving the load during this exercise. The **quadriceps**, **glutes**, and **adductors** will be the main movers, while the **hamstrings**, **psoas**, **abdominals**, and **calf muscles** will help stabilize the pelvis and knee, respectively. The lowering stage is the eccentric action.

Psoas major
Tensor fascia latae
Gluteus maximus
Rectus femoris
Biceps femoris
Knee
Gastrocnemius
Soleus
Tibialis anterior
Peroneus longus
Ankle
Extensor d. lor

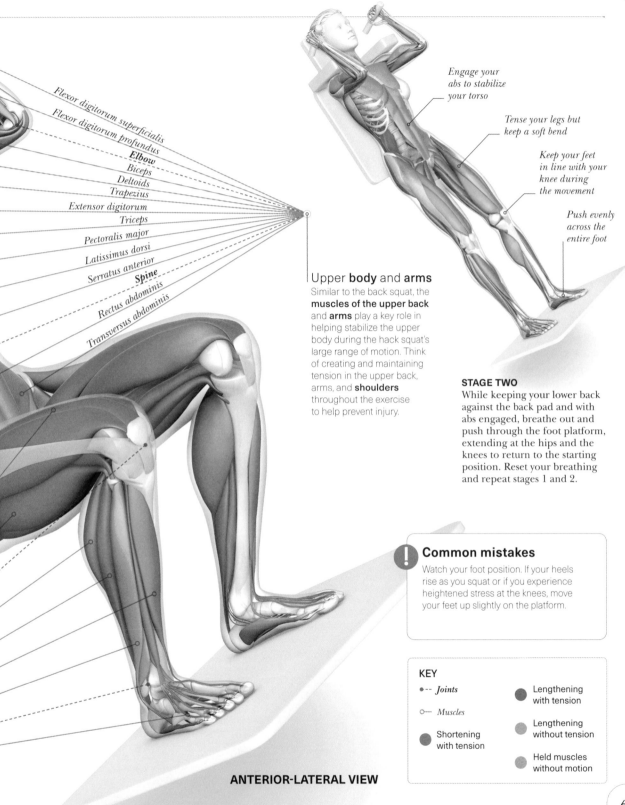

Flexor digitorum superficialis
Flexor digitorum profundus
Elbow
Biceps
Deltoids
Trapezius
Extensor digitorum
Triceps
Pectoralis major
Latissimus dorsi
Serratus anterior
Spine
Rectus abdominis
Transversus abdominis

Engage your
abs to stabilize
your torso

Tense your legs but
keep a soft bend

Keep your feet
in line with your
knee during
the movement

Push evenly
across the
entire foot

Upper **body** and **arms**
Similar to the back squat, the **muscles of the upper back** and **arms** play a key role in helping stabilize the upper body during the hack squat's large range of motion. Think of creating and maintaining tension in the upper back, arms, and **shoulders** throughout the exercise to help prevent injury.

STAGE TWO
While keeping your lower back against the back pad and with abs engaged, breathe out and push through the foot platform, extending at the hips and the knees to return to the starting position. Reset your breathing and repeat stages 1 and 2.

! Common mistakes
Watch your foot position. If your heels rise as you squat or if you experience heightened stress at the knees, move your feet up slightly on the platform.

KEY
- •-- *Joints*
- o— *Muscles*
- ● Shortening with tension
- ● Lengthening with tension
- ● Lengthening without tension
- ● Held muscles without motion

ANTERIOR-LATERAL VIEW

STATIONARY LUNGE WITH DUMBBELLS

The lunge is a useful exercise for training the quadriceps and glutes while also challenging the muscles that stabilize the core. Both legs work hard, but the main focus is on the muscles of the front leg.

THE BIG PICTURE

As you lunge, think downward rather than forward. When in the lunge position, your ear, hip, elbow, and hand should be aligned vertically. Throughout the exercise, ensure your torso is stable, your core is engaged, and your weight is evenly distributed through your front foot and the ball of your back foot. Hold the weights at your side and carry them naturally into the lunge motion. To be sure to exercise both legs evenly, work alternate legs each rep or keep the leg consistent through a set.

Beginners can start with 4 sets of 8–10 reps; discover variations on this exercise on pp.64–65 and other targeted sets within the training programs (see pp.201–214).

Upper **body**
Muscles of the core, upper back, arms, and shoulders help stabilize the upper body. Maintain this tension throughout the exercise to help maximize strength.

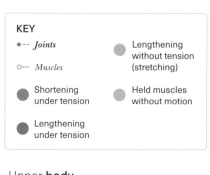

Trapezius
Deltoids
Pectoralis minor
Spine
Triceps
Biceps
Spinal extensors
Rectus abdominis
Transversus abdominis
Gluteus medius
Psoas major
Gluteus maximus
Rectus femoris
Vastus lateralis
Biceps femoris
Knee
Soleus
Extensor digitorum longus
Ankle
Abductor digiti minimi

> **⚠ Common mistakes**
> Taking too big or too small a step forward results in poor form for your lunge. Don't round your upper back.

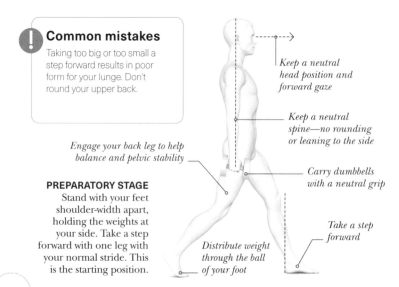

Keep a neutral head position and forward gaze

Engage your back leg to help balance and pelvic stability

Keep a neutral spine—no rounding or leaning to the side

Carry dumbbells with a neutral grip

PREPARATORY STAGE
Stand with your feet shoulder-width apart, holding the weights at your side. Take a step forward with one leg with your normal stride. This is the starting position.

Distribute weight through the ball of your foot

Take a step forward

Back **leg**
Maintaining contact with the ground allows the **quads** to continue working alongside the **gastrocnemius** and **soleus** in helping stabilize the knee. You will feel the tension in the quads, mainly from the **rectus femoris** being challenged.

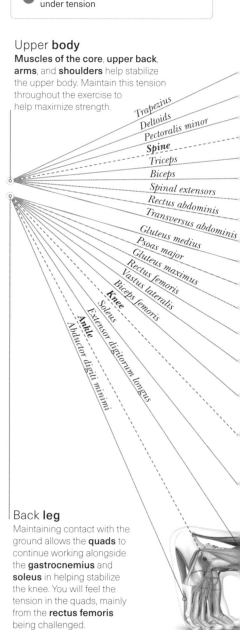

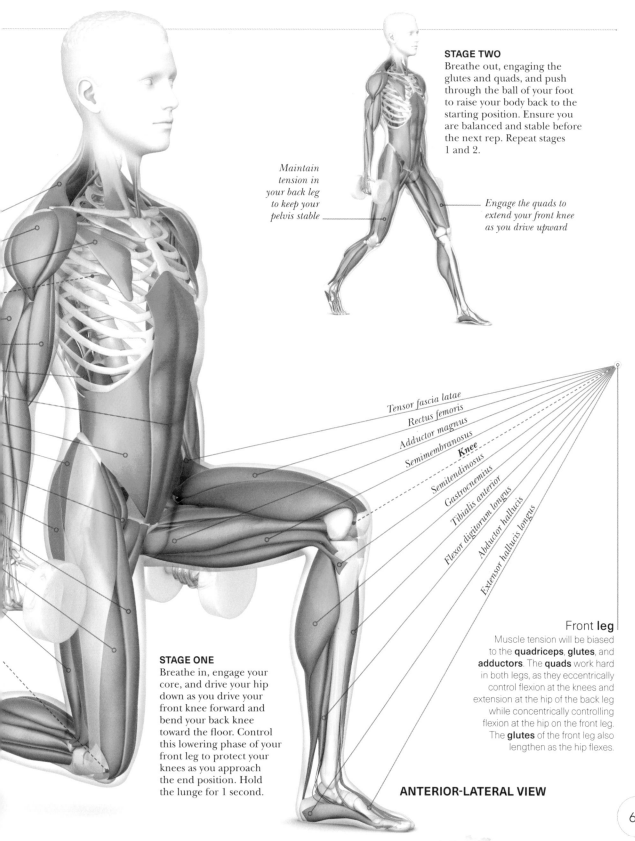

STAGE TWO
Breathe out, engaging the
glutes and quads, and push
through the ball of your foot
to raise your body back to the
starting position. Ensure you
are balanced and stable before
the next rep. Repeat stages
1 and 2.

*Maintain
tension in
your back leg
to keep your
pelvis stable*

*Engage the quads to
extend your front knee
as you drive upward*

Tensor fascia latae
Rectus femoris
Adductor magnus
Semimembranosus
Knee
Semitendinosus
Gastrocnemius
Tibialis anterior
Flexor digitorum longus
Abductor hallucis
Extensor hallucis longus

STAGE ONE
Breathe in, engage your
core, and drive your hip
down as you drive your
front knee forward and
bend your back knee
toward the floor. Control
this lowering phase of your
front leg to protect your
knees as you approach
the end position. Hold
the lunge for 1 second.

Front **leg**
Muscle tension will be biased
to the **quadriceps**, **glutes**, and
adductors. The **quads** work hard
in both legs, as they eccentrically
control flexion at the knees and
extension at the hip of the back leg
while concentrically controlling
flexion at the hip on the front leg.
The **glutes** of the front leg also
lengthen as the hip flexes.

ANTERIOR-LATERAL VIEW

» VARIATIONS

To improve your form through a lunging movement, you may want to practice first without any weights; all lunges target the quads, hamstrings, and glutes. Dumbbells should always be held by your side and carried naturally in and out of the movement.

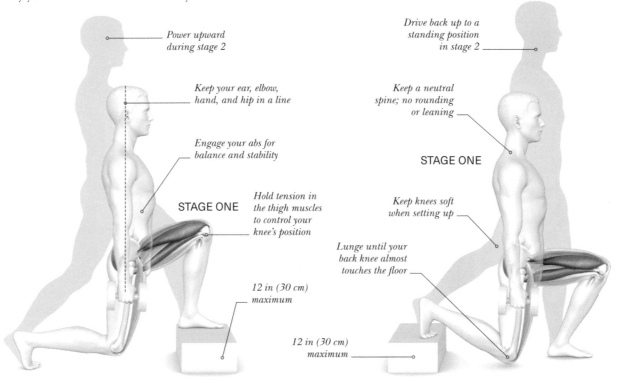

Power upward during stage 2

Keep your ear, elbow, hand, and hip in a line

Engage your abs for balance and stability

STAGE ONE

Hold tension in the thigh muscles to control your knee's position

12 in (30 cm) maximum

Drive back up to a standing position in stage 2

Keep a neutral spine; no rounding or leaning

STAGE ONE

Keep knees soft when setting up

Lunge until your back knee almost touches the floor

12 in (30 cm) maximum

FRONT FOOT ELEVATED SPLIT SQUAT WITH DUMBBELLS

This variation raises the front foot on a step or sturdy box to increase the range of motion while reducing the load on the front knee; keep your legs active to help pelvic stability. Try this easier version if you're new to lunging movements.

PREPARATORY STAGE
Stand with feet shoulder-width apart in a staggered stance. Step your leading leg onto the box. Keep your knees soft and engage your back leg for balance.

STAGE ONE
Breathe in as you drive your hip down and push your front knee forward while your back knee drops toward the floor. Keep your abs activated.

STAGE TWO
Breathe out and power upward using your quads and glutes. Repeat stages 1 and 2 for the desired number of reps, then repeat for the other leg.

BACK FOOT ELEVATED SPLIT SQUAT WITH DUMBBELLS

In this variation, the step or sturdy box increases the amount of hip flexion possible and adds a challenge to your quads; but if the step is too high, your hips may shift out of alignment. Keep your torso still and your arms at your sides.

PREPARATORY STAGE
Stand with your feet shoulder-width apart in front of the box. Step backward with one leg to rest on the ball of your foot. Engage your back leg for stability.

STAGE ONE
Breathe in and press downward with your back knee while your front leg flexes at the knee. Keep the abs engaged and a neutral spine throughout.

STAGE TWO
Exhale to drive back upward using your quads and glutes. Repeat stages 1 and 2 for the desired number of reps, then repeat for the other leg.

WALKING LUNGE
WITH DUMBBELLS

This variations aims to add a challenge and coordination to the stationary lunge. When starting this exercise, use little or no load to ensure you can remain balanced and coordinated as you get used to this walking variation of the lunge. Once you're confident in the movement, then add in more weight.

KEY

● Primary target muscle

● Secondary target muscle

Hold a neutral head position

Engage your core and keep your torso upright

Allow your arms to hang by your sides

Use the quads to drive out of the lunge

Flex your knee so your femur is parallel to the floor

PREPARATORY STAGE
Place your feet shoulder-width apart. Breathe in and stride forward into the lunge position—your front knee is flexed at 90°; your back knee is just off the floor.

STAGE ONE
Power up and out of the lunge, breathing out, and take a stride forward with your other leg. Stand tall and keep your abs engaged throughout.

STAGE TWO
Breathe in as you drive your hip down and your front knee forward, allowing your back knee to flex, as before. Repeat, alternating legs as you move along.

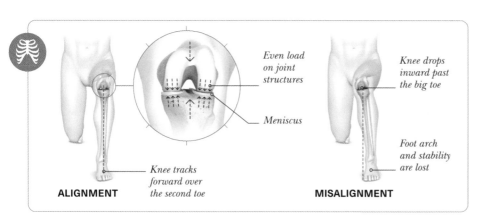

Even load on joint structures

Meniscus

Knee tracks forward over the second toe

ALIGNMENT

Knee drops inward past the big toe

Foot arch and stability are lost

MISALIGNMENT

Knee alignment
A common misalignment happens when the knee tracks inward past the big toe, which can cause problems for the knee and lead to pain and injury. Keep your knee tracking forward in alignment with your second toe—this helps maintain stability around your knee and reduce the risk of injuring yourself.

65

STEP UP WITH DUMBBELLS

This exercise strengthens the quadriceps and glutes while simultaneously challenging the muscles that stabilize the core.

THE BIG PICTURE

You will need an exercise step at least 12 in (30 cm) high. The main focus will be on the front leg, which remains on the step, while you engage your core throughout. Ensure your foot is completely on the step and your feet are shoulder-width apart. You'll drive through the front leg to step up; do not push off with your back foot. To be sure to exercise both legs, work alternate legs each rep or keep the leg consistent through a set.

Beginners can start with 4 sets of 8–10 reps; discover other targeted sets in the training programs (see pp.201–214).

Hip and leg

As you raise yourself up onto the step, focus on the **glutes** and **quads**. This concentric phase of the exercise strengthens the **glutes**, **proximal hamstrings**, and **quadriceps** as you drive through the front leg and fully extend the hip and knee, while the **calf muscles** provide stability. Maintain tension on the **quads** and **glutes** of the front leg during the lowering (eccentric) action rather than allowing the body to drop.

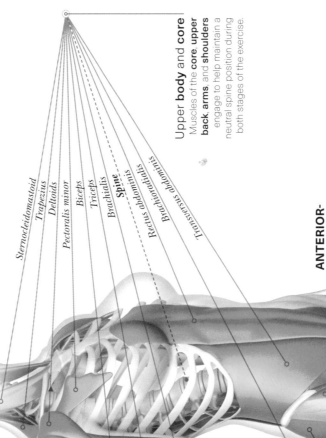

Sternocleidomastoid
Trapezius
Deltoids
Pectoralis minor
Biceps
Triceps
Brachialis
Spine
Rectus abdominis
Brachioradialis
Transversus abdominis

Upper body and core
Muscles of the **core**, upper **back**, **arms**, and **shoulders** engage to help maintain a neutral spine position during both stages of the exercise.

ANTERIOR-LATERAL VIEW

Gluteus medius
Tensor fascia latae
Iliopsoas
Sartorius

KEY

- Lengthening with tension
- Lengthening without tension
- Held muscles without motion
- Shortening with tension
- •--- *Joints*
- O—O *Muscles*

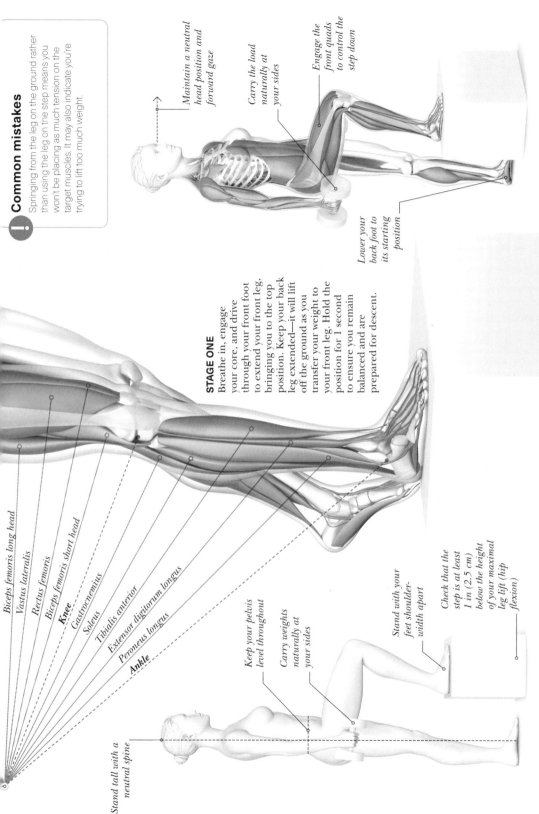

Maintain a neutral head position and forward gaze

Carry the load naturally at your sides

Engage the front quads to control the step down

Lower your back foot to its starting position

STAGE TWO

Breathe out and begin to lower your body by flexing your front hip and knee and by reaching down with your back leg until it touches the ground. Reset your breathing, focus, and core stability. Repeat stages 1 and 2.

STAGE ONE

Breathe in, engage your core, and drive through your front foot to extend your front leg, bringing you to the top position. Keep your back leg extended—it will lift off the ground as you transfer your weight to your front leg. Hold the position for 1 second to ensure you remain balanced and are prepared for descent.

Biceps femoris long head
Vastus lateralis
Rectus femoris
Biceps femoris short head
Knee
Gastrocnemius
Soleus
Tibialis anterior
Extensor digitorum longus
Peroneus longus
Ankle

Stand tall with a neutral spine

Keep your pelvis level throughout

Carry weights naturally at your sides

Stand with your feet shoulder-width apart

Check that the step is at least 1 in (2.5 cm) below the height of your maximal leg lift (hip flexion)

PREPARATORY STAGE

Stand tall with the step in front of you and weights in your hands at your sides. Raise your front leg to place it on the step. Keep your back leg engaged to help maintain balance and pelvic stability.

67

LEG CURL

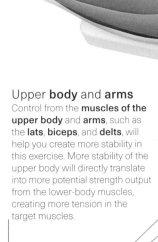

This exercise trains the hamstrings of the thigh and the main calf muscle—the gastrocnemius—both of which help flex the knee. From this fixed, prone position, you can flex at the knee with great force without loading the spine.

THE **BIG PICTURE**

This lying-down movement focuses effort on the knee joint as you curl your leg from straight to bent. It's important to engage your abdominals to stabilize your torso and to avoid any back strain. Before you start, set the weights and check the ankle pad.

Beginners can start with 4 sets of 8–10 reps; discover other variations of this exercise on pp.70–71 and other targeted sets in the training programs (see pp.201–214).

KEY

- •-- *Joints*
- ○-- *Muscles*
- ● Shortening with tension
- ● Lengthening with tension
- ● Lengthening without tension
- ● Held muscles without motion

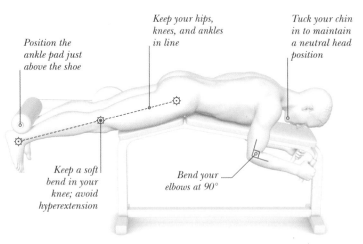

Position the ankle pad just above the shoe

Keep your hips, knees, and ankles in line

Tuck your chin in to maintain a neutral head position

Keep a soft bend in your knee; avoid hyperextension

Bend your elbows at 90°

PREPARATORY STAGE
Lie prone on the machine with your legs extended and the ankle pad just above your shoes. From there, engage your abs and latissimus dorsi by pulling against the handles of the machine and squeeze your glutes to help stabilize your pelvis.

Upper body and arms
Control from the **muscles of the upper body** and arms, such as the **lats**, **biceps**, and **delts**, will help you create more stability in this exercise. More stability of the upper body will directly translate into more potential strength output from the lower-body muscles, creating more tension in the target muscles.

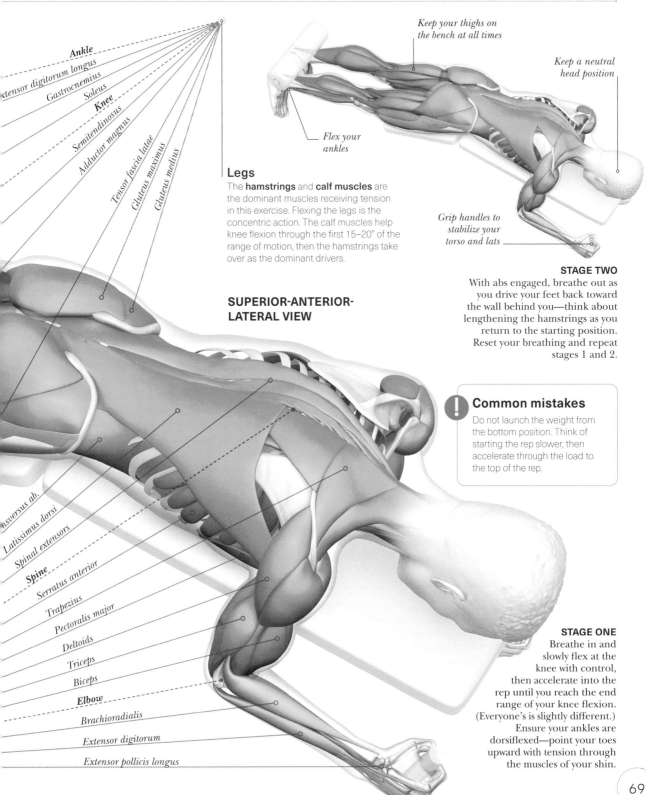

Ankle
Extensor digitorum longus
Gastrocnemius
Soleus
Knee
Semitendinosus
Adductor magnus
Tensor fascia latae
Gluteus maximus
Gluteus medius

Legs
The **hamstrings** and **calf muscles** are the dominant muscles receiving tension in this exercise. Flexing the legs is the concentric action. The calf muscles help knee flexion through the first 15–20° of the range of motion, then the hamstrings take over as the dominant drivers.

SUPERIOR-ANTERIOR-LATERAL VIEW

Transversus ab.
Latissimus dorsi
Spinal extensors
Spine
Serratus anterior
Trapezius
Pectoralis major
Deltoids
Triceps
Biceps
Elbow
Brachioradialis
Extensor digitorum
Extensor pollicis longus

Keep your thighs on the bench at all times

Keep a neutral head position

Flex your ankles

Grip handles to stabilize your torso and lats

STAGE TWO
With abs engaged, breathe out as you drive your feet back toward the wall behind you—think about lengthening the hamstrings as you return to the starting position. Reset your breathing and repeat stages 1 and 2.

! Common mistakes
Do not launch the weight from the bottom position. Think of starting the rep slower, then accelerate through the load to the top of the rep.

STAGE ONE
Breathe in and slowly flex at the knee with control, then accelerate into the rep until you reach the end range of your knee flexion. (Everyone's is slightly different.) Ensure your ankles are dorsiflexed—point your toes upward with tension through the muscles of your shin.

» VARIATIONS

Like the leg curl on the previous pages, all of these variations target
the hamstrings and the gastrocnemius. Being able to perform such
exercises standing up or sitting down opens up possibilities for an
at-home variation or utilizing different machines at the gym.

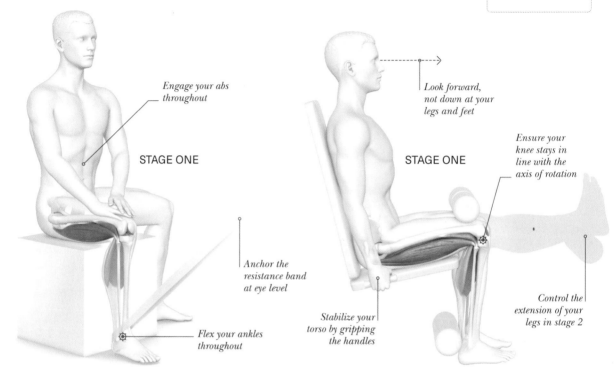

*Engage your abs
throughout*

STAGE ONE

*Anchor the
resistance band
at eye level*

*Flex your ankles
throughout*

*Look forward,
not down at your
legs and feet*

*Ensure your
knee stays in
line with the
axis of rotation*

STAGE ONE

*Control the
extension of your
legs in stage 2*

*Stabilize your
torso by gripping
the handles*

SEATED UNILATERAL BANDED
LEG CURL

Choose an appropriate resistance band (see p.47) and find
a stable anchor point to fix it to; the anchor point should be
at about eye level. This exercise focuses on one leg at a
time, so be sure to alternate your legs.

PREPARATORY STAGE
Fix the resistance band. Sit tall with a wide stance
and your feet flat on the floor. Position the band just
above the back of your shoe on an outstretched leg.

STAGE ONE
Inhale, then breathe out as you curl your lower leg
back toward your seat, keeping your foot off the
floor. Feel the resistance of the band increase.

STAGE TWO
Keeping your abs engaged and ankle dorsiflexed,
breathe in as you extend your leg to the starting
position, with control. Repeat stages 1 and 2.

SEATED LEG CURL

This seated machine-based variation increases the
stabilization of the pelvis while still challenging knee flexion
and the hamstrings in their lengthened position. You can
use this exercise to effectively train the hamstrings and
gastrocnemius via a different gym machine.

PREPARATORY STAGE
Set up the machine. Sit back against the pad with your
knees bent around the end of the seat. Place your
ankles on top of the lower pad and grip the handles.

STAGE ONE
Slowly flex at the knee with control while breathing
out. Continue to flex until you reach the end of
your knee flexion; be sure to dorsiflex your ankles.

STAGE TWO
Breathe in as you extend your legs in a controlled
manner; imagine lengthening your hamstrings as
you do so. Repeat stages 1 and 2.

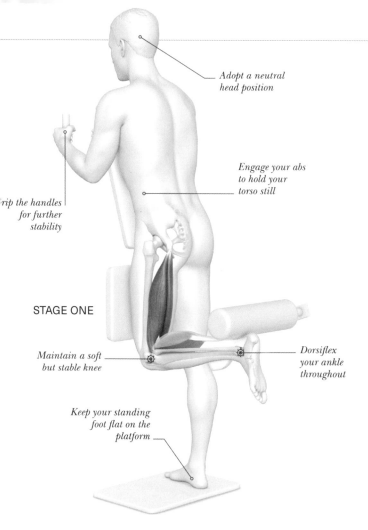

*Adopt a neutral
head position*

*Engage your abs
to hold your
torso still*

*Grip the handles
for further
stability*

STAGE ONE

*Maintain a soft
but stable knee*

*Dorsiflex
your ankle
throughout*

*Keep your standing
foot flat on the
platform*

66 99

*Knee flexion variations
are great for* **challenging
the hamstrings and other
knee flexors** *in a safe and
controlled environment.*

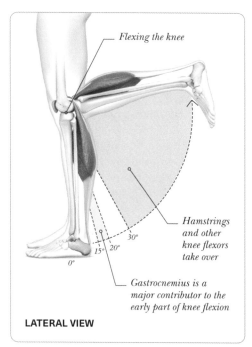

Flexing the knee

*Hamstrings
and other
knee flexors
take over*

30°

15° 20°

0°

*Gastrocnemius is a
major contributor to the
early part of knee flexion*

LATERAL VIEW

STANDING UNILATERAL LEG CURL

You perform this gym-machine-based variation standing up.
Because this movement trains one leg at a time, it's key to
keep track of reps so that you can work each leg equally.
Actively pulling on the handles stabilizes the latissimus dorsi
(in the back), which offers further stability to the pelvis.

PREPARATORY STAGE
Set up the machine. Stand with your thighs pressed
tight to the pad with one leg pushed against the
lower leg pad. Maintain a forward gaze.

STAGE ONE
Inhale, engage your abs, and breathe out while
flexing your knee fully in its range of motion. Tense
the muscles of your shin to dorsiflex your ankle.

STAGE TWO
Breathe in to return to the starting position by
extending your working leg completely, resisting
the weight as you go. Repeat stages 1 and 2.

Role of the **gastrocnemius** in **knee flexion**
The integration of the gastrocnemius and
other knee flexors (such as hamstrings)
allows the knee to have good stability
throughout the range of motion where the
hamstrings lack leverage (between 0 and
15°). To avoid the common mistake of
generating a lot of momentum at the start
of a knee-flexion exercise, it's better to
integrate both calf and hamstrings in a
controlled way, so that flexing your knee
puts tension in all the right muscles.

HAMSTRING BALL CURL

This exercise targets the hamstrings and the gastrocnemius and allows you to train the hamstrings without loading the spine or needing machines. Much work is also done by your core and glutes to support your raised torso during this rolling movement.

THE BIG PICTURE

You will need an exercise ball with a diameter of at least 21½–26 in (55–65 cm). Your back should be flat on the floor and your hips extended, with the contact points of the ball on the lower part of your legs and heels. Then you'll raise your body into a bridge position. One of the greatest challenges of this movement is being able to flex at the knee using your hamstrings while the entire time holding the same body position, with your hips off the floor and your torso stable.

Beginners can start with 4 sets of 8–10 reps; discover other targeted sets in the training programs (see pp.201–214). If your hips start to drop, lower the reps for each set and increase the number of total sets. To push your core muscles further, fold your arms across your chest.

Upper **leg**
The **hamstrings** contract concentrically to flex the knees. Dig your heels into the ball and focus on raising the knees rather than pulling the ball toward you. The **glutes** work to maintain the bridge position and lengthen as your hip flexes. The **hip flexors** engage concentrically to flex your hip. The **gastrocnemius** contracts concentrically to flex the knee and pull the heels up toward the body.

Upper **body**
Your **arms** act as a counterbalance, allowing your upper body to remain stable and prevent rotation. Your **core** works to maintain balance on the ball and to support your lower back.

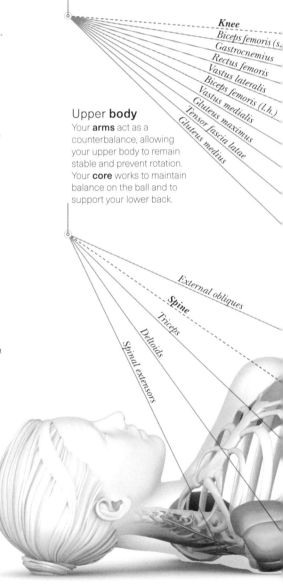

Knee
Biceps femoris (s.
Gastrocnemius
Rectus femoris
Vastus lateralis
Biceps femoris (l.h.)
Vastus medialis
Gluteus maximus
Tensor fascia latae
Gluteus medius

External obliques
Spine
Triceps
Deltoids
Spinal extensors

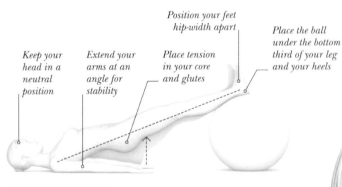

Keep your head in a neutral position

Extend your arms at an angle for stability

Place tension in your core and glutes

Position your feet hip-width apart

Place the ball under the bottom third of your leg and your heels

PREPARATORY STAGE
Lie on the floor on your back with your arms out to the sides and palms facing downward. Position your legs and heels on the ball and place tension in your core and glutes to raise your body into a bridge position. Keep a neutral head and spinal position.

KEY

•-- *Joints*

o— *Muscles*

● Shortening under tension

● Lengthening under tension

● Lengthening without tension (stretching)

● Held muscles without motion

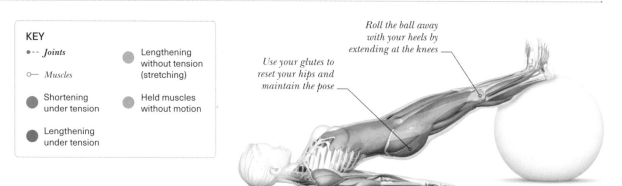

Roll the ball away with your heels by extending at the knees

Use your glutes to reset your hips and maintain the pose

STAGE TWO
Breathe in and slowly roll the ball back to its starting position with your knees and hips extended. Hold this position for a moment to reset your breathing, hip position, and torso stability for the next rep. Repeat stages 1 and 2.

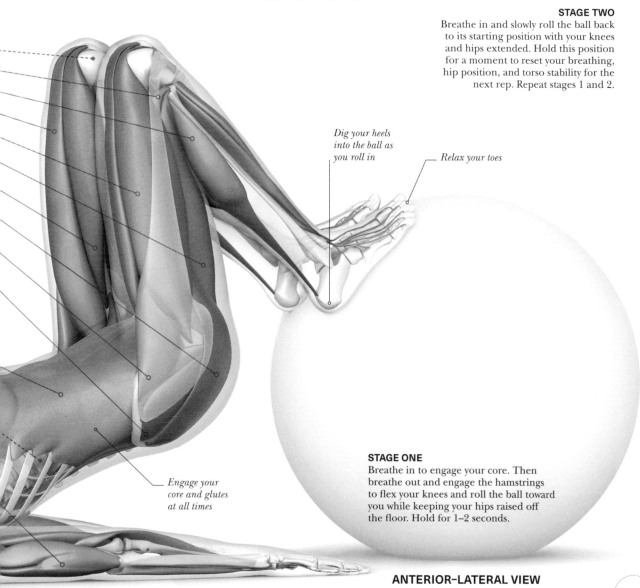

Dig your heels into the ball as you roll in

Relax your toes

Engage your core and glutes at all times

STAGE ONE
Breathe in to engage your core. Then breathe out and engage the hamstrings to flex your knees and roll the ball toward you while keeping your hips raised off the floor. Hold for 1–2 seconds.

ANTERIOR-LATERAL VIEW

73

LEG EXTENSION

This exercise specifically trains the quadriceps as you flex and extend your legs at the knees. It is a great machine-based exercise, even for beginners, because it safely isolates and effectively loads the quadriceps in their shortened position.

THE BIG PICTURE

Adjust the back pad so that, when sitting, your knee wraps naturally around the seat pad; this position aligns your knees with the machine's axis of rotation. Start the rep slowly and accelerate into the top position. The return move should also be controlled.

Beginners can start with 4 sets of 8–10 reps; discover other variations on pp.76–77 and other targeted sets in the training programs (see pp.201–214).

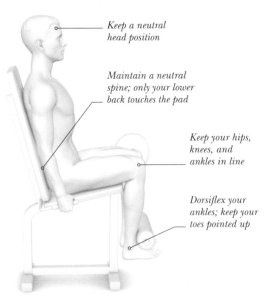

Keep a neutral head position

Maintain a neutral spine; only your lower back touches the pad

Keep your hips, knees, and ankles in line

Dorsiflex your ankles; keep your toes pointed up

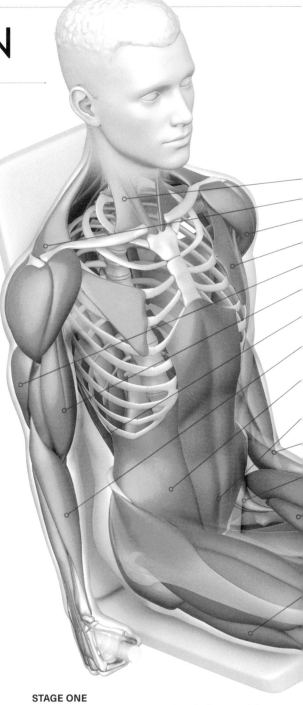

PREPARATORY STAGE
Set the weights and sit in the machine with your knees bent and ankles beneath an ankle pad; adjust the ankle pad so that it touches just above your shoes. Grip the handles and pull down into the seat pad to stabilize your pelvis throughout. Breathe in.

STAGE ONE
Breathe out as you slowly extend at the knees, raising the ankle pad, then accelerate into the rep until you reach the end of your knees' range of extension. (This varies by person.) Dorsiflex your ankles throughout. The goal is fully contracted quadriceps. For an extra challenge, hold at the top for 1–2 seconds.

Torso and arms

Think of creating tension in the **upper back**, **arms**, and **shoulders** (by actively pulling on the handles) to help stabilize your pelvis. The more stability your pelvis receives, the more force your **quadriceps** will be able to produce.

rnocleidomastoid
Trapezius
Deltoids
Pectoralis minor
Triceps
Biceps
Latissimus dorsi
Brachioradialis
Transversus abdominis
Rectus abdominis

Legs

The **quadriceps** receive tension during the exercise. This leg extension also loads the **rectus femoris** (the quadriceps muscle that crosses the hip joint) in its shortened position, which helps stabilize the pelvis. Ensure you control the lowering portion (the eccentric action) of the rep to maintain tension in the quadriceps.

Tensor fascia latae
Iliopsoas
Vastus medialis
Rectus femoris
Biceps femoris
Knee
Adductor magnus
Tibialis anterior
Gastrocnemius
Extensor digitorum longus
Soleus

SUPERIOR-ANTERIOR-LATERAL VIEW

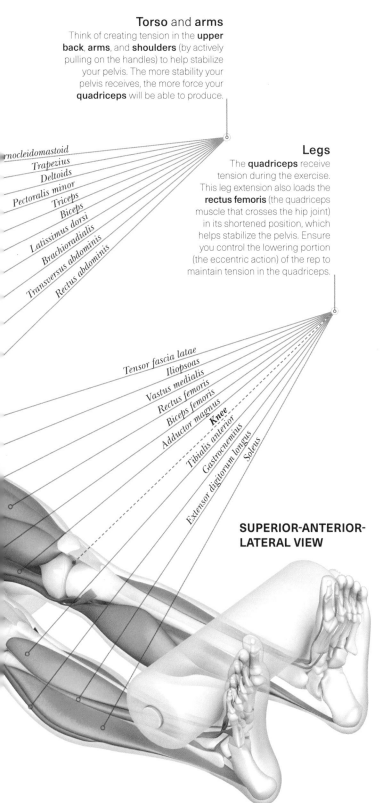

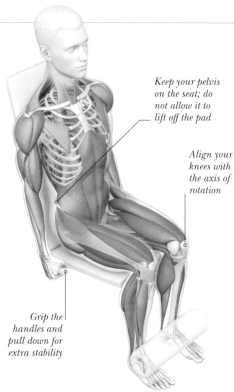

Keep your pelvis on the seat; do not allow it to lift off the pad

Align your knees with the axis of rotation

Grip the handles and pull down for extra stability

STAGE TWO

Keep your abs engaged with your lower back against the pad. Breathe in as you continue to pull yourself down into the seat and slowly flex at the knees in a controlled fashion to return the ankle pad to its starting position. Reset your breathing and repeat stages 1 and 2.

❗ Common mistakes

Rushing the movement—such as by flinging up the ankle pad—opens you up to injury and could take away tension from the target muscles. Coming out of your seat on each rep shows that you're not sufficiently stabilizing your torso and pelvis.

KEY

●-- *Joints*

○— *Muscles*

● Shortening with tension

● Lengthening with tension

● Lengthening without tension

● Held muscles without motion

» VARIATIONS

At first glance, these leg extension variations can look easy. But, when performed correctly, each of these exercises packs a punch, isolating the quadriceps and challenging them in their shortened range—which is not an easy movement to replicate.

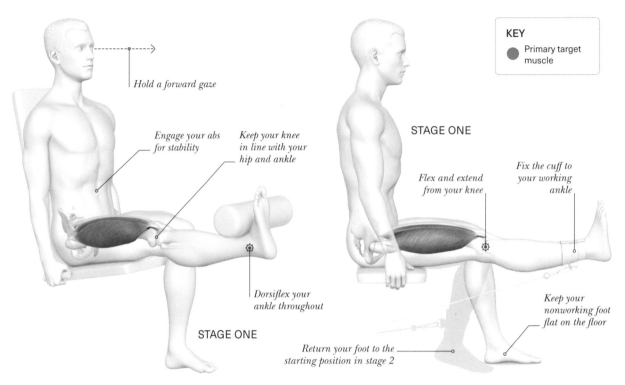

KEY
● Primary target muscle

Hold a forward gaze

Engage your abs for stability

Keep your knee in line with your hip and ankle

Dorsiflex your ankle throughout

STAGE ONE

STAGE ONE

Flex and extend from your knee

Fix the cuff to your working ankle

Keep your nonworking foot flat on the floor

Return your foot to the starting position in stage 2

UNILATERAL LEG EXTENSION

This exercise gives you the ability to challenge one leg at a time. Such unilateral movements can be great for those who are building muscle and strength back after an injury or period off training. As with all single limb movements, be sure to repeat equally on the other side.

PREPARATORY STAGE
Set up the machine. Sit against the back pad with one knee bent around the seat. Place your other foot under the ankle pad. Hold the grips and pull down.

STAGE ONE
Breathe out and, while flexing your ankle, extend the knee of the working leg to lift the ankle pad. Keep a neutral spine and your abs engaged.

STAGE TWO
Breathe in, while continuing to pull down on the handles, to return your working leg to the starting position under control. Repeat on your other leg.

UNILATERAL CUFFED LEG EXTENSION

This exercise uses a cable pulley machine with a cuff but can be swapped out for a free-standing resistance band. The loading reduces as you go through the concentric part (stage 1), which is not ideal. To counteract that, you can add a hold or squeeze for 1–4 seconds at the top position.

PREPARATORY STAGE
Set up the cable from a low setting and attach the cuff to your working ankle. Sit tall with a neutral spine and with your glutes fully on the bench.

STAGE ONE
Breathe out, dorsiflex your ankle, and extend your working leg at the knee to lift your foot, working against the resistance of the cable as you do so.

STAGE TWO
Still gripping the bench, breathe in to slowly return your leg to the starting position. Complete the reps, then switch the cuff and repeat on your other leg.

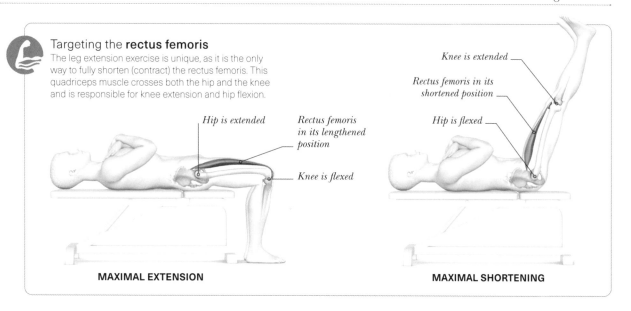

Targeting the **rectus femoris**

The leg extension exercise is unique, as it is the only way to fully shorten (contract) the rectus femoris. This quadriceps muscle crosses both the hip and the knee and is responsible for knee extension and hip flexion.

Hip is extended

Rectus femoris in its lengthened position

Knee is flexed

Knee is extended

Rectus femoris in its shortened position

Hip is flexed

MAXIMAL EXTENSION

MAXIMAL SHORTENING

BANDED LYING
LEG EXTENSION

This machine-free leg extension uses a resistance band and can easily be done at home or in the gym. You'll need to choose an appropriate band (see also p.47) and be sure to find a stable anchor point to fix it to.

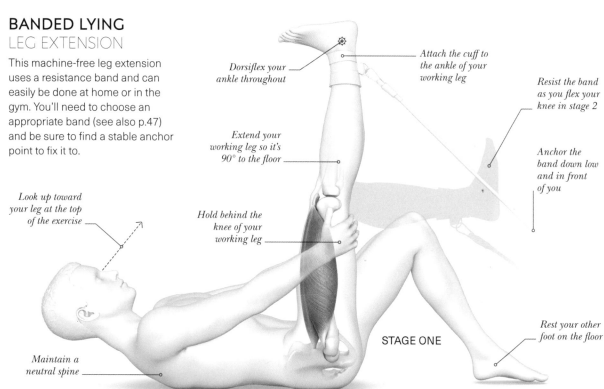

Dorsiflex your ankle throughout

Attach the cuff to the ankle of your working leg

Resist the band as you flex your knee in stage 2

Extend your working leg so it's 90° to the floor

Anchor the band down low and in front of you

Look up toward your leg at the top of the exercise

Hold behind the knee of your working leg

STAGE ONE

Rest your other foot on the floor

Maintain a neutral spine

PREPARATORY STAGE
Fix the resistance band low and in front of you. Lie on your back with your nonworking leg flexed and the band attached to your working leg's ankle.

STAGE ONE
With your ankle flexed and your knee supported, breathe out and extend the knee of your working leg so it's straight up. Hold for 1–4 seconds in this position.

STAGE TWO
Inhale while slowly flexing your leg just at the knee, resisting the band with control. Complete the reps, then switch the ankle cuff and repeat on your other leg.

BARBELL
GLUTE BRIDGE

Upper **body** and **arms**
Muscles of the **abdominals** play a key role
in stabilizing your spine and pelvis during
this exercise and help coordinate the
movement between your upper and lower
body. The muscles of your **arms** and
shoulders help keep the load in position
throughout the range of motion.

Also commonly referred to as the hip thrust, this
exercise trains the glutes as you flex and extend the
hips. Like the leg extension for the quadriceps (see
pp.74–75), this exercise loads the glutes in their
shortened position without the need to load the spine.

THE **BIG PICTURE**

You will need a sturdy bench or step to lean on. You
carry the barbell in your hip crease as you extend and
flex your hips, lifting and lowering your body; if you
find the barbell uncomfortable, add a pad. Correct
alignment of your feet, ankles, and knees is important
for ease of movement and avoiding injury.

Beginners can start with 4 sets of 8–10 reps;
discover other variations on pp.80–81 and other
targeted sets in the training programs (see
pp.201–214).

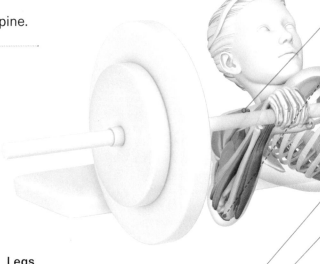

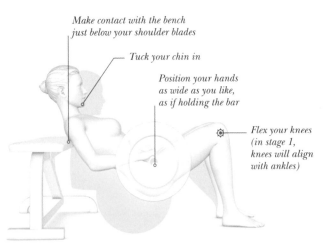

*Make contact with the bench
just below your shoulder blades*

Tuck your chin in

*Position your hands
as wide as you like,
as if holding the bar*

*Flex your knees
(in stage 1,
knees will align
with ankles)*

Legs
The **glutes** are the main
muscles receiving tension.
Think of driving your hips up
through the bar using your
glutes while keeping your **abs**
engaged. The coordination
between your torso and your
pelvis will allow for more tension
to be produced in your glutes.
The **hamstrings**, **adductors**,
and **calf muscles** help
stabilize the load across
your lower body.

Tensor fascia latae
Rectus femoris
Gluteus maximus
Adductor longus
Biceps femoris long head
Vastus lateralis
Adductor magnus
Semimembranosus
Knee
Gastrocnemius
Soleus
Tibialis anterior
Peroneus longus
Peroneus brevis
Ankle
Extensor d. long
Extensor h. long

PREPARATORY STAGE
Sit with your back on the bench with your legs flexed
and feet just outside of shoulder-width apart. With the
barbell in your hip crease, engage your glutes to push
your hips up off the floor into the top starting position.
Breathe in to engage your core.

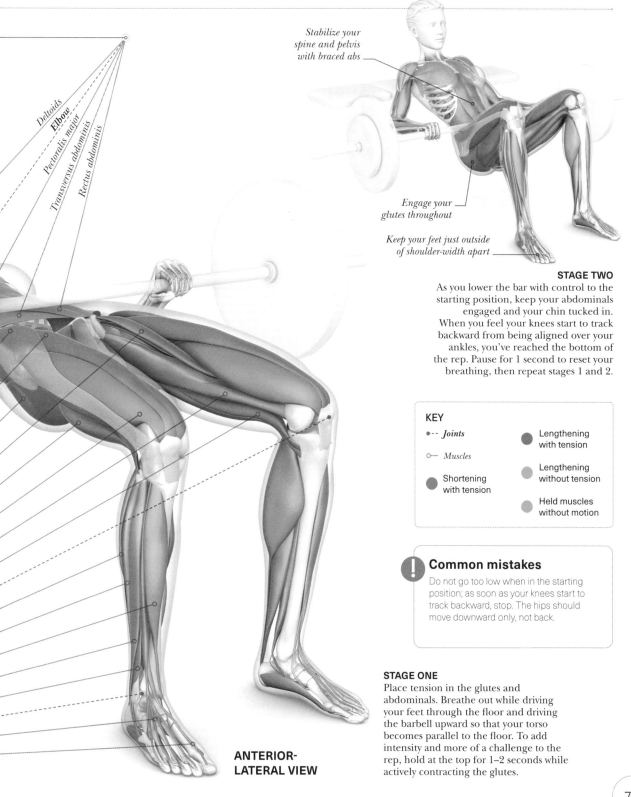

Deltoids
Elbow
Pectoralis major
Transversus abdominis
Rectus abdominis

Stabilize your spine and pelvis with braced abs

Engage your glutes throughout

Keep your feet just outside of shoulder-width apart

ANTERIOR- LATERAL VIEW

STAGE TWO
As you lower the bar with control to the starting position, keep your abdominals engaged and your chin tucked in. When you feel your knees start to track backward from being aligned over your ankles, you've reached the bottom of the rep. Pause for 1 second to reset your breathing, then repeat stages 1 and 2.

KEY
●--- *Joints*

○— *Muscles*

● Shortening with tension

● Lengthening with tension

● Lengthening without tension

● Held muscles without motion

! Common mistakes
Do not go too low when in the starting position; as soon as your knees start to track backward, stop. The hips should move downward only, not back.

STAGE ONE
Place tension in the glutes and abdominals. Breathe out while driving your feet through the floor and driving the barbell upward so that your torso becomes parallel to the floor. To add intensity and more of a challenge to the rep, hold at the top for 1–2 seconds while actively contracting the glutes.

» VARIATIONS

These exercises all target the glutes, as well as isolating the function of hip extension via the hamstrings. Training unilaterally can be particularly effective, as it allows you to increase the intensity of the exercise, putting greater tension on the glutes in your working leg.

KEY
● Primary target muscle
● Secondary target muscle

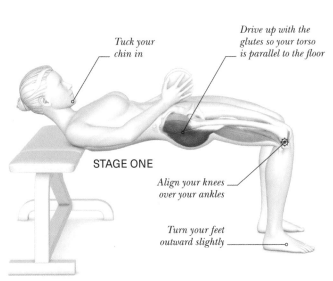

Tuck your chin in

Drive up with the glutes so your torso is parallel to the floor

STAGE ONE

Align your knees over your ankles

Turn your feet outward slightly

Lean forward slightly

STAGE ONE

Extend your working leg by 20–30°

Externally rotate your leg slightly at the hip

Place your weight through the center of your nonworking foot

DUMBBELL GLUTE BRIDGE

Much like the main exercise on the previous pages, this variation follows the same movement but uses a dumbbell instead. Working with a smaller load helps you improve your execution before progressing to heavier weights.

PREPARATORY STAGE
Lean back on the bench with your legs flexed. Place the dumbbell in your hip crease and engage the glutes to lift your hips slightly off the floor.

STAGE ONE
With tension in the glutes and abs, breathe out while driving your torso and the dumbbell upward. Hold at the top for 1–2 seconds, if possible.

STAGE TWO
Keep your abs engaged and chin tucked in as you lower your torso to the starting position. Pause here briefly before repeating stages 1 and 2.

STANDING CABLE GLUTE KICKBACK

Use this variation in conjunction with other glute exercises if you don't have access to free weights or would like to add isolated volume to the glutes. Make sure you do not round at your lower back or use momentum to kick the weight back.

PREPARATORY STAGE
Place the cable strap around your ankle, above the shoe. Stand with your feet hip-width apart and place your hands on the cable machine to stabilize yourself.

STAGE ONE
Breathe in to engage your abs. Then breathe out as you kick your leg back, abducting it to around 20–30°. For an added challenge, hold for 1–2 seconds.

STAGE TWO
Keep your abs engaged and spine neutral as you return to the starting position with control while breathing in. Repeat stages 1 and 2.

SINGLE-LEG GLUTE BRIDGE

If weight is limited or you want to increase the challenge, this single-leg option may be useful. By performing the exercise using one leg at a time, you raise the intensity of the load for your working leg; it can be performed with or without weights. Do keep track of the reps so that you can work each leg equally.

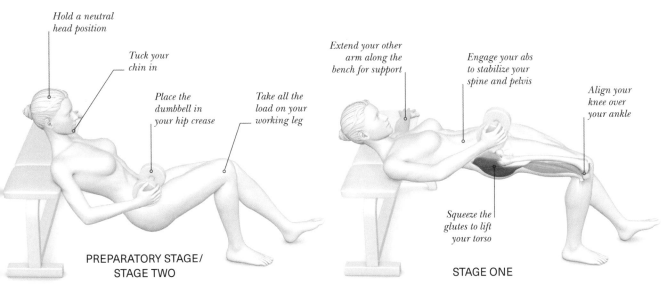

Hold a neutral head position

Tuck your chin in

Place the dumbbell in your hip crease

Take all the load on your working leg

PREPARATORY STAGE/
STAGE TWO

Extend your other arm along the bench for support

Engage your abs to stabilize your spine and pelvis

Align your knee over your ankle

Squeeze the glutes to lift your torso

STAGE ONE

PREPARATORY STAGE
Lean back on the bench with your working leg flexed and the other resting on its heel in front. Engage the glutes to lift your hips slightly off the floor.

STAGE ONE
Keep tension in the glutes and abs and breathe out while driving your torso upward using your working leg only. Hold for 1–2 seconds for an extra challenge.

STAGE TWO
Slowly lower your torso to the starting position while keeping your abs engaged and chin tucked in. Pause here briefly before repeating stages 1 and 2.

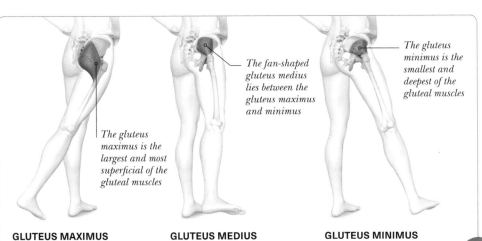

The gluteus maximus is the largest and most superficial of the gluteal muscles

The fan-shaped gluteus medius lies between the gluteus maximus and minimus

The gluteus minimus is the smallest and deepest of the gluteal muscles

GLUTEUS MAXIMUS
This muscle works to extend the hip posteriorly and rotate the leg.

GLUTEUS MEDIUS
This supports g. maximus in extending the hip more laterally and rotating the leg.

GLUTEUS MINIMUS
This muscle supports g. maximus in extending the hip more laterally.

The trio of **gluteal** muscles

The glutes act as key players in hip stability and strength during activities such as walking, jumping, sprinting, and strength training. The gluteus maximus, medius, and minimus help the hip extend, externally and internally rotate, and abduct (see p.50). Strong and functional glutes can help alleviate lower-back pain and make everyday movements—such as standing, walking, and climbing the stairs—that much easier.

CALF RAISE

This machine-based exercise trains the gastrocnemius and soleus muscles of the calf in their role of plantar flexion (standing on tiptoes) and also works the Achilles tendon. Calf strength can help maintain a healthy knee.

THE BIG PICTURE

On the bar, your feet should be parallel and the balls of your feet in full contact with the bar while you raise yourself up onto tiptoes and then lower into a heel drop. Your feet can be parallel or slightly turned out—whatever is most comfortable. Proper execution is crucial, and the movement should be slow and controlled. Keep tension in the leg muscles while allowing a "soft lockout" (a very slight bend in the knees) to avoid hyperextension (fully pushed back position).

Beginners can start with 4 sets of 8–10 reps; discover other variations on pp.84–85 and other targeted sets in the training programs (see pp.201–214).

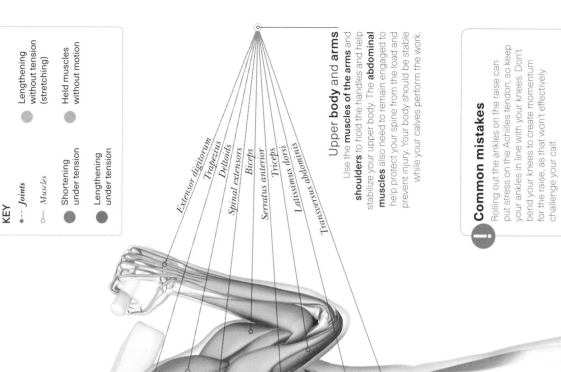

KEY

- - - *Joints*
- ○— *Muscles*
- ● Shortening under tension
- ● Lengthening under tension
- ● Lengthening without tension (stretching)
- ● Held muscles without motion

Extensor digitorum
Trapezius
Deltoids
Spinal extensors
Biceps
Serratus anterior
Triceps
Latissimus dorsi
Transversus abdominis

Upper body and arms

Use the **muscles of the arms** and **shoulders** to hold the handles and help stabilize your upper body. The **abdominal muscles** also need to remain engaged to help protect your spine from the load and prevent injury. Your body should be stable while your calves perform the work.

Common mistakes

Rolling out the ankles on the raise can put stress on the Achilles tendon, so keep your ankles in line with your knees. Don't bend your knees to create momentum for the raise, as that won't effectively challenge your calf.

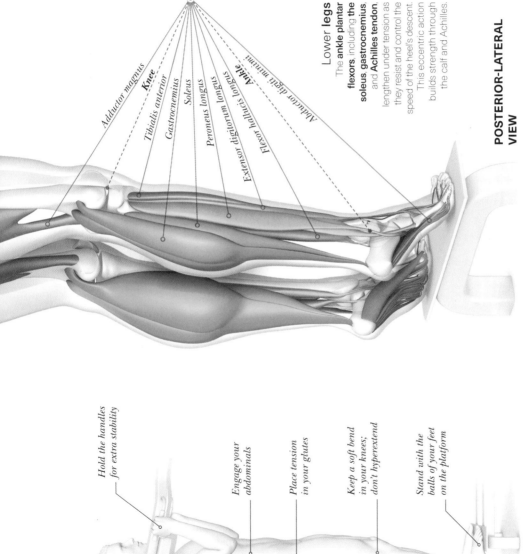

Lower your heels into dorsiflexion

Lower legs

The **ankle plantar flexors**, including the **soleus**, **gastrocnemius**, and **Achilles tendon**, lengthen under tension as they resist and control the speed of the heel's descent. This eccentric action builds strength through the calf and Achilles.

Adductor magnus

Knee

Tibialis anterior

Gastrocnemius

Soleus

Peroneus longus

Extensor digitorum longus

Ankle

Flexor hallucis longus

Abductor digiti minimi

POSTERIOR-LATERAL VIEW

POSTERIOR VIEW

STAGE ONE

Take a breath in to help stabilize your core. Breathe out as you contract your calf to raise your heels in a slow, controlled movement until you're standing on tiptoes. Keep your ankles in line with your knees throughout.

STAGE TWO

Breathe in and slowly lower your heels as far as they will go in a smooth, controlled move. Pause for 1–2 seconds at the bottom to release passive tension in the Achilles tendon. Reset your breathing, then repeat stages 1 and 2 in a rhythmic way.

PREPARATORY STAGE

Set the weights; place your shoulders under the pads; and stand with the balls of your feet on the edge of the step, feet hip-width apart. Ensure your torso and pelvis are stable throughout. Now lower your heels into the starting position.

Hold the handles for extra stability

Engage your abdominals

Place tension in your glutes

Keep a soft bend in your knees; don't hyperextend

Stand with the balls of your feet on the platform

›› VARIATIONS

Strengthening the calf helps maintain a healthy and stable knee joint. As with the calf raise on the previous pages, these variations target the gastrocnemius and soleus muscles and work the Achilles tendon.

KEY
● Primary target muscle

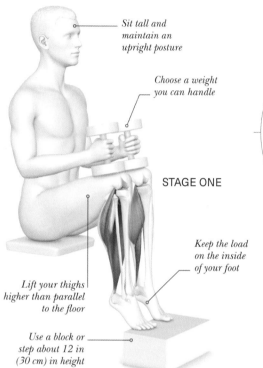

Sit tall and maintain an upright posture

Choose a weight you can handle

STAGE ONE

Keep the load on the inside of your foot

Lift your thighs higher than parallel to the floor

Use a block or step about 12 in (30 cm) in height

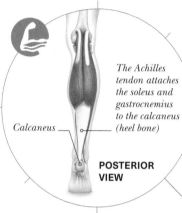

Calcaneus

The Achilles tendon attaches the soleus and gastrocnemius to the calcaneus (heel bone)

POSTERIOR VIEW

Achilles tendon
The Achilles tendon provides elasticity and shock absorbance for the feet and is involved in plantarflexion (see also p.51). Active in walking and running movements, this tendon is strong enough to withstand huge tensile forces—up to 10 times the body's weight.

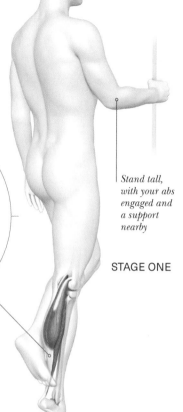

Stand tall, with your abs engaged and a support nearby

STAGE ONE

SEATED CALF RAISE

Performing this exercise in a seated position biases the soleus muscle over the gastrocnemius, because your knees are flexed. This seated calf raise adds variety to your routine whether you're at home or in the gym.

PREPARATORY STAGE
Sit tall with your feet hip-width apart and resting on the balls of your feet on a block or step in front of you. Rest the dumbbells on your knees.

STAGE ONE
Breathe in to engage your core. Breathe out as you contract your calves to raise your heels, driving your feet up and ankles forward, with control.

STAGE TWO
Breathe in and slowly lower your heels, keeping your ankles in line with your knees throughout. Pause at the bottom of each rep. Repeat stages 1 and 2.

SINGLE-LEG CALF RAISE

No extra weights are needed in this unilateral variation because supporting your bodyweight on one leg during its calf raise is enough load. Be sure to work each leg evenly.

PREPARATORY STAGE
Stand tall. Place the ball of one foot on the step and wrap your nonworking leg around the back of the other. Lower your heel into the starting position.

STAGE ONE
Breathe in to engage your core. Breathe out as you raise your heel as you contract your calf. Have a support nearby to hold if balance is an issue.

STAGE TWO
Breathe in and lower your heel in a controlled manner, keeping the load on the inside of your foot. Hold the bottom position, then repeat stages 1 and 2.

" "

*Training the **calf** muscles not only **adds size and strength** to the lower leg, but also aids in **increasing stability at the knee**.*

LEG PRESS CALF RAISE

This variation emulates the calf raise but allows for your body to be in a more stable position and without any load on your spine. It's a great alternative for anyone who may feel unstable or uncomfortable using a standing calf raise machine.

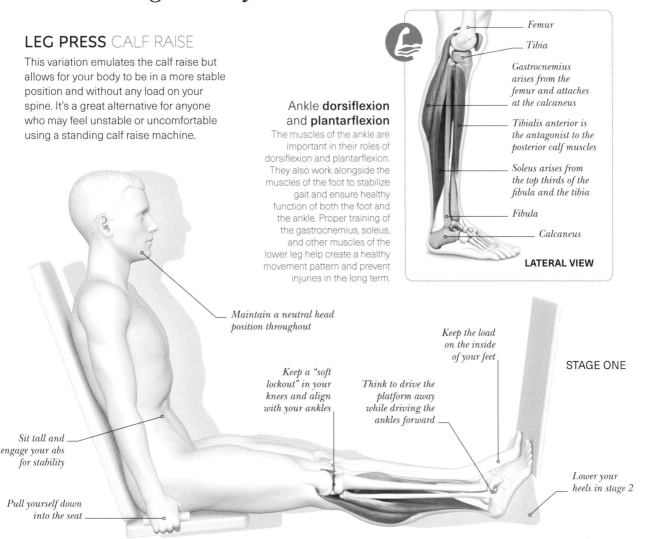

Ankle **dorsiflexion** and **plantarflexion**

The muscles of the ankle are important in their roles of dorsiflexion and plantarflexion. They also work alongside the muscles of the foot to stabilize gait and ensure healthy function of both the foot and the ankle. Proper training of the gastrocnemius, soleus, and other muscles of the lower leg help create a healthy movement pattern and prevent injuries in the long term.

Femur

Tibia

Gastrocnemius arises from the femur and attaches at the calcaneus

Tibialis anterior is the antagonist to the posterior calf muscles

Soleus arises from the top thirds of the fibula and the tibia

Fibula

Calcaneus

LATERAL VIEW

Maintain a neutral head position throughout

Keep the load on the inside of your feet

STAGE ONE

Keep a "soft lockout" in your knees and align with your ankles

Think to drive the platform away while driving the ankles forward

Sit tall and engage your abs for stability

Lower your heels in stage 2

Pull yourself down into the seat

PREPARATORY STAGE
Set the weight. Sit on the seat with the balls of your feet hip-width apart on the platform and your heels lowered.

STAGE ONE
Inhale to engage your core and pull yourself down into the seat. Breathe out as you push the balls of your feet onto the platform so your heels rise.

STAGE TWO
Breathe in and lower your heels to the starting position, maintaining control throughout. Pause at the bottom, then repeat stages 1 and 2.

TRADITIONAL
DEADLIFT

This exercise helps train most of the muscles in the lower body while also challenging many upper-body muscle groups. Hip extension strengthens the glutes and hamstrings (known as the posterior chain), while knee extension trains the quadriceps. To stay safe, work on the mechanics of the movement before upping the load.

THE BIG PICTURE

You will need a barbell with full-size or bumper plates. Rather than thinking of lifting the bar, allow the upward movement generated by the quads, hamstrings, and glutes to raise the bar by driving down. Be sure to control the return move.

Beginners can start with 4 sets of 8–10 reps; discover other variations of this exercise on pp.88–89 and other targeted sets within the training programs (see pp.201–214).

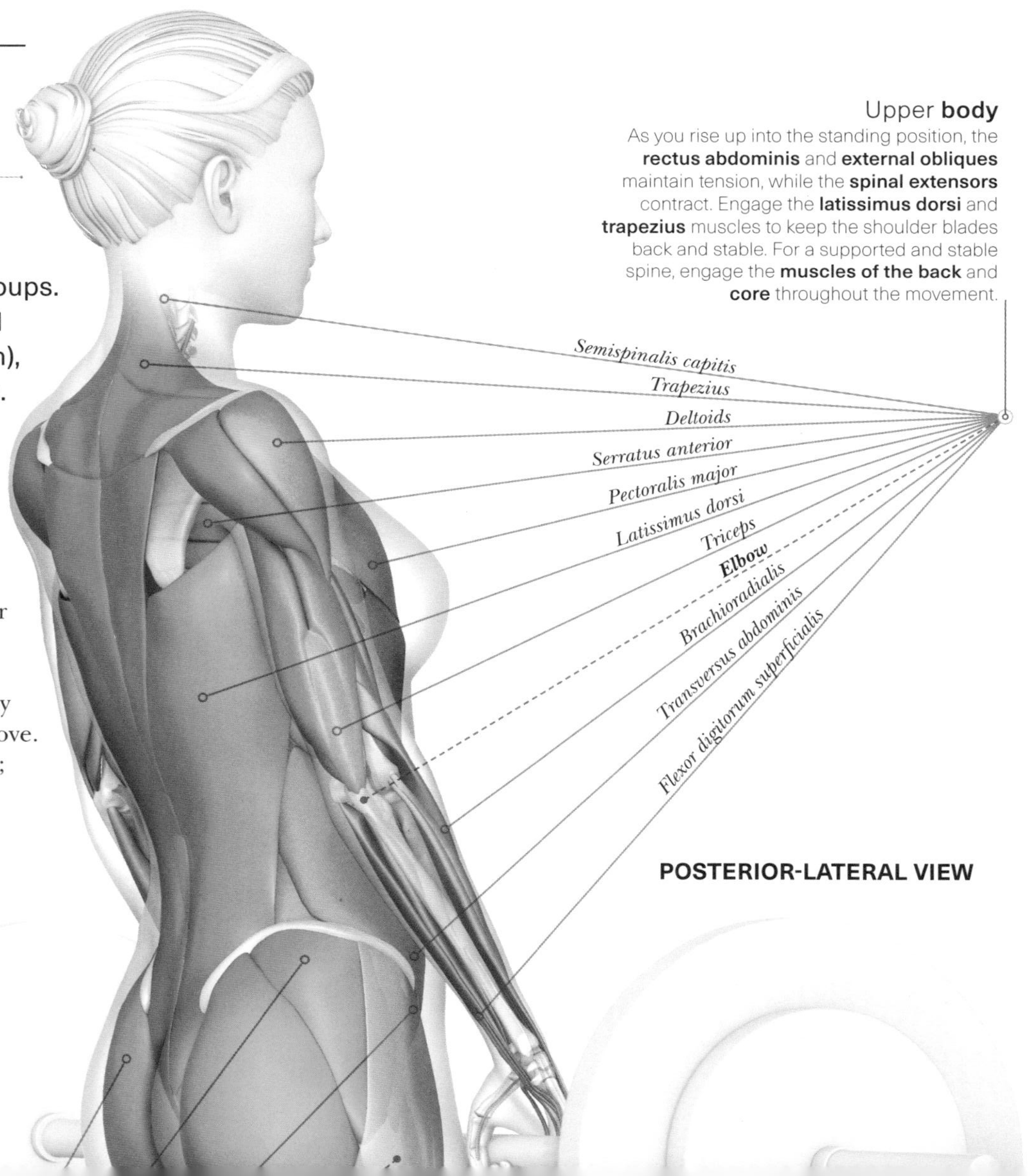

Common mistakes

Not engaging your core and stabilizing your upper body throughout the movement can result in lower-back strain. Be sure to start with a low weight.

Upper body

As you rise up into the standing position, the **rectus abdominis** and **external obliques** maintain tension, while the **spinal extensors** contract. Engage the **latissimus dorsi** and **trapezius** muscles to keep the shoulder blades back and stable. For a supported and stable spine, engage the **muscles of the back and core** throughout the movement.

Semispinalis capitis

Trapezius

Deltoids

Serratus anterior

Pectoralis major

Latissimus dorsi

Triceps

Elbow

Brachioradialis

Transversus abdominis

Flexor digitorum superficialis

POSTERIOR-LATERAL VIEW

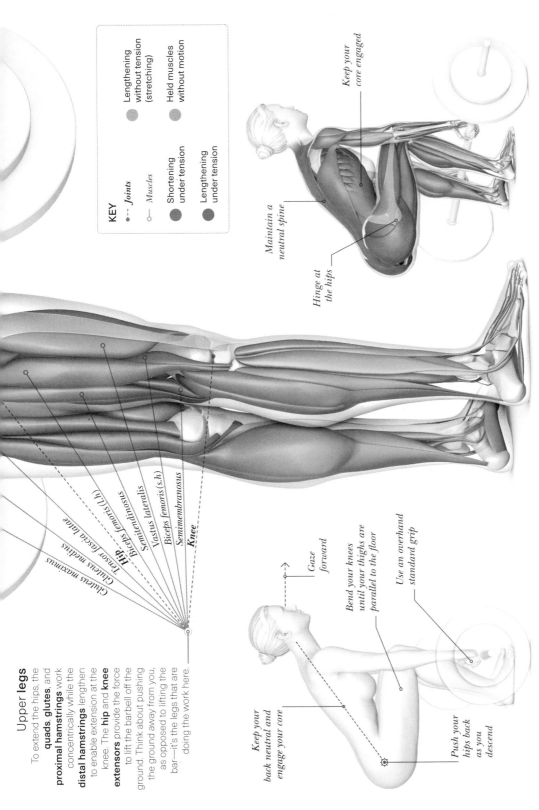

KEY

- - - *Joints*
- *Muscles*
● Shortening under tension
● Lengthening under tension
● Lengthening without tension (stretching)
● Held muscles without motion

Keep your core engaged

Maintain a neutral spine

Hinge at the hips

Upper legs

To extend the hips, the **quads**, **glutes**, and **proximal hamstrings** work concentrically while the **distal hamstrings** lengthen to enable extension at the knee. The **hip** and **knee extensors** provide the force to lift the barbell off the ground. Think about pushing the ground away from you, as opposed to lifting the bar—it's the legs that are doing the work here.

Gluteus maximus

Gluteus medius

Tensor fascia latae

Hip

Biceps femoris (l.h.)

Semitendinosus

Vastus lateralis

Biceps femoris (s.h)

Semimembranosus

Knee

STAGE ONE

Breathe in and brace your upper body and core. Drive through the floor with your quads and power your hips forward as you reach the top of the lift, breathing out as you do so. Hold briefly to check your stability.

STAGE TWO

As you hinge at the hip, controlling the descent of the bar, return to the starting position. Keep a neutral head position, looking forward throughout. Reset your breathing and balance before repeating stages 1 and 2.

Gaze forward

Bend your knees until your thighs are parallel to the floor

Use an overhand standard grip

Keep your back neutral and engage your core

Push your hips back as you descend

PREPARATORY STAGE

Stand centrally along the bar with your feet roughly shoulder-width apart and angled slightly outward. Push your hips back and bend your knees as you reach for the bar; your shins will be close to the bar. Keep a neutral spine, with your shoulders back and your upper-back muscles engaged.

» VARIATIONS

All these variations of the traditional deadlift on the previous pages also work the glutes, quads, spinal erectors, and muscles of the upper back and torso. Such deadlift movement pattern exercises are popular to include in strength training programs because they train so many muscles.

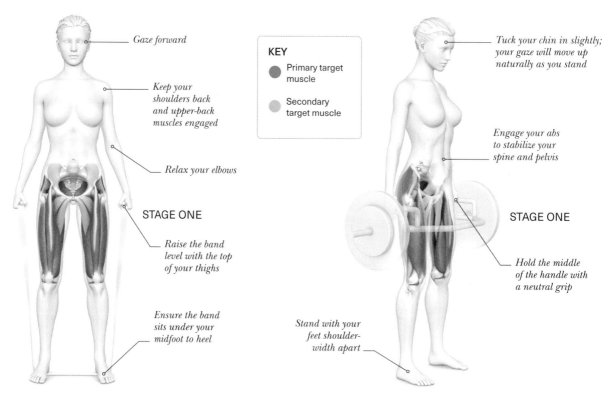

Gaze forward

KEY

● Primary target muscle

● Secondary target muscle

Keep your shoulders back and upper-back muscles engaged

Relax your elbows

STAGE ONE

Raise the band level with the top of your thighs

Ensure the band sits under your midfoot to heel

Tuck your chin in slightly; your gaze will move up naturally as you stand

Engage your abs to stabilize your spine and pelvis

STAGE ONE

Hold the middle of the handle with a neutral grip

Stand with your feet shoulder-width apart

BANDED DEADLIFT

This variation loads the same muscles as the main exercise but allows you to perform the deadlift movement pattern while under resistance. For an extra challenge, you can hold dumbbells with the resistance band (see p.97).

PREPARATORY STAGE
Choose an appropriate resistance band (see also p.47). Stand on the band with your feet shoulder-width apart. Bend to hold the band at knee level.

STAGE ONE
Breathe in and engage your core. Then drive through the floor with your quads while pushing your hips forward, breathing out as you do so.

STAGE TWO
Hinge at the hip to descend into the starting position, keeping a forward gaze and working against the resistance throughout. Repeat stages 1 and 2.

TRAP BAR DEADLIFT

Using a trap bar helps centralize the load throughout and keep the bias on the quads while still challenging the glutes. It's easier on the joints and easier to do, so it can be a great choice for beginners looking to train their quads.

PREPARATORY STAGE
Set the weights and step into the trap bar (hex bar). Stand with feet angled outward slightly. Push your hips back to bend your knees and grip the handle.

STAGE ONE
Breathe in, engage your core, and power your hips forward to stand upright, breathing out as you do so. The bar travels in a straight line at 90° to the floor.

STAGE TWO
Push your hips back to return to the starting position, keeping your shoulders back and holding a forward gaze throughout. Repeat stages 1 and 2.

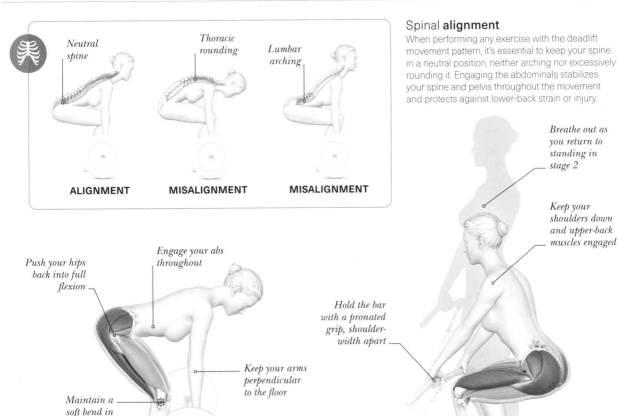

Spinal **alignment**

When performing any exercise with the deadlift movement pattern, it's essential to keep your spine in a neutral position, neither arching nor excessively rounding it. Engaging the abdominals stabilizes your spine and pelvis throughout the movement and protects against lower-back strain or injury.

Neutral spine

Thoracic rounding

Lumbar arching

ALIGNMENT

MISALIGNMENT

MISALIGNMENT

Breathe out as you return to standing in stage 2

Keep your shoulders down and upper-back muscles engaged

Push your hips back into full flexion

Engage your abs throughout

Hold the bar with a pronated grip, shoulder-width apart

Keep your arms perpendicular to the floor

Maintain a soft bend in your knees

Distribute weight evenly through your feet

STAGE ONE

STAGE ONE

Keep your weight on the balls of your feet

ROMANIAN DEADLIFT

This variation starts upright, then descends to the bent-over form. The hamstrings and glutes are the main hip extension muscles, controlling the descent into hip flexion and back into hip extension; the quads play a secondary role.

PREPARATORY STAGE
Stand in front of the barbell with your feet shoulder-width apart. Grip the bar at a comfortable width. Engage your core and drive into an upright position.

STAGE ONE
Breathe in and push your hips back into full flexion. Control the eccentric lowering phase while keeping a neutral head position and strong core.

STAGE TWO
Drive through the floor while pushing your hips forward, breathing out as you return to the upright starting position. Repeat stages 1 and 2.

CABLE DEADLIFT

The loading of this deadlift movement pattern using a cable pulley system will feel slightly different from that using a barbell. You move from a standing position to a squatting one. Be sure to start with a low weight and progress slowly.

PREPARATORY STAGE
Face the pulley machine, pick up the attachment, and step back. Stand with your feet shoulder-width apart, angled slightly outward, and gaze forward.

STAGE ONE
Breathe in and push your hips back into full flexion, controlling the descent. Keep a neutral head position and strong core throughout.

STAGE TWO
From the lower position, power your hips forward and drive through the floor, breathing out as you return to the starting position. Repeat stages 1 and 2.

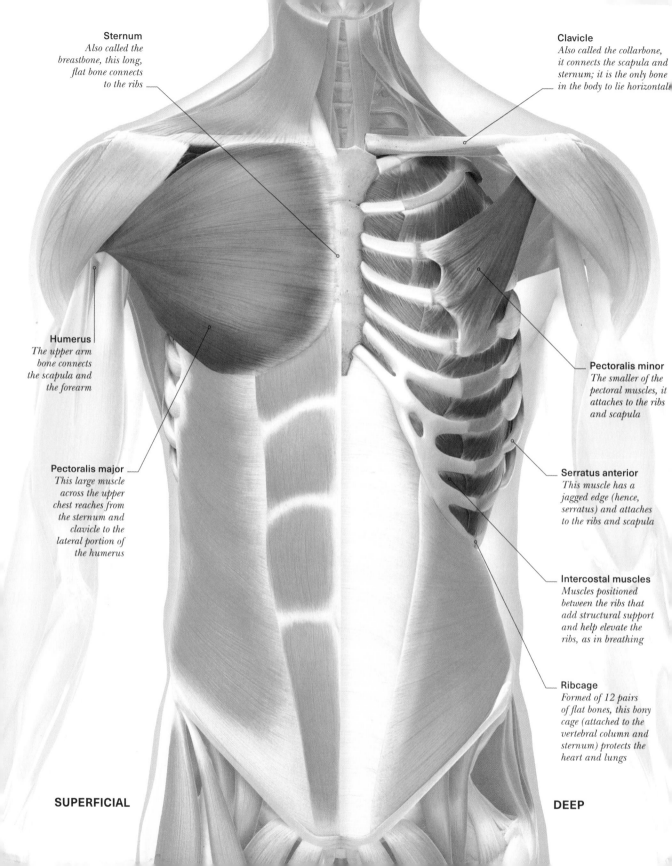

Sternum
Also called the breastbone, this long, flat bone connects to the ribs

Clavicle
Also called the collarbone, it connects the scapula and sternum; it is the only bone in the body to lie horizontally

Humerus
The upper arm bone connects the scapula and the forearm

Pectoralis minor
The smaller of the pectoral muscles, it attaches to the ribs and scapula

Pectoralis major
This large muscle across the upper chest reaches from the sternum and clavicle to the lateral portion of the humerus

Serratus anterior
This muscle has a jagged edge (hence, serratus) and attaches to the ribs and scapula

Intercostal muscles
Muscles positioned between the ribs that add structural support and help elevate the ribs, as in breathing

Ribcage
Formed of 12 pairs of flat bones, this bony cage (attached to the vertebral column and sternum) protects the heart and lungs

SUPERFICIAL

DEEP

CHEST EXERCISES

The main muscles responsible for movement in the chest are: the pectoralis major, the muscle that creates the chest's surface shape; pectoralis minor, positioned deep beneath the pectoralis major and attaching to the ribcage and scapula; and the serratus anterior, also a deep muscle, attaching to the ribcage.

The pectoralis major functions around the shoulder joint, allowing a large and functional range of motion across the upper body. The pectoralis minor and serratus anterior help protract the shoulder forward during pressing and flying motions.

The main role of the pectorals (or pecs) in training is to aid in pulling the upper arm across the chest toward the midline of the body.

- **When performing horizontal pressing** (such as the bench press), you will be integrating the pecs with the help of the deltoids and triceps to complete the range of motion. So rather than think about just getting the load to the top of a movement, instead think how best to combine your pressing and driving actions.

- **When performing flying exercises**, the deltoids and triceps will continue to lend their help but much less so. When flying, don't think about bringing the handles or dumbbells together as much as driving the upper arms in toward the sternum (middle of chest).

Pectoralis minor helps mainly with reaching forward during pressing and flying motions, aided by the serratus anterior. It also helps depress the shoulder in pulldowns.

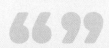

*Training **the chest** is not just about getting the weight to the top, it's **pressing and driving in** the upper arm.*

BARBELL BENCH PRESS

This is a classic chest exercise that involves lifting and lowering a barbell above your chest while lying on a bench. The dominant pressing movement trains muscles of the chest and shoulders, as well as the triceps.

THE BIG PICTURE

For a bench press, it's crucial to set up the rack. Position the bar rack 6–8 in (15–20 cm) from the barbell so you can rack it and unrack it easily. Set the rack to a height that you can easily pick up, and clear rack pins as you get into position.

Beginners can start with 4 sets of 8–10 reps; discover other variations of this exercise on pp.94–95 and targeted sets in the training programs (see pp.201–214).

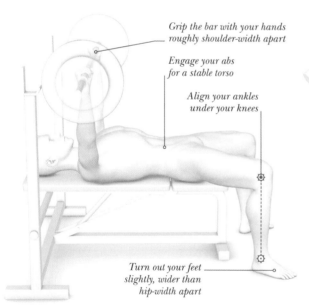

Grip the bar with your hands roughly shoulder-width apart

Engage your abs for a stable torso

Align your ankles under your knees

Turn out your feet slightly, wider than hip-width apart

PREPARATORY STAGE
Having set up the rack, lie flat with your buttocks fully on the bench and your feet flat on the floor. Grip the barbell with an overhand standard grip and lift it straight up. Keep your head in a neutral position throughout.

STAGE ONE
Take a breath in and engage your abs to help stabilize your core and hold. Activate muscles of the upper back and start to bend at the elbow, resisting the load as it moves toward your chest. The bar travels from midchest to lower sternum and can touch your chest or stop just shy of it.

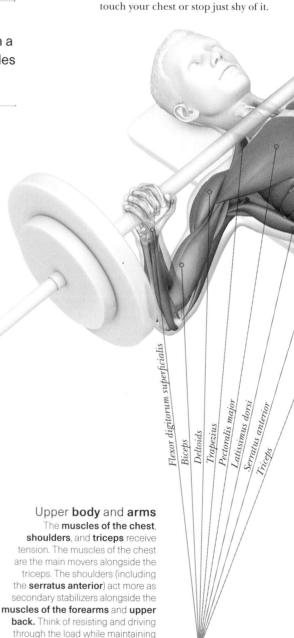

Flexor digitorum superficialis
Biceps
Deltoids
Trapezius
Pectoralis major
Latissimus dorsi
Serratus anterior
Triceps

Upper **body** and **arms**
The **muscles of the chest**, **shoulders**, and **triceps** receive tension. The muscles of the chest are the main movers alongside the triceps. The shoulders (including the **serratus anterior**) act more as secondary stabilizers alongside the **muscles of the forearms** and **upper back.** Think of resisting and driving through the load while maintaining tension on the chest and triceps.

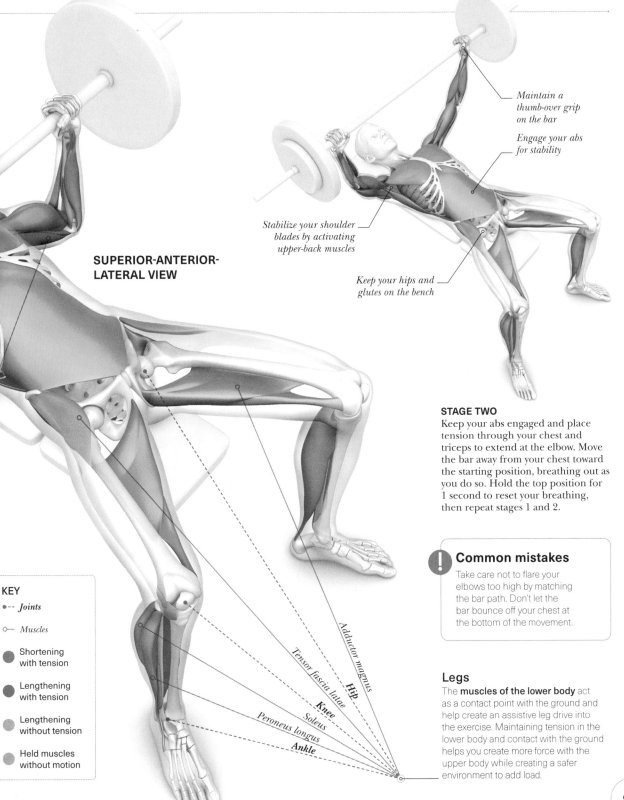

SUPERIOR-ANTERIOR-LATERAL VIEW

Maintain a thumb-over grip on the bar

Engage your abs for stability

Stabilize your shoulder blades by activating upper-back muscles

Keep your hips and glutes on the bench

Adductor magnus
Tensor fascia latae
Hip
Knee
Soleus
Peroneus longus
Ankle

KEY

•-- *Joints*

○— *Muscles*

● Shortening with tension

● Lengthening with tension

● Lengthening without tension

● Held muscles without motion

STAGE TWO
Keep your abs engaged and place tension through your chest and triceps to extend at the elbow. Move the bar away from your chest toward the starting position, breathing out as you do so. Hold the top position for 1 second to reset your breathing, then repeat stages 1 and 2.

! Common mistakes
Take care not to flare your elbows too high by matching the bar path. Don't let the bar bounce off your chest at the bottom of the movement.

Legs
The **muscles of the lower body** act as a contact point with the ground and help create an assistive leg drive into the exercise. Maintaining tension in the lower body and contact with the ground helps you create more force with the upper body while creating a safer environment to add load.

» VARIATIONS

Bench presses are popular strength training exercises because they train so many muscles (pecs, delts, and triceps) at the same time; in fact, a bench press is a full-body workout, as the core, back, and legs are also engaged to support the work of the muscles of the upper body and arms. Building muscle strength in the upper body can be useful for certain sports, such as sprinting, soccer, and tennis.

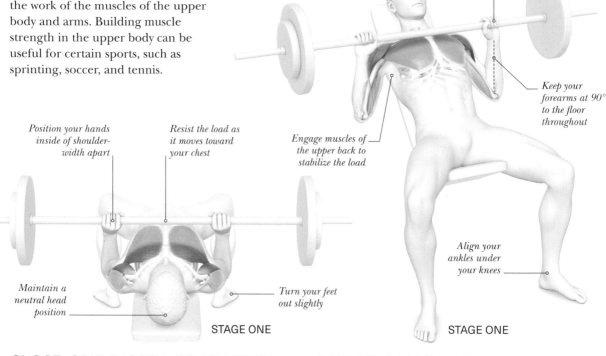

Hold a forward gaze

Position your hands about shoulder-width apart

Keep your forearms at 90° to the floor throughout

Engage muscles of the upper back to stabilize the load

Align your ankles under your knees

Position your hands inside of shoulder-width apart

Resist the load as it moves toward your chest

Maintain a neutral head position

Turn your feet out slightly

STAGE ONE

STAGE ONE

CLOSE-GRIP BARBELL BENCH PRESS

While essentially similar to the wide-grip barbell bench press on the previous pages, shifting the grip inward means this variation is a more dominant triceps exercise. If you experience any joint discomfort during this exercise, try switching to the dumbbell version on pp.96–97.

PREPARATORY STAGE
Set yourself up on the bench as on pp.92–93. Grip the barbell with an overhand grip that's inside shoulder-width. Then lift it level with your eyes.

STAGE ONE
Breathe in and engage your abs before flexing at the elbow and controlling the descent of the bar toward your chest; it might touch or stop just shy of it.

STAGE TWO
As you exhale, place tension through your chest and triceps to extend at the elbow, moving the bar up to the starting position. Repeat stages 1 and 2.

INCLINE BARBELL BENCH PRESS

This seated variation of the bench press offers a similar movement, but the more upright position used here targets more of the middle and upper chest while also training the muscles of the shoulders and the triceps. Set the angle of the bench to about 45°.

PREPARATORY STAGE
Sit on the bench with your back on the back pad and with the barbell across your lap. Lift the barbell above your head so your arms are at 90° to the floor.

STAGE ONE
Breathe in and engage your abs and upper-back muscles while bending your arms at the elbow and resisting the load as it moves toward your chest.

STAGE TWO
Place tension through your chest and triceps to extend at the elbow, lifting the bar up to the starting position while breathing out. Repeat stages 1 and 2.

Working **intensity**

Push-ups are a great overall bodyweight pressing variation. A regular push-up, where you place your feet on the floor, allows you to press 64 percent of your bodyweight. But if you elevate your feet on a 12-in (30-cm) box or bench, the weight you are working with rises to 70 percent of your bodyweight. So elevating your feet is a simple but effective progression if you want an extra challenge.

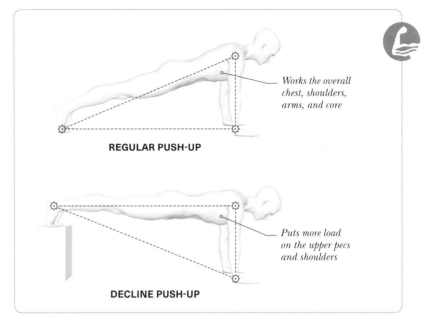

Works the overall chest, shoulders, arms, and core

REGULAR PUSH-UP

KEY

● Primary target muscle

● Secondary target muscle

Puts more load on the upper pecs and shoulders

DECLINE PUSH-UP

PUSH-UP

This variation uses the same pressing movement as the barbell bench press (and so challenges the same muscles) but completes it with bodyweight and in a prone position. It's a "do anytime, anywhere" exercise.

Breathe in as you return to the starting position

Place tension in the triceps to extend your arm at the elbow

Engage your abs throughout; no sagging allowed

Adjust the width of your stance if you need more stability

Look at the floor to keep a neutral head position

Place tension in the shoulders to keep the body in alignment

STAGE ONE

Position your hands flat on the floor

PREPARATORY STAGE
Lie face down on the floor with your feet hip-width apart and your hands just outside of shoulder-width apart. Hold your body as one off the floor slightly.

STAGE ONE
Take a breath in and engage your abs and upper-back muscles. Extend your arms at the elbow, raising your chest and body off the floor while breathing out.

STAGE TWO
Breathe in as you return to the starting position while controlling the descent and keeping your body in alignment throughout. Repeat stages 1 and 2.

DUMBBELL
BENCH PRESS

This exercise trains the chest, triceps, and shoulders.
Using dumbbells rather than a barbell allows for a more
natural and slightly lower arm position—and, consequently,
an increased range of motion and greater degree of
shoulder extension.

THE BIG PICTURE

This move uses the same lying-on-a-bench position as in the
barbell bench press (pp.92–93). Because the weights are above
you, use an overhand grip with thumbs over fingers. Your body
and legs stay still and strong while you lower and lift the load.

Beginners can start with 4 sets of 8–10 reps; discover other
variations on pp.98–99 and other targeted sets in the training
programs (see pp.201–214).

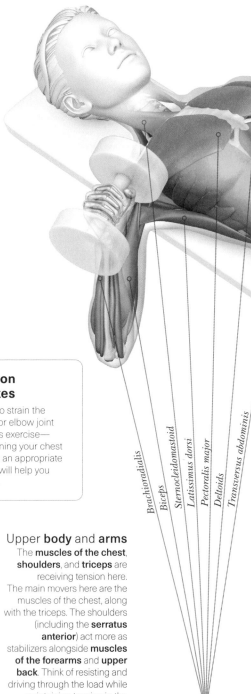

Brachioradialis
Biceps
Sternocleidomastoid
Latissimus dorsi
Pectoralis major
Deltoids
Transversus abdominis

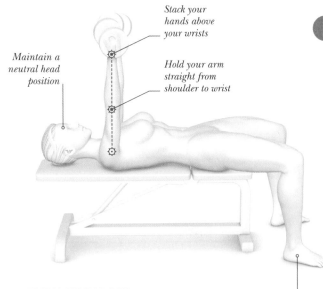

*Stack your
hands above
your wrists*

*Maintain a
neutral head
position*

*Hold your arm
straight from
shoulder to wrist*

ⓘ Common mistakes

It is easy to strain the
shoulder or elbow joint
during this exercise—
strengthening your chest
and using an appropriate
arm path will help you
avoid this.

PREPARATORY STAGE
Lie flat with your buttocks fully on the bench and
your feet flat on the floor. Hold the dumbbells with
an overhand grip, resting them on your legs. Then
lift the weights directly above your shoulders so your
wrists align with your upper arms.

*Place your feet
wider than hip-
width apart*

Upper **body** and **arms**
The **muscles of the chest**,
shoulders, and **triceps** are
receiving tension here.
The main movers here are the
muscles of the chest, along
with the triceps. The shoulders
(including the **serratus
anterior**) act more as
stabilizers alongside **muscles
of the forearms** and **upper
back**. Think of resisting and
driving through the load while
maintaining tension in the
chest and triceps.

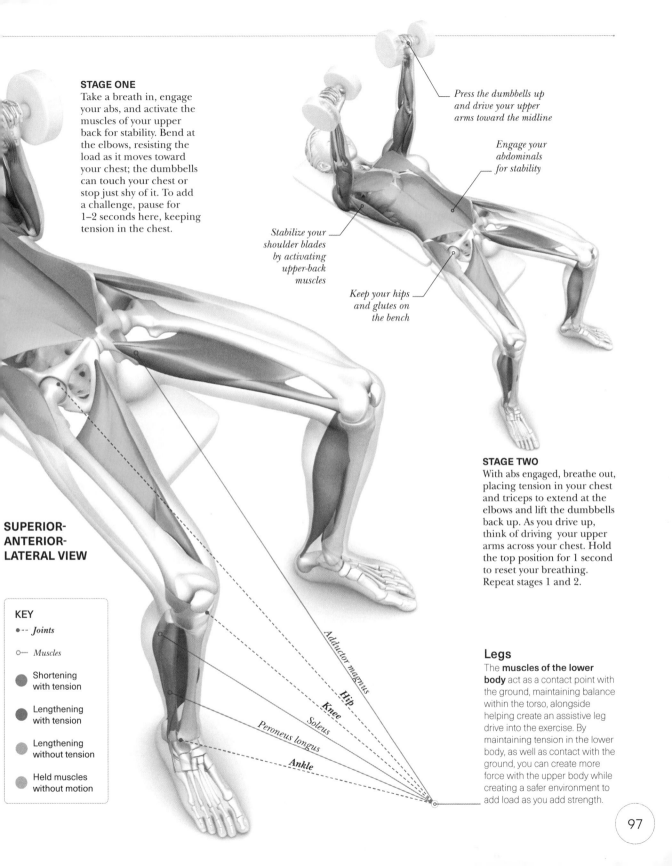

STAGE ONE
Take a breath in, engage your abs, and activate the muscles of your upper back for stability. Bend at the elbows, resisting the load as it moves toward your chest; the dumbbells can touch your chest or stop just shy of it. To add a challenge, pause for 1–2 seconds here, keeping tension in the chest.

Press the dumbbells up and drive your upper arms toward the midline

Engage your abdominals for stability

Stabilize your shoulder blades by activating upper-back muscles

Keep your hips and glutes on the bench

**SUPERIOR-
ANTERIOR-
LATERAL VIEW**

Adductor magnus

Hip

Knee

Soleus

Peroneus longus

Ankle

KEY
- •-- *Joints*
- o— *Muscles*
- ● Shortening with tension
- ● Lengthening with tension
- ● Lengthening without tension
- ● Held muscles without motion

STAGE TWO
With abs engaged, breathe out, placing tension in your chest and triceps to extend at the elbows and lift the dumbbells back up. As you drive up, think of driving your upper arms across your chest. Hold the top position for 1 second to reset your breathing. Repeat stages 1 and 2.

Legs
The muscles of the lower body act as a contact point with the ground, maintaining balance within the torso, alongside helping create an assistive leg drive into the exercise. By maintaining tension in the lower body, as well as contact with the ground, you can create more force with the upper body while creating a safer environment to add load as you add strength.

» VARIATIONS

There's a variation for all situations here with a lying, seated, and standing version of the dumbbell bench press. If you are new to the exercise, you may find it helpful to practice the movement of a bench press while standing or with each arm individually.

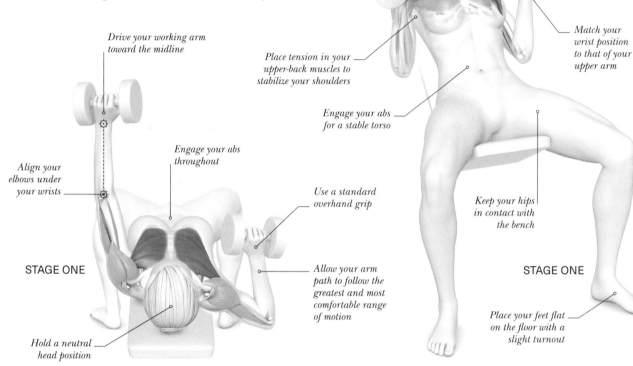

Drive your working arm toward the midline

Place tension in your upper-back muscles to stabilize your shoulders

Match your wrist position to that of your upper arm

Engage your abs for a stable torso

Align your elbows under your wrists

Engage your abs throughout

Use a standard overhand grip

Keep your hips in contact with the bench

STAGE ONE

Allow your arm path to follow the greatest and most comfortable range of motion

STAGE ONE

Hold a neutral head position

Place your feet flat on the floor with a slight turnout

UNILATERAL DUMBBELL BENCH PRESS

This lying variation targets the chest, shoulders, and triceps. But performing the movement one arm at a time also challenges your core and hip stability, as well as adding variety to your pressing options. Be sure to work each arm evenly; alternate each time or do reps on one side and swap.

PREPARATORY STAGE
Set yourself up on the bench as on pp.96–97. Hold the dumbbells with a standard overhand grip. Drive your upper arms toward the midline to lift the load.

STAGE ONE
Take a breath in, engage your abs, and activate your upper-back muscles. Bend at the elbow of your working arm to resist the load as it descends.

STAGE TWO
With abs engaged and tension in your triceps and chest, extend your working arm to press the weight away as you breathe out. Repeat stages 1 and 2.

INCLINE DUMBBELL BENCH PRESS

This seated variation is related to the incline barbell bench press (see p.94) but has the versatility of using a more individualized arm path, with the freedom that a dumbbell offers over a barbell. You'll also work more of the upper and middle chest, along with the shoulders and triceps.

PREPARATORY STAGE
Set yourself up as on p.96 but with the dumbbells in your lap. Using a standard overhand grip, press the dumbbells up and toward the midline.

STAGE ONE
Take a breath in, engage your abs, and activate your upper-back muscles. Bend at the elbows and resist the load as it moves toward your chest.

STAGE TWO
With your abs engaged and tension in your triceps and chest, extend your arm to press the weight away, breathing out as you do so. Repeat stages 1 and 2.

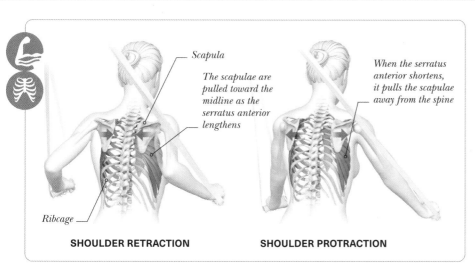

Scapula

The scapulae are pulled toward the midline as the serratus anterior lengthens

When the serratus anterior shortens, it pulls the scapulae away from the spine

Ribcage

SHOULDER RETRACTION

SHOULDER PROTRACTION

The role of the serratus anterior

Often known as the "boxer's muscle" because it relates to the reaching and punching movement, the serratus anterior is a deep, fan-shaped muscle that sits under the scapula and wraps around the ribcage. It anchors the scapula, so it is key in the protraction of the scapula and the lifting of the ribcage. The serratus anterior also plays a vital role in stabilizing the shoulder during overhead pressing movements.

BANDED CHEST PRESS

This standing variation allows you to train the movement of the pressing pattern. Your intent should be to drive your arms back out away from the midline by using your upper-back muscles to help pull your arm back, all the while keeping tension in your chest.

PREPARATORY STAGE
Choose an appropriate resistance band (see p.47) and anchor high up. Adopt a staggered stance with the band in your hands and your elbows flexed.

STAGE ONE
Take a breath in and engage your abs. Activate your upper-back muscles to pull your arms back, bending at the elbows and resisting the band.

STAGE TWO
Place tension in your triceps and chest, then extend your arm to press away toward the midline, breathing out as you do so. Repeat stages 1 and 2.

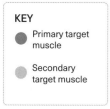

KEY

● Primary target muscle

● Secondary target muscle

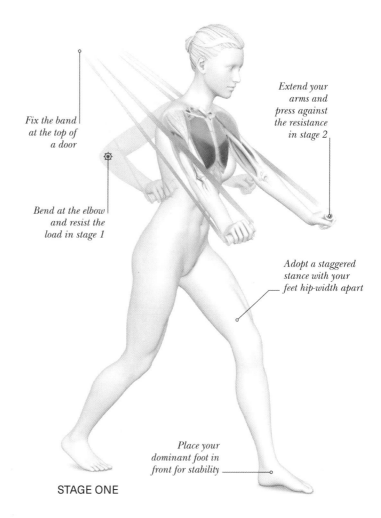

Fix the band at the top of a door

Bend at the elbow and resist the load in stage 1

Extend your arms and press against the resistance in stage 2

Adopt a staggered stance with your feet hip-width apart

Place your dominant foot in front for stability

STAGE ONE

HIGH–LOW CABLE **CHEST FLY**

This exercise uses a high-to-low flying movement to strengthen the muscles of the chest and the shoulders, particularly the serratus anterior and pectoralis minor. The cable machine offers you the freedom to follow your own arm path.

THE **BIG PICTURE**

This movement works the lower division of the pecs, so set the cable high. If you experience joint discomfort, try adjusting the setting; the path of the cable should match your arm path.

Beginners can start with 4 sets of 8–10 reps; discover variations on pp.102–103 and other targeted sets in the training programs (see pp.201–214).

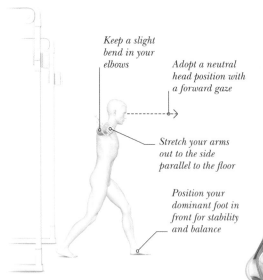

Keep a slight bend in your elbows

Adopt a neutral head position with a forward gaze

Stretch your arms out to the side parallel to the floor

Position your dominant foot in front for stability and balance

ANTERIOR-LATERAL VIEW

PREPARATORY STAGE
Set the weights and cable height. Grasp the handles (if you have shoulder discomfort, grab one handle at a time), then adopt a staggered stance, facing away at the middle of the machine, with your hips square. Engage your core.

STAGE ONE
Breathe in and activate the muscles of your upper back. Breathe out as you engage your chest and shoulder muscles to drive your upper arms smoothly toward the midline; your arms will naturally straighten. Hold for 1 second.

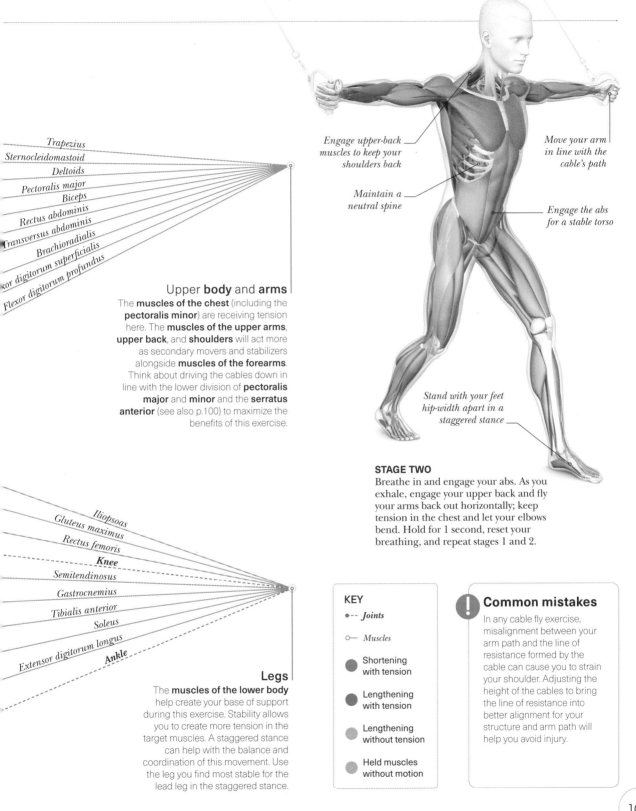

Engage upper-back
muscles to keep your
shoulders back

Maintain a
neutral spine

Move your arm
in line with the
cable's path

Engage the abs
for a stable torso

Stand with your feet
hip-width apart in a
staggered stance

Trapezius
Sternocleidomastoid
Deltoids
Pectoralis major
Biceps
Rectus abdominis
Transversus abdominis
Brachioradialis
Flexor digitorum superficialis
Flexor digitorum profundus

Upper **body** and **arms**

The **muscles of the chest** (including the
pectoralis minor) are receiving tension
here. The **muscles of the upper arms**,
upper back, and **shoulders** will act more
as secondary movers and stabilizers
alongside **muscles of the forearms**.
Think about driving the cables down in
line with the lower division of **pectoralis
major** and **minor** and the **serratus
anterior** (see also p.100) to maximize the
benefits of this exercise.

Iliopsoas
Gluteus maximus
Rectus femoris
Knee
Semitendinosus
Gastrocnemius
Tibialis anterior
Soleus
Extensor digitorum longus
Ankle

Legs

The **muscles of the lower body**
help create your base of support
during this exercise. Stability allows
you to create more tension in the
target muscles. A staggered stance
can help with the balance and
coordination of this movement. Use
the leg you find most stable for the
lead leg in the staggered stance.

STAGE TWO

Breathe in and engage your abs. As you
exhale, engage your upper back and fly
your arms back out horizontally; keep
tension in the chest and let your elbows
bend. Hold for 1 second, reset your
breathing, and repeat stages 1 and 2.

KEY

- •-- *Joints*
- ○-- *Muscles*
- ● Shortening with tension
- ● Lengthening with tension
- ● Lengthening without tension
- ● Held muscles without motion

⚠ Common mistakes

In any cable fly exercise,
misalignment between your
arm path and the line of
resistance formed by the
cable can cause you to strain
your shoulder. Adjusting the
height of the cables to bring
the line of resistance into
better alignment for your
structure and arm path will
help you avoid injury.

›› VARIATIONS

Varying the starting and end positions of the cable in a chest fly allows you to target different muscle areas. A change in starting position will affect the position of the arms—which in turn directly impacts where the resistance moves across the chest and which division of the pectoralis major is used. There is also a high-to-low option that doesn't require cables, using bands to provide resistance instead, making it ideal for at-home training.

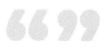

*Target chest muscles safely and effectively **using cables**. The cable machine keeps tension on your pecs for **both the lifting and the lowering parts** of each rep.*

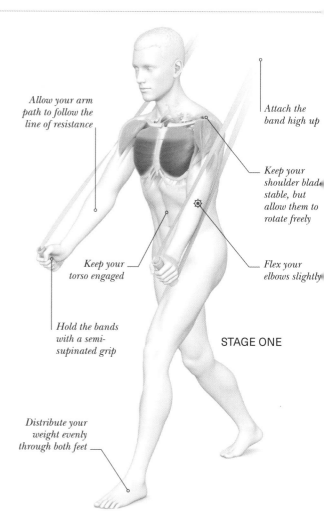

Allow your arm path to follow the line of resistance

Attach the band high up

Keep your shoulder blade stable, but allow them to rotate freely

Keep your torso engaged

Flex your elbows slightly

Hold the bands with a semi-supinated grip

STAGE ONE

Distribute your weight evenly through both feet

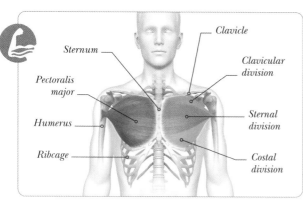

Clavicle

Sternum

Clavicular division

Pectoralis major

Sternal division

Humerus

Ribcage

Costal division

The three divisions of **pectoralis major**
Pectoralis major is divided into three main divisions: costal (lower), sternal (mid), and clavicular (upper). Your arm path and the line of resistance (formed by the cable or bands you are working with) will determine which of these divisions is most challenged during a pressing or a flying movement.

HIGH–LOW BANDED CHEST FLY

This at-home option allows you to train the movement pattern of the fly without the need for free weights or cables; it is a more effective way to challenge the chest muscles compared to a push-up or press.

PREPARATORY STAGE
Secure two bands on top of a door or other anchor. Adopt the starting position on pp.100–101, with your dominant foot forward, and hold onto the bands.

STAGE ONE
Breathe in and engage your core. Breathe out as you drive your arms down and toward the midline, following the path of the bands. Hold for 1 second.

STAGE TWO
Breathe in to engage your core, then breathe out to drive your arms back and away from the midline, using the upper-back muscles. Repeat stages 1 and 2.

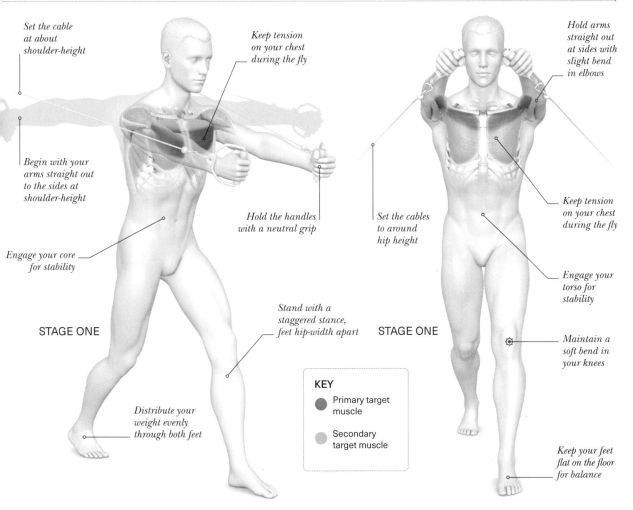

Set the cable at about shoulder-height

Keep tension on your chest during the fly

Begin with your arms straight out to the sides at shoulder-height

Hold the handles with a neutral grip

Engage your core for stability

STAGE ONE

Stand with a staggered stance, feet hip-width apart

Distribute your weight evenly through both feet

Hold arms straight out at sides with slight bend in elbows

Set the cables to around hip height

Keep tension on your chest during the fly

Engage your torso for stability

STAGE ONE

Maintain a soft bend in your knees

Keep your feet flat on the floor for balance

KEY

● Primary target muscle

● Secondary target muscle

MID-CABLE CHEST FLY

Keep a slight bend at the elbows during this cable exercise to reduce the strain on your biceps. Your arms should line up with the line of resistance from the cable. Avoid rounding your shoulders as you fly forward.

PREPARATORY STAGE
Set the cable starting position at shoulder height and adopt the starting pose used on pp.100–101. Hold your arms straight out to the sides.

STAGE ONE
Breathe in to brace your core, then breathe out as you drive your arms together so they are parallel out in front of you; your arms will straighten out.

STAGE TWO
Breathe in again to engage your core, then breathe out to fly your arms back to the starting position, flexing slightly at the elbows. Repeat stages 1 and 2.

LOW–HIGH CABLE CHEST FLY

This variation targets the upper muscle fibers of the chest while also training the front deltoids. Your shoulder blades should be stable, with tension in your upper back, but still able to rotate freely through the range of motion.

PREPARATORY STAGE
Set the cable starting position at around hip height or slightly lower and adopt the same pose used on pp.100–101, arms at your sides.

STAGE ONE
Breathe in to engage your core, then breathe out as you drive your arms up and toward the midline, using the muscles of the upper chest and front delts.

STAGE TWO
Breathe in to engage your core again, hold, then breathe out to drive your arms back out, engaging the upper-back muscles. Repeat stages 1 and 2.

MACHINE
CHEST FLY

This exercise—also known as the pec deck—trains muscles of the chest and shoulders. Performing the movement using a machine allows you to operate within a safe and effective training environment.

THE BIG PICTURE

It is important to position the seat correctly to best fit your body structure and desired arm path, to minimize any shoulder discomfort during the exercise. Your arms should be able to move easily between the midline and out wide at the sides, parallel to the floor, in a controlled flying motion.

Beginners can start with 4 sets of 8–10 reps; discover other targeted sets in the training programs (see pp.201–214).

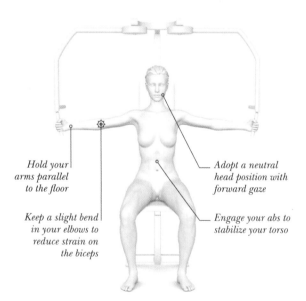

Hold your arms parallel to the floor

Keep a slight bend in your elbows to reduce strain on the biceps

Adopt a neutral head position with forward gaze

Engage your abs to stabilize your torso

PREPARATORY STAGE
Set the weights and adjust the height of the seat. Sit down and take up a stable, comfortable stance with your feet flat on the floor and your back flat against the pad. Stretch your arms out to the sides and grasp the handles. (If you have shoulder discomfort, grab one handle at a time.)

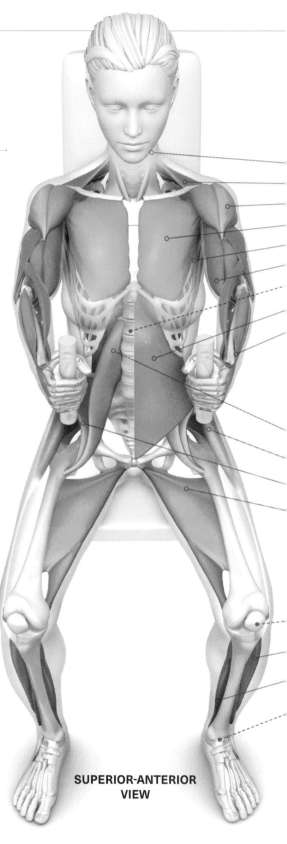

SUPERIOR-ANTERIOR VIEW

STAGE ONE

Inhale and activate your abs and upper-back muscles. Breathe out as you engage the muscles of your chest and shoulders to drive your upper arms across your chest toward your sternum; your arms will naturally straighten. To add a challenge, pause for 1–2 seconds, keeping tension in the chest.

KEY

●-- *Joints*

○— *Muscles*

● Shortening with tension

● Lengthening with tension

● Lengthening without tension

● Held muscles without motion

Common mistakes

Straining at the shoulder joint—due to not correctly aligning the machine to your arm path—is commonly seen. Those who think about driving the handles or hands together should be instead focusing on driving the upper arms toward the midline to target the correct muscles.

rnocleidomastoid
Trapezius
Deltoids
Pectoralis major
Serratus anterior
Biceps
Spine
ransversus abdominis
Extensor digitorum

Upper **body** and **arms**

The **muscles of the chest** are receiving tension here. The muscles of the **arms**, **upper back**, and **shoulders** (including the **serratus anterior**) act more as secondary movers and stabilizers alongside the **muscles of the forearms**. Think about driving your upper arms toward the midline to maximize tension placed in the chest.

Engage your upper-back muscles to keep your shoulders back

Ensure your back is flat against the pad

Psoas major
Tensor fascia latae
Iliacus
Adductor magnus

Knee
Peroneus longus
Soleus
Ankle

STAGE TWO

Breathe in to engage your abs. As you exhale, engage the muscles of your upper back to aid in flying your arms back to the starting point, bending your elbows and keeping tension in your chest; keep the muscles of your upper back engaged. Reset your breathing, then repeat stages 1 and 2.

Legs

The **muscles of the lower body** will help provide your base of support during this move. Being stable allows you to create more tension in the target muscles. If you are a shorter individual, try putting down a step or small box for your feet to rest on so that they maintain contact with the ground during the exercise.

Keep your feet flat on the floor for even weight distribution

DUMBBELL
CHEST FLY

STAGE ONE
Breathe in and engage your core and upper back for stability. Breathe out as you fly your arms out to the sides, keeping tension in your chest and shoulders. The dumbbells should remain parallel to your torso. To add a challenge, pause for 1–2 seconds.

This exercise is isolation based—it places tension on just one area, the chest and front deltoids. Moving the weights far away from the midline allows gravity's effect to kick in, offering a greater challenge in the eccentric contraction (lower phase) than other versions of the chest fly.

THE BIG PICTURE

You might find you have to work harder to perform a chest fly while lying down; it's also crucial to get the technique right to avoid injury. Ensure you decelerate at the bottom of the rep to avoid strain to muscles or joints. If you experience joint discomfort during this exercise, switch to the cable or machine versions (see pp.100–101 and pp.104–105).

Beginners can start with 4 sets of 8–10 reps; discover other targeted sets in the training programs (see pp.201–214).

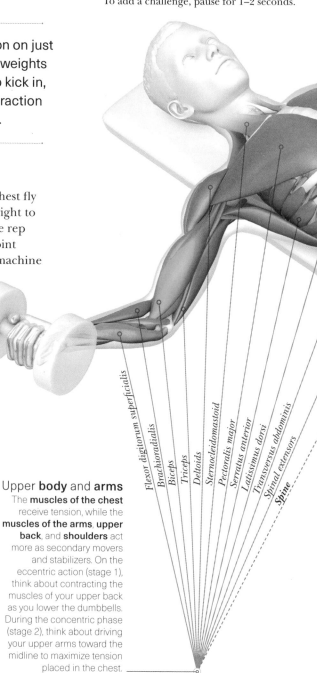

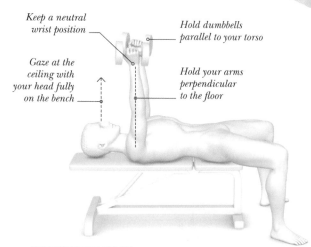

Keep a neutral wrist position

Hold dumbbells parallel to your torso

Gaze at the ceiling with your head fully on the bench

Hold your arms perpendicular to the floor

PREPARATORY STAGE
Lie flat with your buttocks fully on the bench and your feet flat on the floor, wider than hip-width apart. Hold the dumbbells at the sides of your body. Then raise the weights up above your chest while keeping your head in a neutral position.

Upper **body** and **arms**
The **muscles of the chest** receive tension, while the **muscles of the arms**, **upper back**, and **shoulders** act more as secondary movers and stabilizers. On the eccentric action (stage 1), think about contracting the muscles of your upper back as you lower the dumbbells. During the concentric phase (stage 2), think about driving your upper arms toward the midline to maximize tension placed in the chest.

Flexor digitorum superficialis
Brachioradialis
Biceps
Triceps
Deltoids
Sternocleidomastoid
Pectoralis major
Serratus anterior
Latissimus dorsi
Transversus abdominis
Spinal extensors
Spine

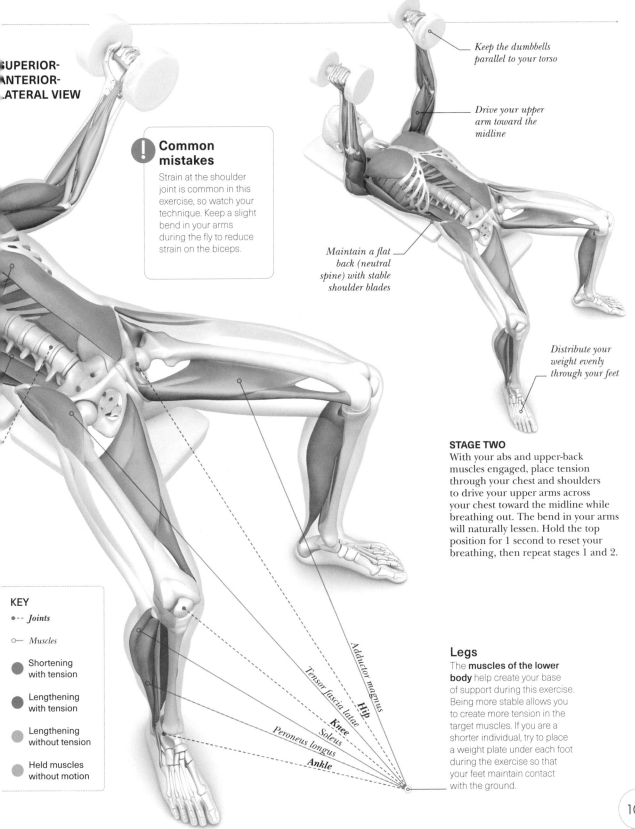

SUPERIOR-ANTERIOR-LATERAL VIEW

! Common mistakes

Strain at the shoulder joint is common in this exercise, so watch your technique. Keep a slight bend in your arms during the fly to reduce strain on the biceps.

Keep the dumbbells parallel to your torso

Drive your upper arm toward the midline

Maintain a flat back (neutral spine) with stable shoulder blades

Distribute your weight evenly through your feet

KEY

●--- *Joints*

○— *Muscles*

● Shortening with tension

● Lengthening with tension

● Lengthening without tension

● Held muscles without motion

Adductor magnus

Tensor fascia latae

Hip

Knee

Soleus

Peroneus longus

Ankle

STAGE TWO

With your abs and upper-back muscles engaged, place tension through your chest and shoulders to drive your upper arms across your chest toward the midline while breathing out. The bend in your arms will naturally lessen. Hold the top position for 1 second to reset your breathing, then repeat stages 1 and 2.

Legs

The **muscles of the lower body** help create your base of support during this exercise. Being more stable allows you to create more tension in the target muscles. If you are a shorter individual, try to place a weight plate under each foot during the exercise so that your feet maintain contact with the ground.

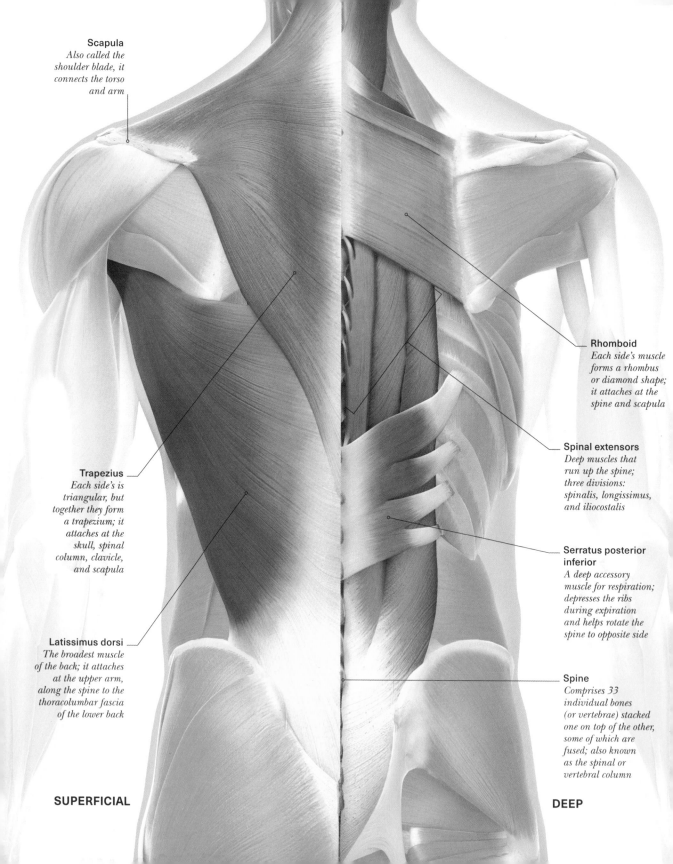

Scapula
Also called the shoulder blade, it connects the torso and arm

Rhomboid
Each side's muscle forms a rhombus or diamond shape; it attaches at the spine and scapula

Trapezius
Each side's is triangular, but together they form a trapezium; it attaches at the skull, spinal column, clavicle, and scapula

Spinal extensors
Deep muscles that run up the spine; three divisions: spinalis, longissimus, and iliocostalis

Serratus posterior inferior
A deep accessory muscle for respiration; depresses the ribs during expiration and helps rotate the spine to opposite side

Latissimus dorsi
The broadest muscle of the back; it attaches at the upper arm, along the spine to the thoracolumbar fascia of the lower back

Spine
Comprises 33 individual bones (or vertebrae) stacked one on top of the other, some of which are fused; also known as the spinal or vertebral column

SUPERFICIAL

DEEP

BACK EXERCISES

The main muscles responsible for movement in the back are: the latissimus dorsi (lats), the largest among the muscles nearest to the surface; the trapezius (traps), the other main superficial muscle; the rhomboids, positioned deep beneath the trapezius; and the spinal extensors, deep beneath the rhomboids.

The lats attach to the upper arms and connective tissue around the lower back, while the traps and rhomboids attach to the scapulae and spine in the upper back. The spinal extensors attach to the pelvis, spine, and ribcage.

The muscles of the back enable extension, vertical and horizontal adduction, depression, and retraction of the shoulder and extension and lateral flexion of the spine. They act as antagonists to muscles of the chest and torso, helping stabilize and protect the spine in squats and deadlifts.

- **When performing rowing variations**, muscles with a more horizontal fiber alignment, such as the middle division of the traps and upper lats, help bring the arms back and around toward the midline.

- **When performing pulldown variations**, muscles with a more vertical fiber alignment, such as the lower lats and upper and lower traps, help in bringing the arms down, back, and around toward the midline.

When performing any movement focusing on the back, you will be using any number of muscles in combination to complete the full range of motion, alongside muscles of the shoulders and arms.

❝❞

*Strong back muscles enable a **wide range of movement patterns** in perfect **synchronicity**.*

WIDE-GRIP VERTICAL PULLDOWN

Vertical pulling is a great exercise for supporting good posture and general mobility. The wide grip used in this variation of the exercise puts the focus on the muscles of the upper back and the latissimus dorsi, as well as training the biceps and rear deltoid muscles of the upper arm and shoulder.

THE BIG PICTURE

A wide grip on the bar targets the upper back, whereas a more neutral grip works the lats and biceps more; to discover how a change of grip tweaks the muscles worked, see pp.112–113. If you experience joint discomfort during this exercise, try adjusting your range of motion in stage 2 to place less stress on the shoulder joint.

Beginners can start with 4 sets of 8–10 reps; discover other variations to practice at home on pp.112–113 and other targeted sets in the training programs (see pp.201–214).

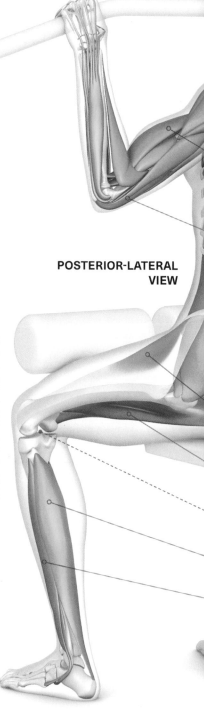

POSTERIOR-LATERAL VIEW

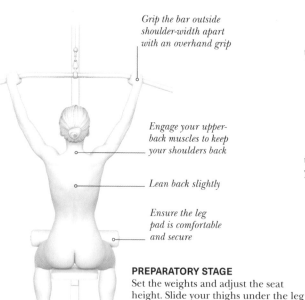

Grip the bar outside shoulder-width apart with an overhand grip

Engage your upper-back muscles to keep your shoulders back

Lean back slightly

Ensure the leg pad is comfortable and secure

PREPARATORY STAGE
Set the weights and adjust the seat height. Slide your thighs under the leg pad and sit with your knees bent and feet flat on the floor. Take hold of the bar and lean your torso back a little, slightly extending your upper back.

STAGE ONE
Breathe in and engage your abs to stabilize and tighten your core. As you breathe out, pull the bar down by flexing at the elbows and contracting the muscles of your upper/mid back; your elbows will be driven outward. Keep your chest high and pull the bar toward the top of your sternum. (It doesn't have to touch you.)

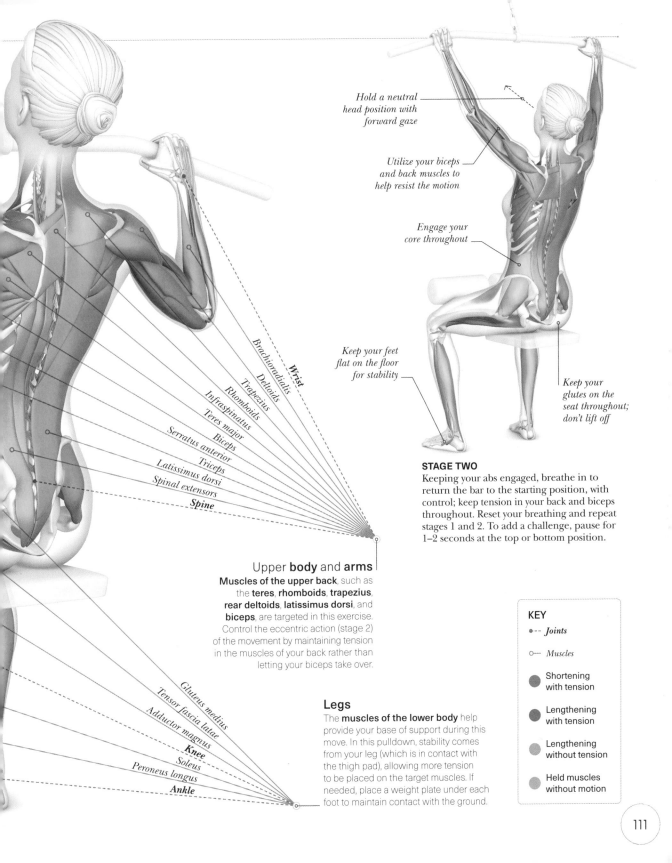

Hold a neutral head position with forward gaze

Utilize your biceps and back muscles to help resist the motion

Engage your core throughout

Keep your feet flat on the floor for stability

Keep your glutes on the seat throughout; don't lift off

STAGE TWO
Keeping your abs engaged, breathe in to return the bar to the starting position, with control; keep tension in your back and biceps throughout. Reset your breathing and repeat stages 1 and 2. To add a challenge, pause for 1–2 seconds at the top or bottom position.

Brachioradialis
Deltoids
Trapezius
Rhomboids
Infraspinatus
Teres major
Biceps
Serratus anterior
Triceps
Latissimus dorsi
Spinal extensors
Wrist
Spine

Gluteus medius
Tensor fascia latae
Adductor magnus
Knee
Soleus
Peroneus longus
Ankle

Upper **body** and **arms**
Muscles of the upper back, such as the **teres, rhomboids, trapezius, rear deltoids, latissimus dorsi**, and **biceps**, are targeted in this exercise. Control the eccentric action (stage 2) of the movement by maintaining tension in the muscles of your back rather than letting your biceps take over.

Legs
The **muscles of the lower body** help provide your base of support during this move. In this pulldown, stability comes from your leg (which is in contact with the thigh pad), allowing more tension to be placed on the target muscles. If needed, place a weight plate under each foot to maintain contact with the ground.

KEY
•--- *Joints*
○--- *Muscles*

● Shortening with tension
● Lengthening with tension
● Lengthening without tension
● Held muscles without motion

» VARIATIONS

The motion of a vertical pulldown can be adapted to various pieces of equipment. Adjusting your grip will alter the specific muscles being targeted, including the lats, traps, and delts. Again, take care not to place too much stress on your shoulder joints during these moves.

KEY
● Primary target muscle
● Secondary target muscle

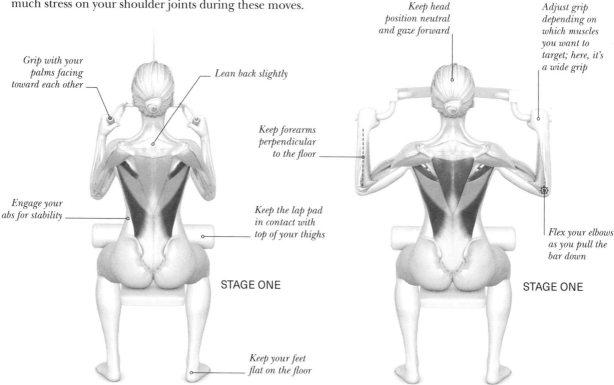

Grip with your palms facing toward each other

Lean back slightly

Keep forearms perpendicular to the floor

Engage your abs for stability

Keep the lap pad in contact with top of your thighs

STAGE ONE

Keep your feet flat on the floor

Keep head position neutral and gaze forward

Adjust grip depending on which muscles you want to target; here, it's a wide grip

Flex your elbows as you pull the bar down

STAGE ONE

NEUTRAL-GRIP VERTICAL PULLDOWN

Where the wider, pronated grip on the pulldown on the previous pages targets the upper-back muscles, this variation with a neutral grip—with palms facing each other—helps bias the latissimus dorsi.

PREPARATORY STAGE
Position your body as for a wide-grip pulldown. Your hands should be shoulder-width apart in a neutral grip. Lean your torso back slightly.

STAGE ONE
Breathe in and engage your abdominal muscles. Breathe out as you pull the bar down by flexing at the elbows and contracting the lats.

STAGE TWO
Breathe in again and engage your abdominal muscles. Return the bar to the starting position, maintaining control. Repeat stages 1 and 2.

MACHINE VERTICAL PULLDOWN

This machine variation allows for either a pronated wide grip or a neutral grip while providing a fixed path of resistance from the machine. This wide-grip version targets more of the traps than the neutral-grip one.

PREPARATORY STAGE
Set up the machine. Sit with your thighs under the leg pad, knees bent, and with your feet on the floor. Hold onto the handles using your preferred grip.

STAGE ONE
Breathe in and engage your abdominals, then breathe out as you pull the bar down, contracting the muscles of your upper/midback.

STAGE TWO
Breathe in again and engage your core, then, maintaining control, breathe out to return the bar to its starting position. Repeat stages 1 and 2.

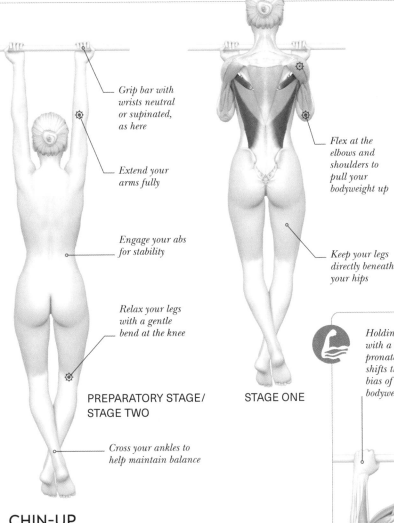

Grip bar with wrists neutral or supinated, as here

Extend your arms fully

Engage your abs for stability

Relax your legs with a gentle bend at the knee

PREPARATORY STAGE/ STAGE TWO

Cross your ankles to help maintain balance

Flex at the elbows and shoulders to pull your bodyweight up

Keep your legs directly beneath your hips

STAGE ONE

> *Your grip will influence which **muscles will be more biased** over others during a **pulldown** variation.*

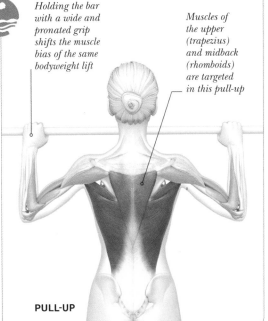

Holding the bar with a wide and pronated grip shifts the muscle bias of the same bodyweight lift

Muscles of the upper (trapezius) and midback (rhomboids) are targeted in this pull-up

PULL-UP

CHIN-UP

This exercise trains the upper back, lats, and biceps. Bodyweight vertical pulling is a great addition to every strength program, and this neutral-grip variation trains a large portion of the back with each rep.

PREPARATORY STAGE
Start in a hanging position with your core stabilized. You can cross one foot over the other at your ankle to help maintain balance and coordination.

STAGE ONE
Breathe out as you flex your elbows to pull yourself off the ground. To make the exercise more challenging, pause in this position for 1–2 seconds.

STAGE TWO
Breathe in as you extend your elbows to lower your body, keeping your core engaged. Do not swing to create momentum. Repeat stages 1 and 2.

A matter of **grip**
Having your hands close together and in a more neutral, semi-, or supinated grip will allow you to perform a chin-up, which involves more lats and biceps relative to the upper back. The wider and more pronated grip results in a pull-up, with more upper-back focus while still training the biceps, but less lats overall.

NEUTRAL-GRIP
HORIZONTAL ROW

Horizontal pulling fits well into any strength training program; this neutral-grip variation trains a large portion of the upper back, lats, and biceps. Finding the correct position on the bench—not too close to the apparatus—is key to ensuring you are working with a full range of motion.

THE **BIG PICTURE**

Place your feet low down on the foot platform to allow for more flexibility at the hip. If you experience any shoulder discomfort, try adjusting your range of motion in stage 2.

Beginners can start with 4 sets of 8–10 reps; discover other variations to practice on pp.116–117 and other targeted sets in the training programs (see pp.201–214).

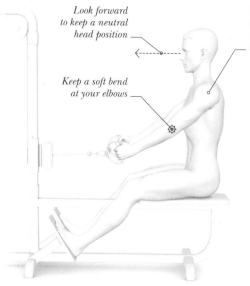

Look forward to keep a neutral head position

Engage your upper-back muscles to keep your shoulders back

Keep a soft bend at your elbows

! Common mistakes

Many people make the mistake of generating momentum at the hip and torso, which will cause you to lean back rather than rowing back. Aim to keep your core in a fixed position throughout.

PREPARATORY STAGE
Set the weights and adjust the seat height, then sit on the bench, facing the machine; your feet should be low down on the platform and your legs softly bent. Hold the attachment with your hands shoulder-width apart and sit back, arms extended and back upright.

STAGE ONE
Breathe in and engage your abs. As you exhale, flex your elbows and contract your upper/mid back muscles to row the attachment toward your upper abdomen; your elbows will be driven back. Stop just before your shoulders start to round forward.

POSTERIOR-LATERAL VIEW

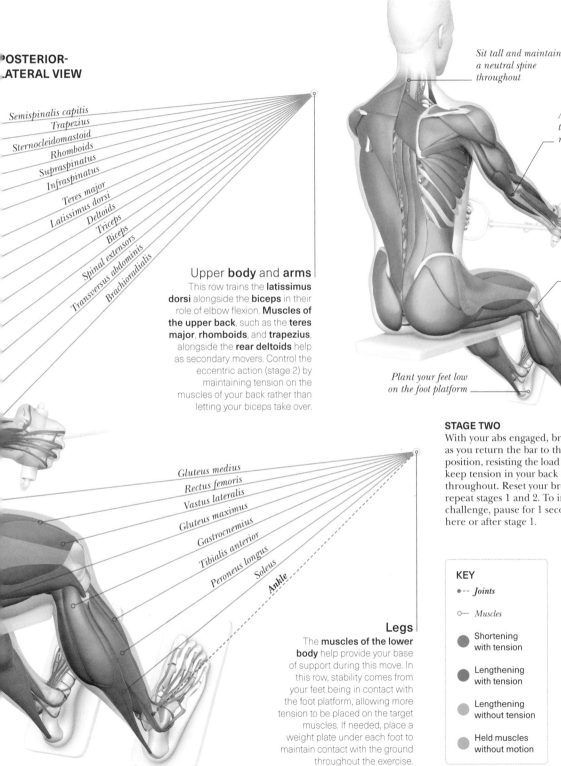

Semispinalis capitis
Trapezius
Sternocleidomastoid
Rhomboids
Supraspinatus
Infraspinatus
Teres major
Latissimus dorsi
Deltoids
Triceps
Biceps
Spinal extensors
Transversus abdominis
Brachioradialis

Sit tall and maintain a neutral spine throughout

Allow your arms to extend as you resist the load

Keep a soft bend at your knee

Plant your feet low on the foot platform

Upper body and arms
This row trains the **latissimus dorsi** alongside the **biceps** in their role of elbow flexion. **Muscles of the upper back**, such as the **teres major**, **rhomboids**, and **trapezius**, alongside the **rear deltoids** help as secondary movers. Control the eccentric action (stage 2) by maintaining tension on the muscles of your back rather than letting your biceps take over.

STAGE TWO
With your abs engaged, breathe in as you return the bar to the starting position, resisting the load with control; keep tension in your back and biceps throughout. Reset your breathing and repeat stages 1 and 2. To increase the challenge, pause for 1 second either here or after stage 1.

Gluteus medius
Rectus femoris
Vastus lateralis
Gluteus maximus
Gastrocnemius
Tibialis anterior
Peroneus longus
Soleus
Ankle

Legs
The **muscles of the lower body** help provide your base of support during this move. In this row, stability comes from your feet being in contact with the foot platform, allowing more tension to be placed on the target muscles. If needed, place a weight plate under each foot to maintain contact with the ground throughout the exercise.

KEY
- •-- *Joints*
- ○— *Muscles*
- ● Shortening with tension
- ● Lengthening with tension
- ● Lengthening without tension
- ● Held muscles without motion

» VARIATIONS

A rowing movement targets the latissimus dorsi, other back muscles, and the biceps. You can adapt this exercise to your range of equipment. Keep your torso stable and move your shoulders and arms back in a fluid motion on each rep.

KEY
● Primary target muscle
● Secondary target muscle

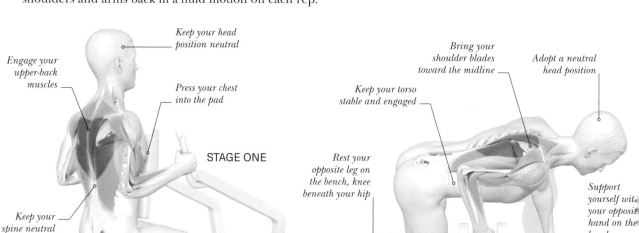

Engage your upper-back muscles

Keep your head position neutral

Press your chest into the pad

STAGE ONE

Keep your spine neutral

Place your feet flat against the platform or floor

Bring your shoulder blades toward the midline

Keep your torso stable and engaged

Adopt a neutral head position

Rest your opposite leg on the bench, knee beneath your hip

Support yourself with your opposite hand on the bench

STAGE ONE

Slightly bend your supporting leg

Lower the weight in stage 2

MACHINE HORIZONTAL ROW

This alternative machine-based variation trains the upper- and midback muscles. The chest support provided by the machine creates a stable and safe environment. For more of a challenge, hold at the top position for 1–2 seconds.

PREPARATORY STAGE
Sit on the machine and place your feet against the platform if there is one. Lean forward and place your chest against the pad.

STAGE ONE
Inhale to engage your abs. Breathe out as you pull the attachment toward you, bringing your shoulders back and arms behind you in one continuous motion.

STAGE TWO
Breathe in as you return the bar to its starting position, controlling the movement throughout. Repeat stages 1 and 2.

DUMBBELL BENT-OVER ROW

Using dumbbells allows you to perform the movement either unilaterally, with one leg supported on a bench as here, or bilaterally, with both legs flexed at the knees and your hips flexed at 90°. For more of a challenge, hold the top position for 1–2 seconds.

PREPARATORY STAGE
Place your opposite knee on the bench and position your other leg beneath your hip. Lean forward so your back is flat and breathe in to brace your core.

STAGE ONE
Breathe out as you retract your shoulder blades and drive your arm up, flexing your elbow between 30° and 75°; the angle changes the muscle bias.

STAGE TWO
Breathe in as you lower the dumbbell in a controlled movement, keeping your abs engaged. Repeat stages 1 and 2.

BARBELL BENT-OVER ROW

This popular barbell variation targets the muscles of the core in addition to those of the upper and midback. Be aware that your range of motion may decrease when standing. As with the other variations, hold at the top position for 1–2 seconds for an added challenge.

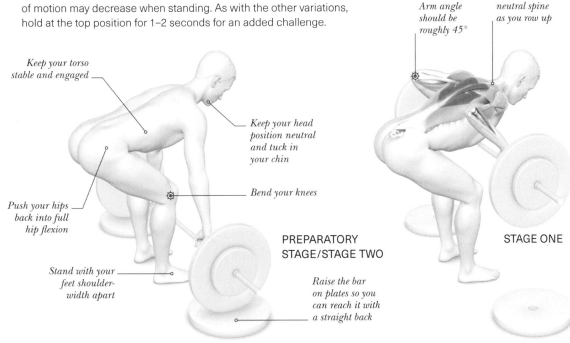

Keep your torso stable and engaged

Keep your head position neutral and tuck in your chin

Push your hips back into full hip flexion

Bend your knees

Stand with your feet shoulder-width apart

PREPARATORY STAGE/STAGE TWO

Raise the bar on plates so you can reach it with a straight back

Arm angle should be roughly 45°

Maintain a neutral spine as you row up

STAGE ONE

PREPARATORY STAGE
Stand bending forward and hold the barbell in your hands with a pronated grip without sacrificing your neutral spine position.

STAGE ONE
Breathe in to brace your core, then breathe out as you row up, lifting the bar toward your chest and bringing your elbows back behind your body.

STAGE TWO
Breathe in as you lower the barbell to its starting position, maintaining control in your arms, shoulders, back, and core. Repeat stages 1 and 2.

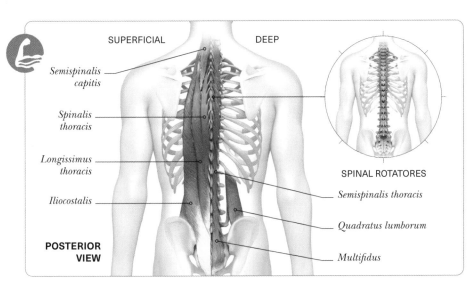

SUPERFICIAL   DEEP

Semispinalis capitis

Spinalis thoracis

Longissimus thoracis

Iliocostalis

POSTERIOR VIEW

SPINAL ROTATORES

Semispinalis thoracis

Quadratus lumborum

Multifidus

Spinal **extensors**

The superficial extensors (erector spinae) muscle group extends up the vertebral column and is made up of three divisions: spinalis, longissimus, and iliocostalis. The deep extensor muscles (including the rotatores) support the mobility work of the erector spinae and crucially help stabilize the spine and the pelvis. Together, these muscles work tirelessly to keep the body from falling forward and help maintain good posture.

DUMBBELL
TRAP SHRUG

This exercise trains the upper trapezius muscles (or traps) in a safe and effective way. The extra load of two dumbbells makes your muscles work even harder.

THE BIG PICTURE

Using dumbbells rather than a barbell removes the constraints of the bar so you can adapt your form to your individual mechanics and mobility limitations. If you have access to a machine, the cable variation allows for the greatest individualization and best resistance.

Beginners can start with 4 sets of 8–10 reps; discover other variations on pp.120–121 and other targeted sets in the training programs (see pp.201–214). If you experience discomfort during this exercise, try the cable or resistance-band variations overleaf.

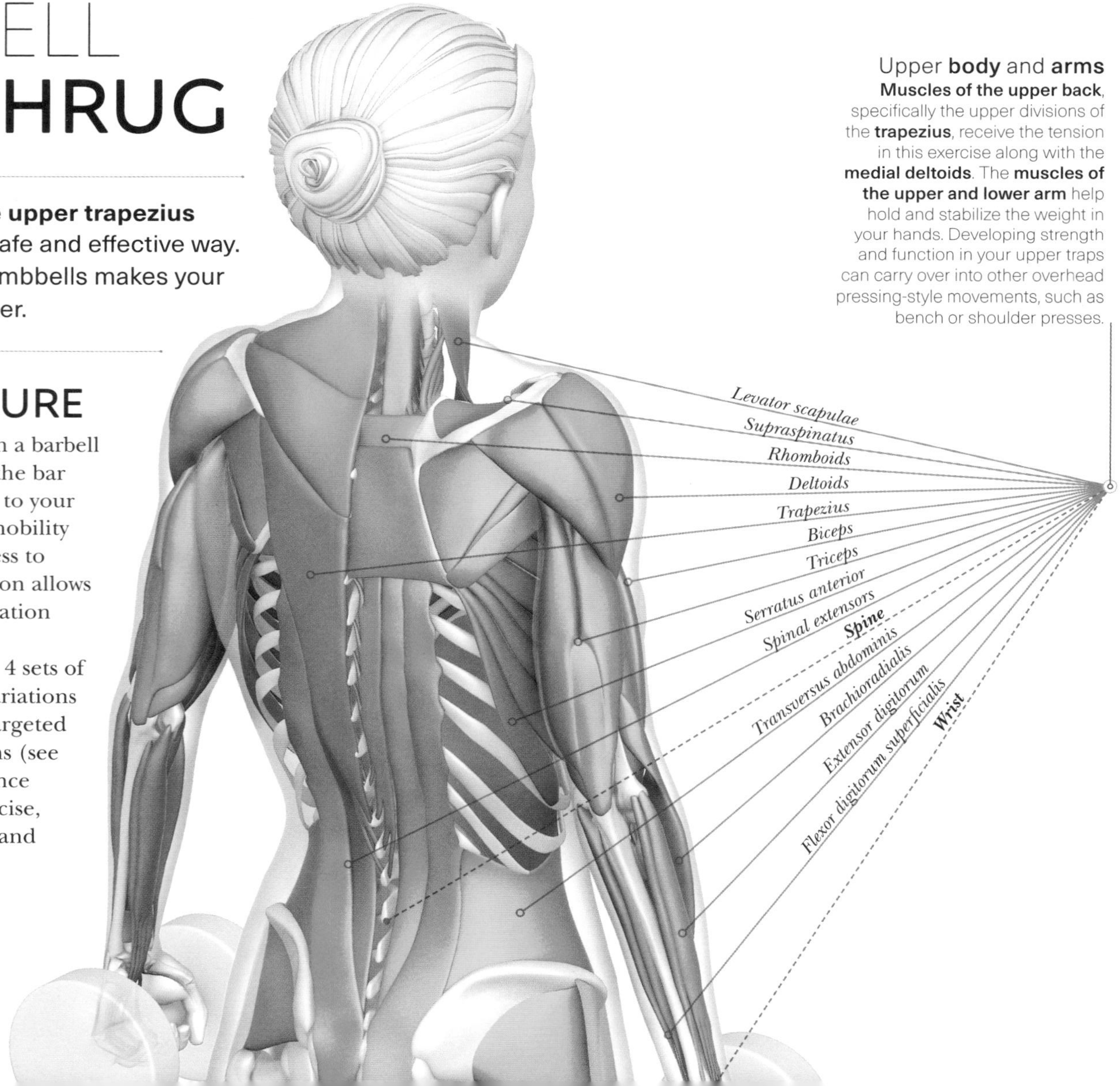

Upper **body** and **arms**
Muscles of the upper back, specifically the upper divisions of the **trapezius**, receive the tension in this exercise along with the **medial deltoids**. The **muscles of the upper and lower arm** help hold and stabilize the weight in your hands. Developing strength and function in your upper traps can carry over into other overhead pressing-style movements, such as bench or shoulder presses.

Levator scapulae
Supraspinatus
Rhomboids
Deltoids
Trapezius
Biceps
Triceps
Serratus anterior
Spinal extensors
Spine
Transversus abdominis
Brachioradialis
Extensor digitorum
Flexor digitorum superficialis
Wrist

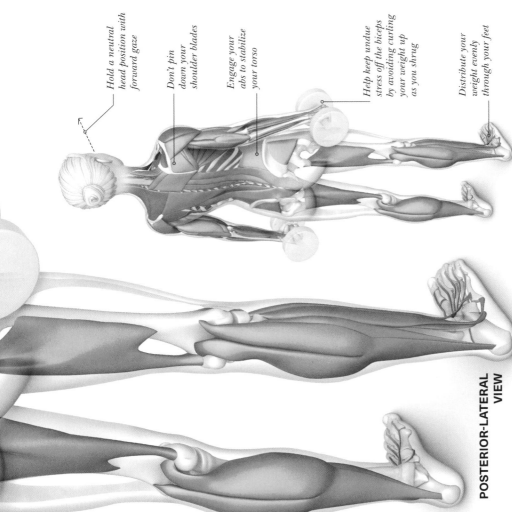

Hold a neutral head position with forward gaze

Don't pin down your shoulder blades

Engage your abs to stabilize your torso

Help keep undue stress off the biceps by avoiding curling your weight up as you shrug

Distribute your weight evenly through your feet

POSTERIOR-LATERAL VIEW

STAGE ONE

Take a breath in and engage your abs. Keeping your torso stable, exhale as you shrug your shoulders up toward your ears, taking both dumbbells upward. Stand still without any movement at your hips or torso. Hold for 1–2 seconds.

STAGE TWO

Keeping your core engaged, breathe in as you return the weights to the starting position, resisting the lowering motion of the dumbbells with your upper traps. Reset your breathing and repeat stages 1 and 2.

KEY

--- Joints
—○ Muscles

● Shortening with tension
● Lengthening with tension
● Lengthening without tension
● Held muscles without motion

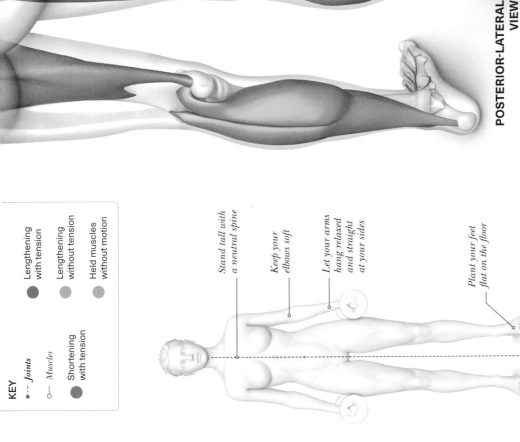

Stand tall with a neutral spine

Keep your elbows soft

Let your arms hang relaxed and straight at your sides

Plant your feet flat on the floor

PREPARATORY STAGE

Stand with your feet shoulder-width apart. Grip the dumbbells with a neutral wrist position (palms facing inward) and hold them at the sides of your body. Keep a neutral head position—do not look up or down.

≫ VARIATIONS

These versions of the trap shrug, which still target
the trapezius and medial deltoid, use cables or
resistance bands and can be easier on the neck
and biceps. Cables also allow you to adapt the
movement to suit your needs.

BANDED UPRIGHT ROW

This variation uses a resistance band to train the
upper traps and muscles of the shoulders. For an added
challenge, hold for 1–2 seconds at the top position.

Working the **upper traps**

The upper division of
the trapezius has a role
in opposing the force
that the medial delt
exhibits on the scapula.
This makes the trap
shrug great for training
both of these muscles
in one movement.

Upper trapezius

Medial deltoid

LATERAL VIEW

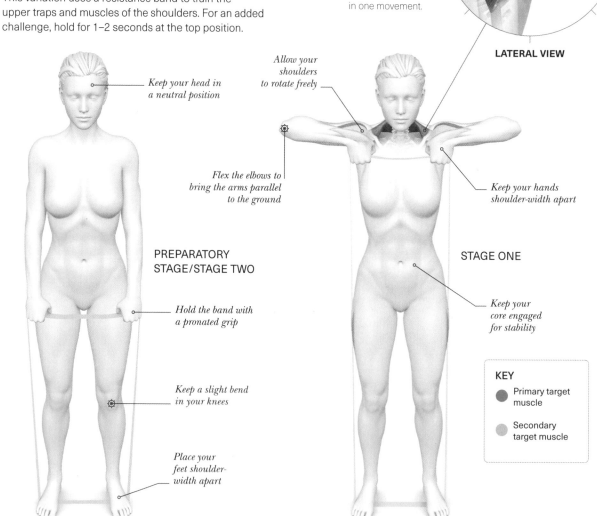

*Keep your head in
a neutral position*

*Allow your
shoulders
to rotate freely*

*Flex the elbows to
bring the arms parallel
to the ground*

**PREPARATORY
STAGE/STAGE TWO**

*Hold the band with
a pronated grip*

*Keep a slight bend
in your knees*

*Place your
feet shoulder-
width apart*

*Keep your hands
shoulder-width apart*

STAGE ONE

*Keep your
core engaged
for stability*

KEY

● Primary target
muscle

○ Secondary
target muscle

PREPARATORY STAGE
Place the resistance band beneath your
feet and hold it with a pronated grip,
hands shoulder-width apart. Stand tall
with your shoulders relaxed.

STAGE ONE
Breathe in to engage your core, then
breathe out as you row up, lifting your
shoulders and bringing your hands
upward as you flex your elbows.

STAGE 2
Breathe in as you lower your shoulders
and extend your arms back to your
starting position, with control. Repeat
stages 1 and 2.

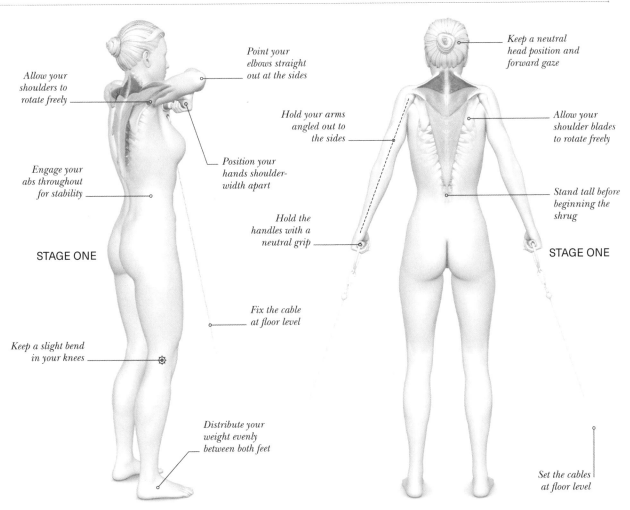

Allow your
shoulders to
rotate freely

Point your
elbows straight
out at the sides

Hold your arms
angled out to
the sides

Keep a neutral
head position and
forward gaze

Allow your
shoulder blades
to rotate freely

Engage your
abs throughout
for stability

Position your
hands shoulder-
width apart

Hold the
handles with a
neutral grip

Stand tall before
beginning the
shrug

STAGE ONE

STAGE ONE

Fix the cable
at floor level

Keep a slight bend
in your knees

Distribute your
weight evenly
between both feet

Set the cables
at floor level

CABLE UPRIGHT ROW

This cable-based variation trains the upper traps and
the muscles of the shoulders. The cables keep tension
on your shoulders. Hold the cable at chin height for
1–2 seconds for a more intense workout.

PREPARATORY STAGE
Stand tall with your feet shoulder-width apart and
a slight bend in your knees. Hold the cable handle
with both hands in a pronated grip.

STAGE ONE
Breathe in and engage your abs, then breathe out to
row the cable up to chin height, flexing your elbows
outward to bring your arms parallel to the floor.

STAGE TWO
Breathe in as you lower the cable with control
back to the starting position. Keep tension in your
shoulders throughout. Repeat stages 1 and 2.

CABLE TRAP SHRUG

This variation, using bilateral cables, is ideal for training
the upper traps, the muscle fibers of which line up well
with the line of resistance formed by the cable. For an
added challenge, hold at the top position for 1–2 seconds.

PREPARATORY STAGE
Stand with your feet shoulder-width apart and a
slight bend in your knees. Bend over to grasp the
cable handles, then stand up straight.

STAGE ONE
Breathe in and engage your core. Breathe out as
you shrug your shoulders up and in toward your
ears without rolling them forward or back.

STAGE TWO
Breathe in as you lower your shoulders back to
the starting position, keeping your core and traps
engaged for control. Repeat stages 1 and 2.

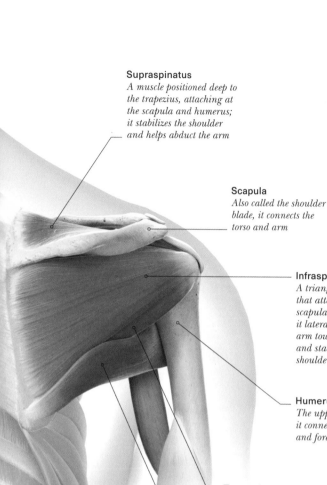

Supraspinatus
A muscle positioned deep to the trapezius, attaching at the scapula and humerus; it stabilizes the shoulder and helps abduct the arm

Clavicle
Also called the collarbone, it connects the scapula and sternum

Deltoids
A triangular muscle (delta is triangle in Greek) in three primary divisions; it attaches at the clavicle, scapula, and humerus

Scapula
Also called the shoulder blade, it connects the torso and arm

Infraspinatus
A triangular muscle that attaches at the scapula and humerus; it laterally rotates the arm toward the midline and stabilizes the shoulder

Humerus
The upper arm bone; it connects the scapula and forearm

Teres minor
A muscle that attaches to the scapula and humerus; it externally rotates and extends the arm and stabilizes the shoulder

Coracobrachialis
An upper-arm muscle that reaches from the scapula to the humerus; it flexes and adducts the arm at the shoulder

Teres major
A muscle that attaches to the scapula and humerus; it extends and medially rotates the arm and stabilizes the shoulder

Subscapularis
A triangular muscle that attaches to the scapula and humerus; it medially rotates the arm and stabilizes the shoulder

POSTERIOR VIEW

ANTERIOR VIEW

SHOULDER
EXERCISES

The main muscle responsible for moving the shoulders is the deltoid, the muscle that wraps around the shoulder, front to back, and gives the shoulders much of their shape. Other muscles are key for stabilizing the shoulder joint, including teres major, teres minor, supraspinatus, and subscapularis.

The main role of the deltoids (or delts) in training is to help raise or extend your arms; there are three primary divisions of the deltoid. The front (anterior) delt enables flexion, raising your arm up in front of your body; the medial (lateral) delt enables abduction, raising your arm away from your body; and the rear (posterior) delt enables extension, rotating your arm behind you.

You use delts repetitively in your day-to-day life and in training, so it's key to train them via different loading methods and rep counts.

- **When pressing**, the shoulders integrate with the triceps and muscles of the upper back to help in driving the weight up as the deltoid brings the arm closer to the midline.

- **When raising**, the shoulders work almost in isolation, with some assistance from the traps. Don't just think about getting the resistance to a certain destination—remember the function and anatomy of the portion of the deltoid you want to target and move appropriately through the full range of motion.

Use pressing and raising movements to target the front and middle deltoids and rowing and flying to work the rear delts.

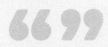

*Having a strong upper body **improves posture**, **mobility**, **flexibility**, and **range of motion**.*

BARBELL OVERHEAD SHOULDER PRESS

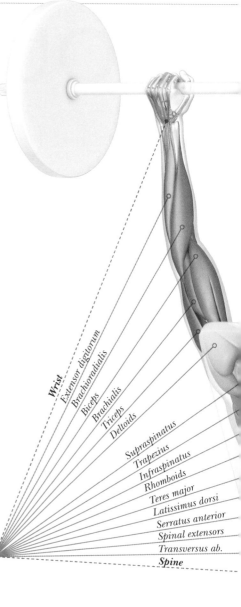

This dominant vertical pressing movement trains the muscles of the shoulders and the triceps while also targeting the upper back and challenging core stability. The overhead press can be performed seated or standing; keep the barbell even and the movements controlled.

THE **BIG PICTURE**

Your knees should be bent at 90° for this seated shoulder press, so adjust the seat height of the machine accordingly. Most machines set the bar just above and behind your head so you can easily reach and then lift the bar off to bring it into position. If you experience any joint discomfort, try switching to the dumbbell variation (see p.127).

Beginners can start with 4 sets of 8–10 reps; discover other variations on pp.126–127 and other targeted sets in the training programs (see pp.201–214).

Wrist
Extensor digitorum
Brachioradialis
Biceps
Brachialis
Triceps
Deltoids
Supraspinatus
Trapezius
Infraspinatus
Rhomboids
Teres major
Latissimus dorsi
Serratus anterior
Spinal extensors
Transversus ab.
Spine

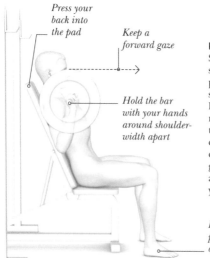

Press your back into the pad

Keep a forward gaze

Hold the bar with your hands around shoulder-width apart

Place your feet parallel and flat on the floor

PREPARATORY STAGE
Set up the machine and sit with your back on the pad, knees bent and feet shoulder-width apart. Keep your head in a neutral position. Rest the barbell under your chin and against your chest using a thumb-over grip. Engage your glutes and core to help stabilize your upper body.

Upper **body and arms**
This exercise places tension on the **muscles of the front and medial parts of the shoulder**, as well as the **triceps**. The **core** is important to ensure the torso and the pelvis remain stable, helping prevent injury to the spine or lower back. Remember to keep your lower back in contact with the pad to prevent any straining.

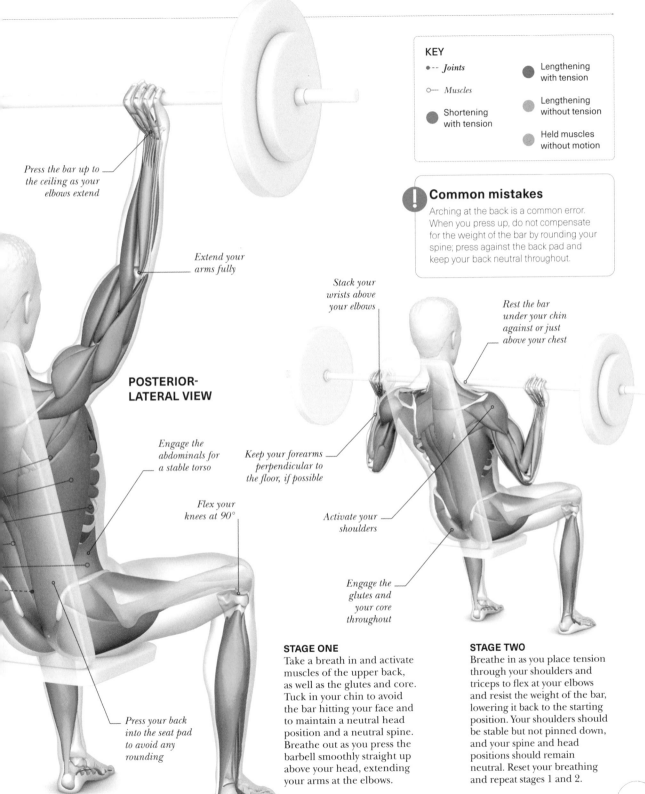

Press the bar up to
the ceiling as your
elbows extend

Extend your
arms fully

**POSTERIOR-
LATERAL VIEW**

Engage the
abdominals for
a stable torso

Flex your
knees at 90°

Press your back
into the seat pad
to avoid any
rounding

KEY

●-- *Joints*

○— *Muscles*

● Shortening
with tension

● Lengthening
with tension

● Lengthening
without tension

● Held muscles
without motion

❗ Common mistakes

Arching at the back is a common error.
When you press up, do not compensate
for the weight of the bar by rounding your
spine; press against the back pad and
keep your back neutral throughout.

Stack your
wrists above
your elbows

Rest the bar
under your chin
against or just
above your chest

Keep your forearms
perpendicular to
the floor, if possible

Activate your
shoulders

Engage the
glutes and
your core
throughout

STAGE ONE
Take a breath in and activate
muscles of the upper back,
as well as the glutes and core.
Tuck in your chin to avoid
the bar hitting your face and
to maintain a neutral head
position and a neutral spine.
Breathe out as you press the
barbell smoothly straight up
above your head, extending
your arms at the elbows.

STAGE TWO
Breathe in as you place tension
through your shoulders and
triceps to flex at your elbows
and resist the weight of the bar,
lowering it back to the starting
position. Your shoulders should
be stable but not pinned down,
and your spine and head
positions should remain
neutral. Reset your breathing
and repeat stages 1 and 2.

»VARIATIONS

Target the delts and triceps while performing an overhead press on various pieces of equipment; standing versions will work your core harder. All three exercises here reduce strain on the shoulders, as the shoulder blades can freely rotate.

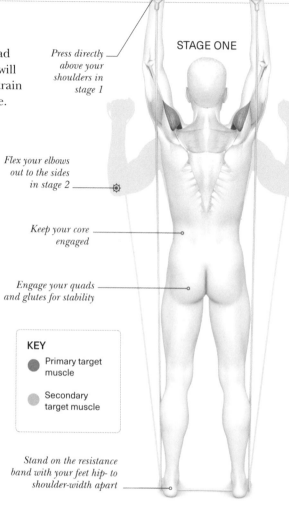

Press directly above your shoulders in stage 1

STAGE ONE

Flex your elbows out to the sides in stage 2

Keep your core engaged

Engage your quads and glutes for stability

Stand on the resistance band with your feet hip- to shoulder-width apart

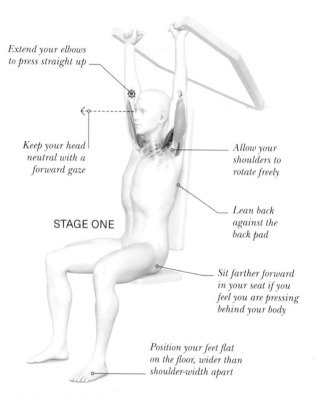

Extend your elbows to press straight up

Keep your head neutral with a forward gaze

Allow your shoulders to rotate freely

Lean back against the back pad

STAGE ONE

Sit farther forward in your seat if you feel you are pressing behind your body

Position your feet flat on the floor, wider than shoulder-width apart

KEY

● Primary target muscle

● Secondary target muscle

MACHINE SHOULDER PRESS

This machine-based variation is great for adding variety to your shoulder training; it works well as either a stand-alone exercise or part of a combination. The machine offers a safe and effective environment for vertical pressing.

PREPARATORY STAGE
Sit in position (adjust the seat height if needed) and grasp the attachment handles, with your elbows flexed out to the sides and hands in a pronated grip.

STAGE ONE
Inhale to engage your core, then exhale as you extend your elbows to drive your arms upward, focusing on driving your upper arms toward your ears.

STAGE TWO
Breathe in to lower your arms, maintaining control, to return the attachment to its starting point. Adjust your position if needed. Repeat stages 1 and 2.

BANDED SHOULDER PRESS

This resistance-band-based variation trains the vertical press while allowing for more individualization based on shoulder mobility and preference. Your arm path as you drive up will depend on your shoulder mobility.

PREPARATORY STAGE
Place the resistance band beneath your feet and grasp the handles in a pronated grip. Stand tall, with your arms flexed and hands at ear height.

STAGE ONE
Breathe in to engage your abs, then breathe out to drive your arms up, pressing your upper arms in toward your ears.

STAGE TWO
Breathe in as you lower your arms with control, flexing your elbows to lower your hands to their starting position. Repeat stages 1 and 2.

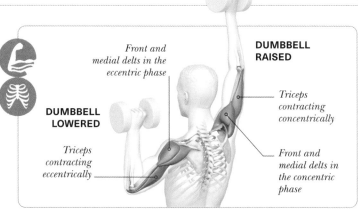

DUMBBELL RAISED

Front and medial delts in the eccentric phase

Triceps contracting concentrically

DUMBBELL LOWERED

Triceps contracting eccentrically

Front and medial delts in the concentric phase

Combining forces

Muscles work in synchronicity with one another. As you can see, in vertical pressing, the triceps works together with the front and medial deltoids to drive the dumbbells up and in.

DUMBBELL
SHOULDER PRESS

This is another useful variation for customization based on shoulder mobility—which will determine the angle of the dumbbells and your arm path—and preference. It also provides greater core engagement and reduces pressure on the shoulders.

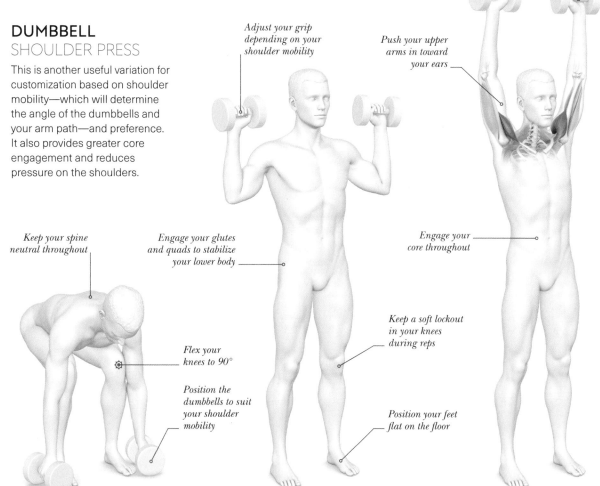

Adjust your grip depending on your shoulder mobility

Push your upper arms in toward your ears

Keep the dumbbells parallel to the floor

Keep your spine neutral throughout

Engage your glutes and quads to stabilize your lower body

Engage your core throughout

Flex your knees to 90°

Keep a soft lockout in your knees during reps

Position the dumbbells to suit your shoulder mobility

Position your feet flat on the floor

PICKING UP THE WEIGHTS SAFELY
Stand with your feet hip- to shoulder-width apart and flex at the knees and hips to reach the dumbbells, which should be on either side of your feet.

PREPARATORY STAGE/STAGE TWO
Straighten your knees and raise the dumbbells to above shoulder height, with your elbows flexed. Keep your core engaged as you prepare to press up.

STAGE ONE
Breathe in to brace your abdominals, then breathe out as you drive the dumbbells upward. Breathe in to return to stage 2. Repeat stages 1 and 2.

127

DUMBBELL LATERAL RAISE

Common mistakes

If you are moving your lower body and bending your knees, you could be lifting too heavy a weight. Avoid lowering the weights quickly without control: you miss out on the powerful eccentric contraction.

The middle part of the deltoid muscle is the focus of this exercise, along with the supraspinatus and the upper part of the trapezius, which stabilize your shoulder blades. The lateral raise is a safe and effective way to train your shoulders using minimal equipment.

THE BIG PICTURE

Raising and lowering dumbbells laterally—out to the sides of your body—isolates and trains the medial division of the deltoid. Keep the movement smooth and controlled at all times; don't throw the weights up and let them fall down.

Beginners can start with 4 sets of 8–10 reps; discover other variations on pp.130–131 and other targeted sets in the training programs (see pp.201–214).

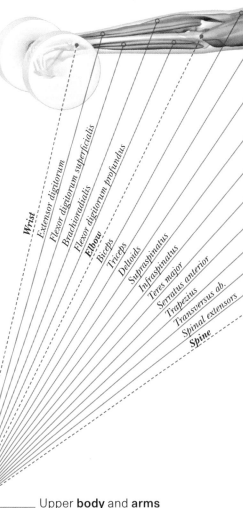

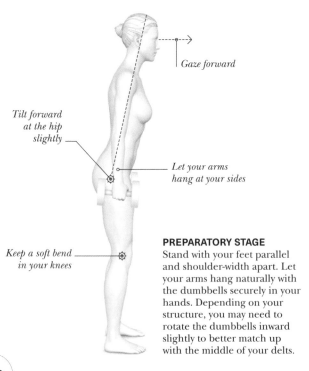

Gaze forward

Tilt forward at the hip slightly

Let your arms hang at your sides

Keep a soft bend in your knees

PREPARATORY STAGE
Stand with your feet parallel and shoulder-width apart. Let your arms hang naturally with the dumbbells securely in your hands. Depending on your structure, you may need to rotate the dumbbells inward slightly to better match up with the middle of your delts.

Upper **body** and **arms**
The **supraspinatus** helps the abduction of the shoulder (raising the arm out to the side) alongside the **front deltoid** and the **upper division of the trapezius**—both of which help stabilize the shoulder blade, as well as contributing to the move. Think of driving the dumbbells, or your fists, out as you drive your arms up during the concentric action (stage 1).

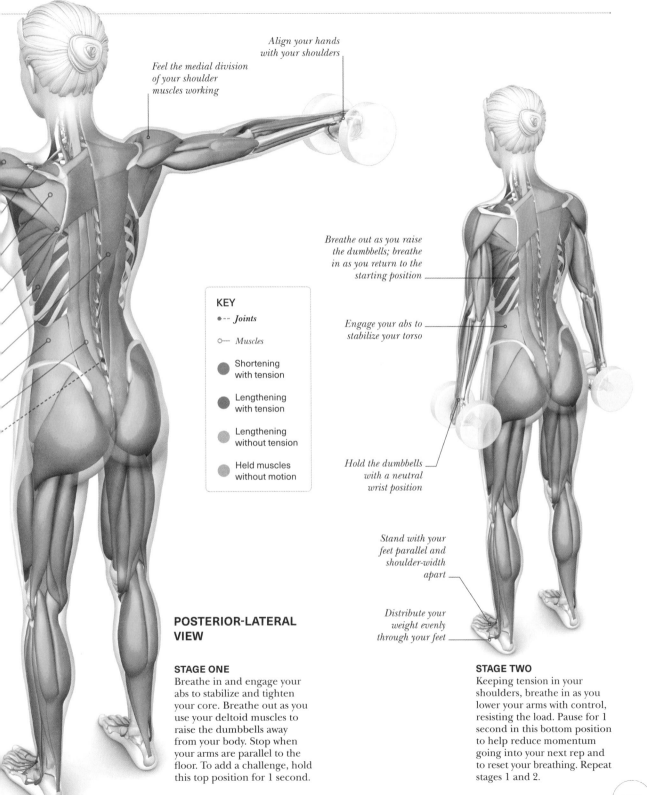

Feel the medial division of your shoulder muscles working

Align your hands with your shoulders

Breathe out as you raise the dumbbells; breathe in as you return to the starting position

Engage your abs to stabilize your torso

Hold the dumbbells with a neutral wrist position

Stand with your feet parallel and shoulder-width apart

Distribute your weight evenly through your feet

KEY

●-- *Joints*

○— *Muscles*

● Shortening with tension

● Lengthening with tension

● Lengthening without tension

● Held muscles without motion

POSTERIOR-LATERAL VIEW

STAGE ONE
Breathe in and engage your abs to stabilize and tighten your core. Breathe out as you use your deltoid muscles to raise the dumbbells away from your body. Stop when your arms are parallel to the floor. To add a challenge, hold this top position for 1 second.

STAGE TWO
Keeping tension in your shoulders, breathe in as you lower your arms with control, resisting the load. Pause for 1 second in this bottom position to help reduce momentum going into your next rep and to reset your breathing. Repeat stages 1 and 2.

» VARIATIONS

Using bands or cables helps vary the resistance demands of these exercises that target the delts. The tension in the bands will increase as you go through the rep, while the cable will provide fairly even resistance, increasing toward the top of the movement.

BANDED LATERAL RAISE

In this variation, the resistance provided by the bands increases as you approach the top position. Your stance width also affects the difficulty of the exercise—the wider apart your feet, the more resistance there is from the band.

*These exercises are a great way to **better isolate** tension on **the deltoids**.*

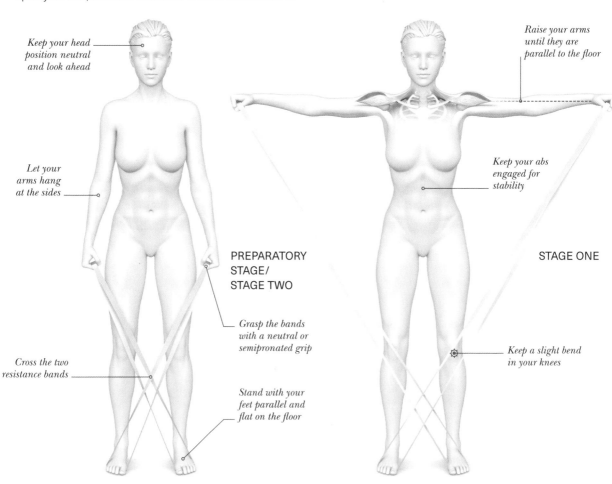

Keep your head position neutral and look ahead

Let your arms hang at the sides

Cross the two resistance bands

PREPARATORY STAGE/ STAGE TWO

Grasp the bands with a neutral or semipronated grip

Stand with your feet parallel and flat on the floor

Raise your arms until they are parallel to the floor

Keep your abs engaged for stability

STAGE ONE

Keep a slight bend in your knees

PREPARATORY STAGE
Place a band beneath each foot and hold them with opposite hands. Lean your torso forward slightly to line up the delt with the line of resistance.

STAGE ONE
Inhale to brace your core. Breathe out as you raise your arms to shoulder-height, keeping your elbows extended. For an added challenge, hold for 1–2 seconds.

STAGE TWO
Breathe in while lowering your arms, ensuring the movement is controlled. Return your arms to your sides, elbows extended. Repeat stages 1 and 2.

UNILATERAL CABLE
LATERAL RAISE

The cable pulley used in this variation provides continuous resistance during the raise. This exercise also allows you to work each side of the body in isolation, allowing for more variety within your shoulder training.

PREPARATORY STAGE
Stand tall, leaning your torso forward slightly to help line up the division of your delt with the line of resistance. Hold the cable with your arm at your side.

STAGE ONE
Inhale to engage your core, then breathe out as you raise your arm to shoulder level, keeping your elbow extended. For an added challenge, hold for 1–2 seconds.

STAGE TWO
Breathe in as you lower your arm, keeping tension in your shoulders to control the movement. Repeat stages 1 and 2.

KEY

● Primary target muscle ● Secondary target muscle

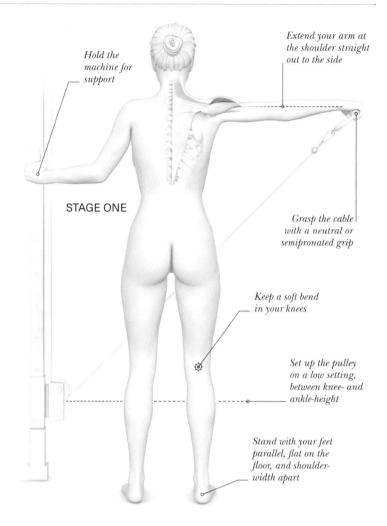

Hold the machine for support

Extend your arm at the shoulder straight out to the side

STAGE ONE

Grasp the cable with a neutral or semipronated grip

Keep a soft bend in your knees

Set up the pulley on a low setting, between knee- and ankle-height

Stand with your feet parallel, flat on the floor, and shoulder-width apart

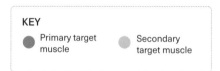

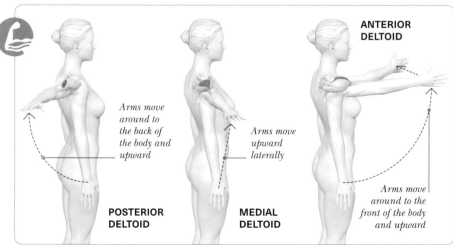

POSTERIOR DELTOID

Arms move around to the back of the body and upward

MEDIAL DELTOID

Arms move upward laterally

ANTERIOR DELTOID

Arms move around to the front of the body and upward

Targeting divisions of the **deltoids**

Each division of the delts—anterior (front), medial (side), and posterior (rear)—performs different muscle actions and has a different line of pull. Because of this, it is important that you choose exercises that best challenge the role of each specific division of the deltoid. Pressing and pulling exercises tend to have good overlap with the front and rear delt muscles. The medial delt needs to be isolated the most with exercises such as the lateral raise.

131

DUMBBELL
FRONT RAISE

The front (anterior) part of the deltoid muscle is the principle focus of this exercise. As with the lateral raise (see pp.128–129), you can also perform this movement using cables or resistance bands (see pp.134–135).

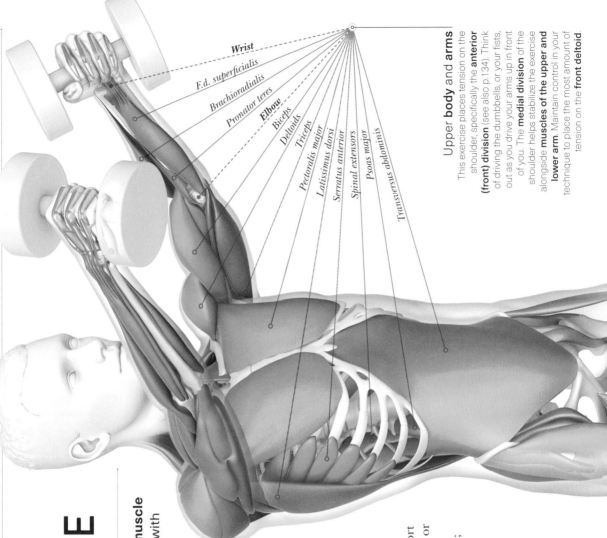

Wrist

F.d. superficialis

Brachioradialis

Pronator teres

Elbow

Biceps

Deltoids

Triceps

Pectoralis major

Latissimus dorsi

Serratus anterior

Spinal extensors

Psoas major

Transversus abdominis

Upper **body** and arms

This exercise places tension on the shoulder, specifically the **anterior (front) division** (see also p.134). Think of driving the dumbbells, or your fists, out as you drive your arms up in front of you. The **medial division** of the shoulder helps stabilize the exercise alongside **muscles of the upper and lower arm.** Maintain control in your technique to place the most amount of tension on the **front deltoid**

THE **BIG PICTURE**

Raising and lowering dumbbells directly in front of your body targets the front division of the deltoid. Ensure a smooth, controlled movement throughout; don't throw the weights up and let them fall down. Your arms will naturally move slightly inward as you raise to best align with the inward pull of the front delts. If you experience any shoulder discomfort during this exercise, try switching to the cable or the resistance-band variation (overleaf).

Beginners can start with 4 sets of 8–10 reps; discover other variations on pp.134–135 and other targeted sets in the training programs (see pp.201–214).

Common mistakes

Lift the weights too high and you will shift the muscle target to the upper trapezius; keep too low, and you won't get a powerful enough contraction on the front deltoid. Avoid leaning back, too.

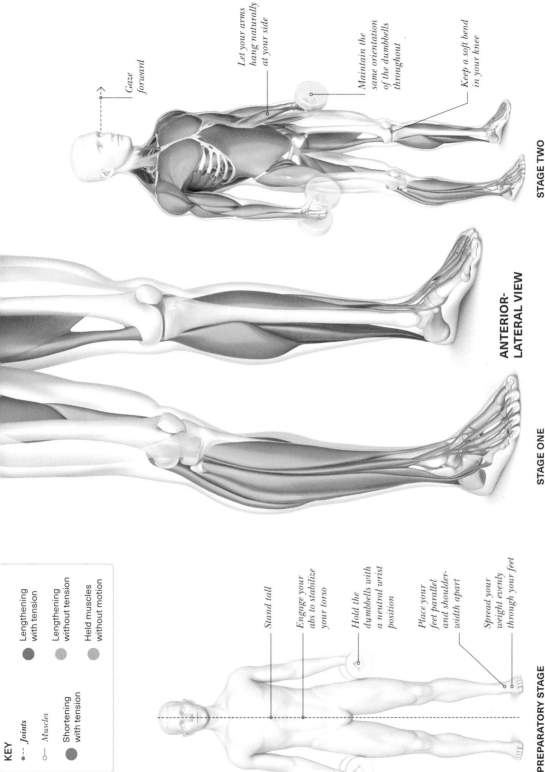

Gaze forward

Let your arms hang naturally at your side

Maintain the same orientation of the dumbbells throughout

Keep a soft bend in your knee

STAGE TWO

Keeping tension in your shoulders, breathe in to lower your arms with control, resisting the load. Pause for 1 second here to help reduce momentum going into your next rep and to reset your breathing. Repeat stages 1 and 2.

ANTERIOR-LATERAL VIEW

STAGE ONE

Breathe in and engage your core. Exhale and, using your front deltoids, flex at the shoulders to raise the dumbbells directly in front of you. Stop when your arms are at or just above parallel to the floor. To add a challenge, hold for 1 second.

KEY

- ●-- **Joints**
- ○— **Muscles**

- ● Shortening with tension
- ● Lengthening with tension
- ● Lengthening without tension
- ● Held muscles without motion

PREPARATORY STAGE

Stand with your feet parallel and shoulder-width apart. Let your arms hang naturally at the side of your body with the dumbbells securely in your hands. Ensure that your head position is neutral.

Stand tall

Engage your abs to stabilize your torso

Hold the dumbbells with a neutral wrist position

Place your feet parallel and shoulder-width apart

Spread your weight evenly through your feet

›› VARIATIONS

Variations of the front raise using a resistance band or cables are useful alternatives to the dumbbell version on pp.132–133, while a seated shoulder press that targets the anterior (front) deltoids is an effective way to practice the pressing motion. As with the dumbbell front raise, raise and lower your arms with smooth, controlled movements; the cable pulley variation will make this easier to achieve.

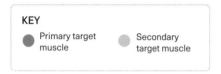

KEY

● Primary target muscle

● Secondary target muscle

Differences in **resistance**

Each piece of training equipment challenges muscles differently. Dumbbells are directly impacted by gravity and so place most tension on the muscle at the bottom of the range of motion. Resistance bands gain more tension as they are stretched, reaching peak challenge at the top of the range of movement. Cables provide the most even form of resistance.

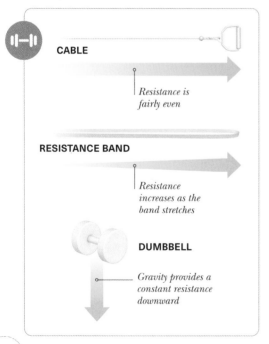

CABLE

Resistance is fairly even

RESISTANCE BAND

Resistance increases as the band stretches

DUMBBELL

Gravity provides a constant resistance downward

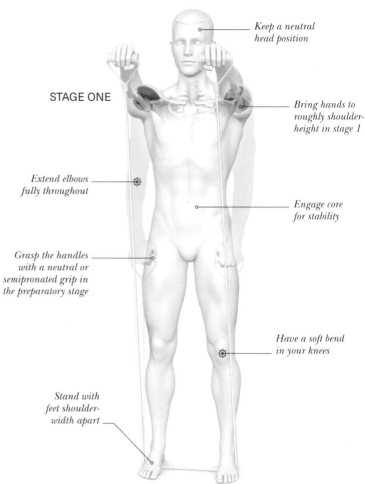

STAGE ONE

Keep a neutral head position

Bring hands to roughly shoulder-height in stage 1

Extend elbows fully throughout

Engage core for stability

Grasp the handles with a neutral or semipronated grip in the preparatory stage

Have a soft bend in your knees

Stand with feet shoulder-width apart

BANDED FRONT RAISE

If you experience any shoulder discomfort when practicing the dumbbell front raise, this variation using a resistance band could be a useful alternative. For an added challenge, hold the top position for 1–2 seconds.

PREPARATORY STAGE
Place the band beneath your feet and take hold of the handles. Stand tall with your arms hanging relaxed at your sides.

STAGE ONE
Breathe in to engage your abs, then breathe out as you raise your arms straight in front of your body while flexing at the shoulders.

STAGE TWO
Breathe in to lower your arms to the starting position, maintaining control throughout. Repeat stages 1 and 2.

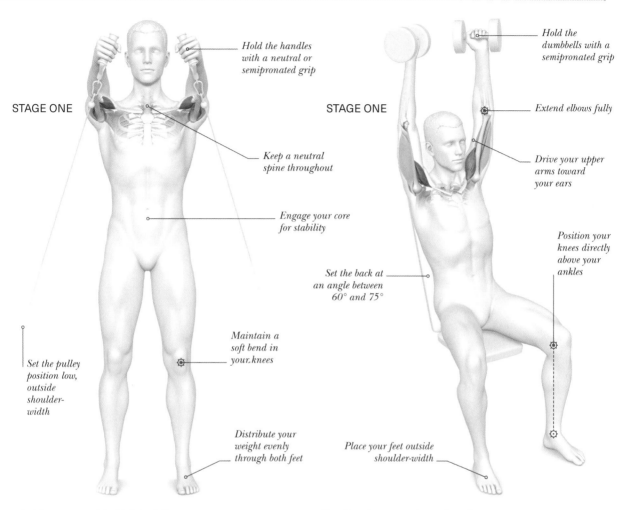

STAGE ONE

Hold the handles with a neutral or semipronated grip

Keep a neutral spine throughout

Engage your core for stability

Set the pulley position low, outside shoulder-width

Maintain a soft bend in your knees

Distribute your weight evenly through both feet

STAGE ONE

Hold the dumbbells with a semipronated grip

Extend elbows fully

Drive your upper arms toward your ears

Position your knees directly above your ankles

Set the back at an angle between 60° and 75°

Place your feet outside shoulder-width

CABLE FRONT RAISE

This variation allows for a more continuous, even resistance from the cable pulley, which should line up with the fibers of your front deltoids. To increase the challenge of the exercise, hold at the top position for 1–2 seconds.

PREPARATORY STAGE
Stand with feet shoulder-width apart; you can also stagger your feet for more stability. Grasp the cable handles and relax your shoulders so your arms hang.

STAGE ONE
Breathe in to brace your core, then breathe out as you raise your arms until your hands are at ear-height, keeping your elbows extended.

STAGE TWO
Breathe in to lower the cables to their starting position, controlling the movement and with straight arms throughout. Repeat stages 1 and 2.

FRONT DELTOID SHOULDER PRESS

This exercise trains the vertical pressing motion, working your triceps and elbow flexors, as well as your front delts. This variation is better aligned to the front delt than a standard seated shoulder press (see pp.124–125).

PREPARATORY STAGE
Position yourself on the bench. Take hold of the dumbbells with a semipronated grip and hold them just above shoulder-height with your elbows flexed.

STAGE ONE
Breathe in to engage your core. Breathe out as you extend your arms to raise the weights above your head, stacking your wrists above your elbows.

STAGE TWO
Breathe in to lower your arms with control, returning them to the starting position. Repeat stages 1 and 2.

DUMBBELL **REAR** DELTOID FLY

> **❗ Common mistakes**
>
> Lifting too much weight makes it harder to get the mechanics of the action right; a better bet for harder work is to boost your sets. The rear deltoid is a small muscle, so it takes focus to feel the work.

This fly exercise trains the rear deltoid muscle while also challenging the muscles of the upper back. As with the front raise (see pp.132–133), you can also perform this movement with cables or resistance bands (see pp.138–139).

THE **BIG PICTURE**

Raising and lowering dumbbells from low to high and from the front to the side of your body (in a flying movement) targets the rear division of your deltoid. Move the weights with control rather than throwing them out and letting them fall back. If you experience any shoulder discomfort, try switching to the cable or the resistance-band variation (overleaf).

Beginners can start with 4 sets of 8–10 reps; discover other variations on pp.138–139 and other targeted sets in the training programs (see pp.201–214).

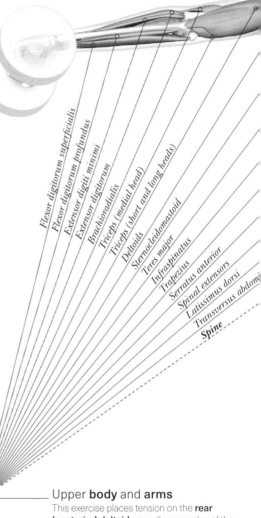

Flexor digitorum superficialis
Flexor digitorum profundus
Extensor digiti minimi
Extensor digitorum
Brachioradialis
Triceps (medial head)
Triceps (short and long heads)
Deltoids
Sternocleidomastoid
Teres major
Infraspinatus
Trapezius
Serratus anterior
Spinal extensors
Latissimus dorsi
Transversus abdomi—
Spine

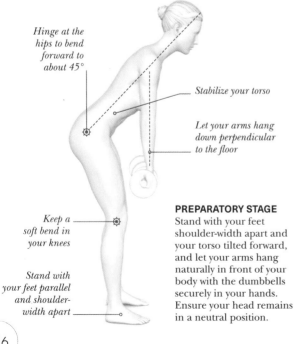

Hinge at the hips to bend forward to about 45°

Stabilize your torso

Let your arms hang down perpendicular to the floor

Keep a soft bend in your knees

Stand with your feet parallel and shoulder-width apart

PREPARATORY STAGE
Stand with your feet shoulder-width apart and your torso tilted forward, and let your arms hang naturally in front of your body with the dumbbells securely in your hands. Ensure your head remains in a neutral position.

Upper **body** and **arms**
This exercise places tension on the **rear (posterior) deltoid**, as well as muscles of the upper back, such as the **trapezius**. The **core muscles** alongside the **spinal extensors** will play an important role in stabilizing your torso and spine. This exercise is most challenging toward the top of the movement, so ensure you use a weight that you can control and perform with good technique.

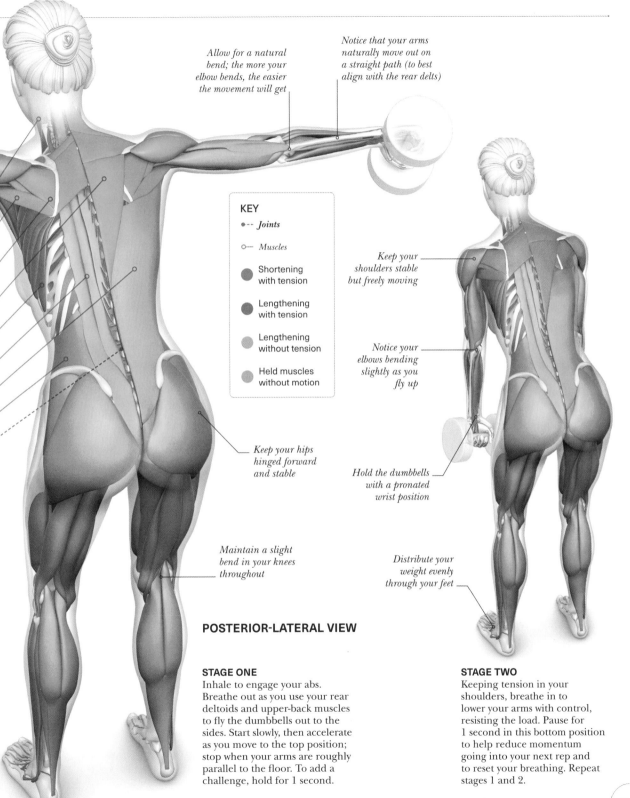

Allow for a natural bend; the more your elbow bends, the easier the movement will get

Notice that your arms naturally move out on a straight path (to best align with the rear delts)

KEY

●-- *Joints*

○— *Muscles*

● Shortening with tension

● Lengthening with tension

● Lengthening without tension

● Held muscles without motion

Keep your shoulders stable but freely moving

Notice your elbows bending slightly as you fly up

Keep your hips hinged forward and stable

Hold the dumbbells with a pronated wrist position

Maintain a slight bend in your knees throughout

Distribute your weight evenly through your feet

POSTERIOR-LATERAL VIEW

STAGE ONE
Inhale to engage your abs. Breathe out as you use your rear deltoids and upper-back muscles to fly the dumbbells out to the sides. Start slowly, then accelerate as you move to the top position; stop when your arms are roughly parallel to the floor. To add a challenge, hold for 1 second.

STAGE TWO
Keeping tension in your shoulders, breathe in to lower your arms with control, resisting the load. Pause for 1 second in this bottom position to help reduce momentum going into your next rep and to reset your breathing. Repeat stages 1 and 2.

» VARIATIONS

These variations can be useful alternatives if you experience shoulder discomfort from the dumbbell rear deltoid fly. The prone bench rear deltoid raise and banded deltoid row also offer a closer alignment between the line of resistance and the fibers of the rear delt. The arm path will be around 45° in both, with the trapezius providing support.

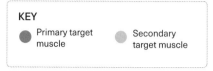

KEY

● Primary target muscle

○ Secondary target muscle

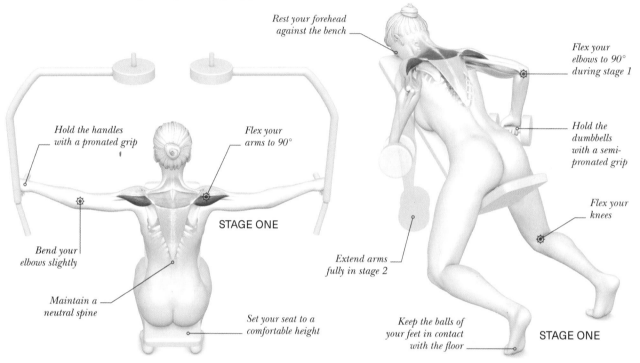

Rest your forehead against the bench

Flex your elbows to 90° during stage 1

Hold the handles with a pronated grip

Flex your arms to 90°

STAGE ONE

Hold the dumbbells with a semi-pronated grip

Bend your elbows slightly

Flex your knees

Maintain a neutral spine

Extend arms fully in stage 2

Set your seat to a comfortable height

Keep the balls of your feet in contact with the floor

STAGE ONE

MACHINE REAR DELTOID FLY

This is an effective machine-based variation. Don't use too heavy a weight or retract your scapulae during the fly, as it will bias your rhomboids and traps instead of your delts. For an added challenge, hold at the top position for 1–2 seconds.

PREPARATORY STAGE
Sit with your chest and abdomen pressed against the pad. Hold onto the handles of the attachment with your arms directly in front of your shoulders.

STAGE ONE
Breathe in to brace your core, then breathe out as you fly your arms out to the sides. Keep your elbows slightly flexed and your arms parallel to the floor.

STAGE TWO
Breathe in to return your arms to the starting position, ensuring the movement is smooth and controlled. Repeat stages 1 and 2.

PRONE BENCH REAR DELTOID RAISE

Being positioned prone on the bench creates an opposing force to push through as you row, increasing your stability and allowing you to lift greater loads. For an added challenge, hold at the top position for 1–2 seconds.

PREPARATORY STAGE
Lie on the bench and place your feet touching the floor, wider than shoulder-width apart. Hang your arms beneath your shoulders, weights in your hands.

STAGE ONE
Inhale to engage your abs. Breathe out as you row up, flexing your elbows and retracting your shoulder blades to bring the dumbbells to waist height.

STAGE TWO
Breathe in to lower the dumbbells back to the starting position, with control, so your elbows are fully extended again. Repeat stages 1 and 2.

66 99

*The **deltoid row and rear delt raise** train the rear delt through **a larger range of motion** than the rear delt fly.*

Targeting **the rear delts**

It is common to see the cable or banded deltoid row used for training the upper back. While still useful in this capacity, this exercise is even more effective at bringing focus to the rear delts; the arm path of the row and rear delt raise aligns better with the direct line of pull of the rear delt fibers than the rear delt fly.

BANDED DELTOID ROW

This resistance-band-based variation targets the rear deltoid and muscles of the upper back without the need for free weights. For more of a challenge, hold at the top position for 1–2 seconds.

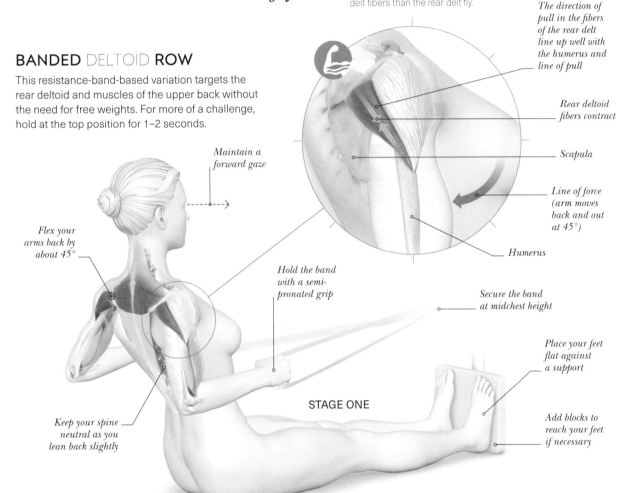

The direction of pull in the fibers of the rear delt line up well with the humerus and line of pull

Rear deltoid fibers contract

Scapula

Line of force (arm moves back and out at 45°)

Humerus

Maintain a forward gaze

Flex your arms back by about 45°

Hold the band with a semi-pronated grip

Secure the band at midchest height

Place your feet flat against a support

Keep your spine neutral as you lean back slightly

Add blocks to reach your feet if necessary

STAGE ONE

PREPARATORY STAGE

Sit with your legs flat on the ground, feet against a stable support or surface, and lean back slightly. Hold the ends of the band with your arms out in front of you.

STAGE ONE

Breathe in to engage your core, then breathe out as you row back, flexing your elbows out and back as you do so without moving your spine.

STAGE TWO

Breathe in to return your arms to the starting position, maintaining control throughout the movement. Repeat stages 1 and 2.

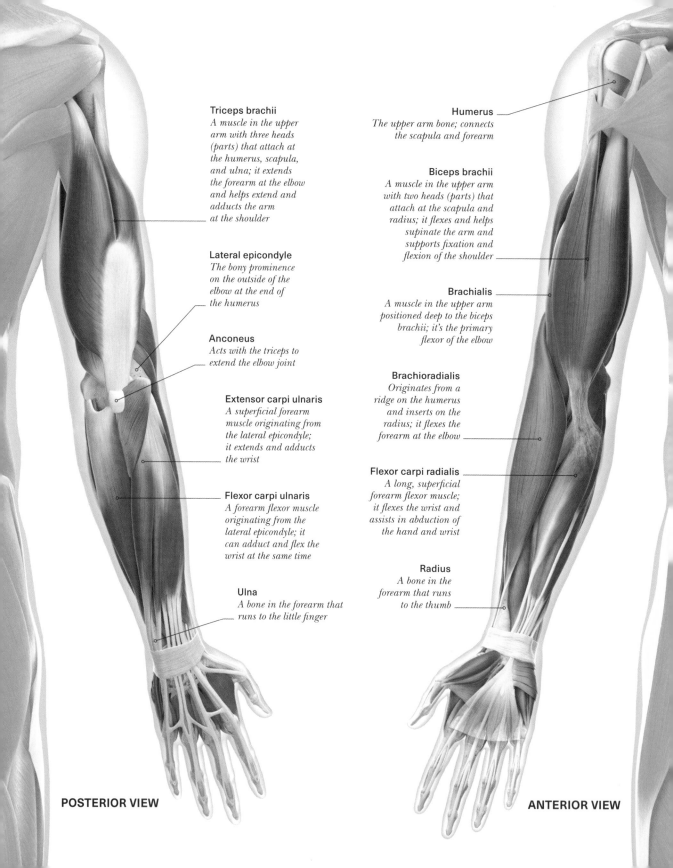

Triceps brachii
*A muscle in the upper
arm with three heads
(parts) that attach at
the humerus, scapula,
and ulna; it extends
the forearm at the elbow
and helps extend and
adducts the arm
at the shoulder*

Lateral epicondyle
*The bony prominence
on the outside of the
elbow at the end of
the humerus*

Anconeus
*Acts with the triceps to
extend the elbow joint*

Extensor carpi ulnaris
*A superficial forearm
muscle originating from
the lateral epicondyle;
it extends and adducts
the wrist*

Flexor carpi ulnaris
*A forearm flexor muscle
originating from the
lateral epicondyle; it
can adduct and flex the
wrist at the same time*

Ulna
*A bone in the forearm that
runs to the little finger*

Humerus
*The upper arm bone; connects
the scapula and forearm*

Biceps brachii
*A muscle in the upper arm
with two heads (parts) that
attach at the scapula and
radius; it flexes and helps
supinate the arm and
supports fixation and
flexion of the shoulder*

Brachialis
*A muscle in the upper arm
positioned deep to the biceps
brachii; it's the primary
flexor of the elbow*

Brachioradialis
*Originates from a
ridge on the humerus
and inserts on the
radius; it flexes the
forearm at the elbow*

Flexor carpi radialis
*A long, superficial
forearm flexor muscle;
it flexes the wrist and
assists in abduction of
the hand and wrist*

Radius
*A bone in the
forearm that runs
to the thumb*

POSTERIOR VIEW

ANTERIOR VIEW

ARM EXERCISES

The main muscles responsible for movement in the arms are: the biceps brachii, positioned at the front of the upper arms; the triceps brachii, at the back of the upper arms; and the muscles of the forearms, which help in gripping weights and allow for control of your grip position.

The biceps and triceps muscles both attach to the forearm, the humerus, and the scapula. The biceps allows for flexion and supination at the elbow and for fixation at the shoulder (helping maintain its position). It also stabilizes the elbow and shoulder during exercises where they aren't in motion. The triceps aids in extension at the elbow and has a large role in supporting the chest and shoulders in pressing movements.

Other elbow flexors, including the brachialis and brachioradialis, aid the biceps in coordinating elbow flexion throughout a large range of motion.

● When performing flexion and extension-based exercises, remember to keep your elbow and shoulder positions fixed. Doing so will increase the amount of tension being placed on the target muscle, as well as helping prevent stress to the elbow or shoulder joint.

*Equally as important as leg strength, **good arm strength facilitates higher loads** in other exercises.*

DUMBBELL
BICEPS CURL

This seated exercise safely trains the biceps while also challenging other elbow-flexor muscles. The use of dumbbells over a barbell allows for better adaptation to your individual mechanics; you can also use cables or resistance bands (see pp.144–145).

THE **BIG PICTURE**

The classic biceps curl involves lifting and lowering a weight while hinging at the elbow. Working seated on an incline bench or a chair with an adjustable back support rather than standing allows a greater range of movement and more muscle isolation. If you experience discomfort at the wrist, elbow, or shoulder, try switching to the cable or resistance-band variations (overleaf).

Beginners can start with 4 sets of 8–10 reps; discover other variations on pp.144–145 and other targeted sets in the training programs (see pp.201–214).

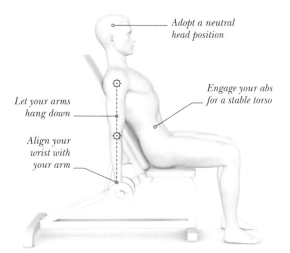

Adopt a neutral head position

Let your arms hang down

Engage your abs for a stable torso

Align your wrist with your arm

PREPARATORY STAGE
Sit on an incline bench with your back on the seat pad and your feet flat on the floor, shoulder-width apart. Grasp the dumbbells using an overhand standard grip and let your arms hang. Your wrist position will match the angle of your upper arm.

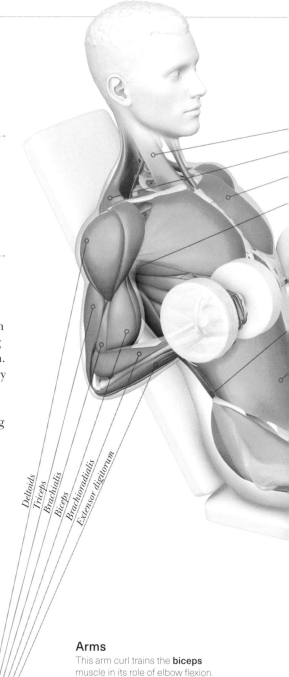

Deltoids
Triceps
Brachialis
Biceps
Brachioradialis
Extensor digitorum

Arms

This arm curl trains the **biceps** muscle in its role of elbow flexion. Maintain a consistent shoulder position and focus on flexing and extending at the elbow. Think of driving your forearm into your biceps at the top as you curl up. This exercise helps build muscle and strength in the biceps, which carries over into helping other strength training exercises.

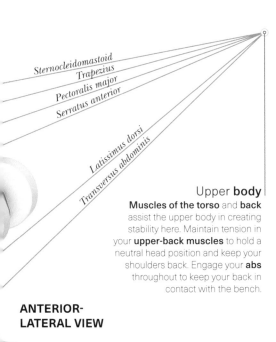

Sternocleidomastoid
Trapezius
Pectoralis major
Serratus anterior

Latissimus dorsi
Transversus abdominis

Upper **body**
Muscles of the torso and **back**
assist the upper body in creating
stability here. Maintain tension in
your **upper-back muscles** to hold a
neutral head position and keep your
shoulders back. Engage your **abs**
throughout to keep your back in
contact with the bench.

**ANTERIOR-
LATERAL VIEW**

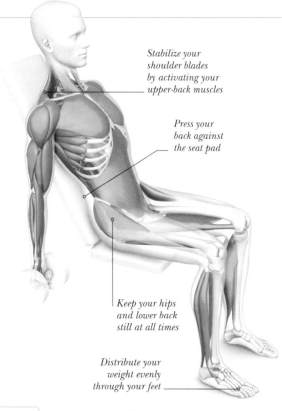

*Stabilize your
shoulder blades
by activating your
upper-back muscles*

*Press your
back against
the seat pad*

*Keep your hips
and lower back
still at all times*

*Distribute your
weight evenly
through your feet*

KEY

●-- *Joints*

○— *Muscles*

● Shortening
with tension

● Lengthening
with tension

● Lengthening
without tension

● Held muscles
without motion

STAGE TWO
While keeping tension in your core
and your elbows still, breathe in to
return the dumbbells to the starting
position, resisting the weight with
your biceps. Reset your breathing
and repeat stages 1 and 2.

STAGE ONE
Take a breath in and engage your
abs to help stabilize your core.
Breathe out as you flex at the
elbows and curl the dumbbells up
toward your shoulders, keeping
your shoulders still. Your feet
should remain flat on the floor
without any movement in your
hips or torso.

❗ Common mistakes
Instability in the shoulder, hips, or
lower back can create momentum
and allow other muscles, such as
the front deltoid, to help move the
dumbbells instead, so stabilizing
muscles is key. Rather than starting
with a heavy weight, go light until
you've mastered the mechanics
of the move, then increase
incrementally.

» VARIATIONS

The biceps curl is easily adaptable to different pieces of equipment. Make sure your upper-back muscles are engaged throughout to keep your shoulders from rounding, to protect them from injury, and to create more tension in the biceps brachii and elbow flexors during the movement.

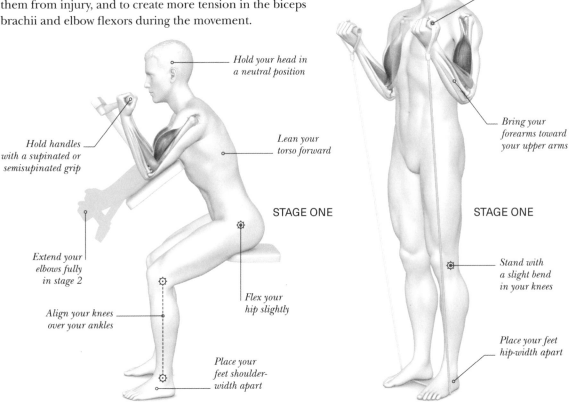

Hold your head in a neutral position

Hold handles with a supinated or semisupinated grip

Lean your torso forward

STAGE ONE

Extend your elbows fully in stage 2

Align your knees over your ankles

Flex your hip slightly

Place your feet shoulder-width apart

Hold the handles with a supinated grip

Bring your forearms toward your upper arms

STAGE ONE

Stand with a slight bend in your knees

Place your feet hip-width apart

MACHINE BICEPS CURL

Using a machine to perform this exercise allows for a fixed arm path, making this variation a useful way to practice the biceps curl movement. It works well either as a standalone exercise or within a combination.

PREPARATORY STAGE
Sit leaning forward slightly and place your arms over the pad to grasp the handles. (The angle of the pad and the angle of the legs will vary by machine.)

STAGE ONE
Breathe in to engage your core, then breathe out as you curl up, pressing your upper arms down onto the pad. Avoid rounding your shoulders.

STAGE TWO
Breathe in as you lower your arms, extending your elbows fully. Engage your core and keep your spine neutral throughout. Repeat stages 1 and 2.

BANDED BICEPS CURL

This variation, which makes use of a resistance band, is useful if you experience discomfort in your joints when using weights. The band can help you achieve a smooth, even movement throughout the exercise.

PREPARATORY STAGE
Place the band midway beneath your feet and stand tall with your arms down in front of your hips and your hands holding the handles.

STAGE ONE
Breathe in to engage your core, then breathe out as you curl up. Keep some tension in your upper back so your shoulders don't round forward.

STAGE TWO
Breathe in as you lower your arms with control, returning them to their starting position in front of your hips. Repeat stages 1 and 2.

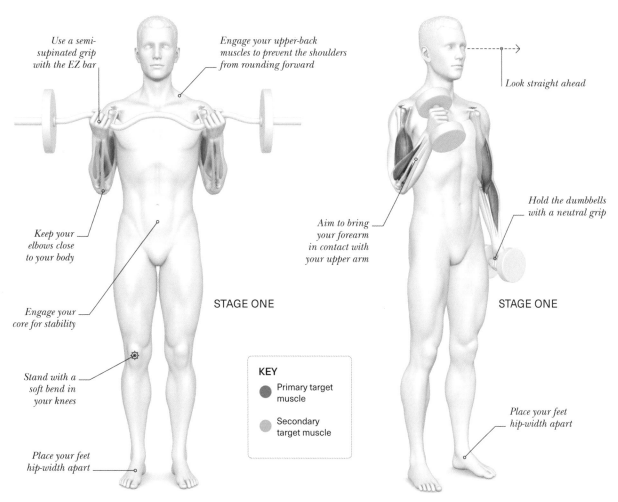

Use a semi-supinated grip with the EZ bar

Engage your upper-back muscles to prevent the shoulders from rounding forward

Look straight ahead

Keep your elbows close to your body

Aim to bring your forearm in contact with your upper arm

Hold the dumbbells with a neutral grip

Engage your core for stability

Stand with a soft bend in your knees

STAGE ONE

STAGE ONE

KEY

● Primary target muscle

● Secondary target muscle

Place your feet hip-width apart

Place your feet hip-width apart

EZ BAR BICEPS CURL

An EZ bar is a type of barbell with an undulating bar, designed to take pressure off your wrists during biceps curls; you could use a straight barbell. For an added challenge, hold at the top position for 1–2 seconds.

PREPARATORY STAGE
Hold the bar with your arms in front of you, elbows fully extended. Use a semisupinated grip with an EZ bar or a supinated grip with a straight barbell.

STAGE ONE
Breathe in, engage your core, then exhale as you curl up. Your elbows should remain in position, tight to the body.

STAGE TWO
Breathe in during the lowering phase, keeping your core engaged. Return your arms to the starting position. Repeat stages 1 and 2.

HAMMER CURL

This variation has the advantage of also challenging other elbow flexors, including the brachioradialis and brachialis. You can perform it bilaterally or unilaterally (as above). Hold for 1–2 seconds at the top position for more of a challenge.

PREPARATORY STAGE
Hold a dumbbell in each hand and stand tall with your arms hanging at your sides. Keep your wrist in a neutral position.

STAGE ONE
Breathe in, engage your core, then breathe out as you curl up (either with one arm or both), flexing your elbow to the top position.

STAGE TWO
Breathe in as you lower your arm(s). Repeat stages 1 and 2, being sure to work both arms equally if performing the exercise unilaterally.

DUMBBELL
TRICEPS EXTENSION

Keep your upper arm position fixed through the entire range of motion

Also known as "the skull crusher," this exercise builds muscle and strength in the triceps in the upper arm in a movement that can benefit other strength exercises. You can perform this lying either on a bench or on the floor—all you need is a pair of dumbbells.

THE **BIG PICTURE**

Your core and legs stay still and strong while you bend your elbows to lower and lift the weights above your head. Because the weights are above you, a secure overhand standard grip is best. If you experience any joint discomfort, try switching to a cable-based or resistance-band variation (see overleaf).

Beginners can start with 4 sets of 8–10 reps; discover other variations on pp.148–149 and other targeted sets in the training programs (see pp.201–214).

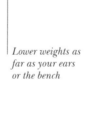

Lower weights as far as your ears or the bench

Extensor digitorum superficialis
Flexor digitorum superficialis
Brachioradialis
Triceps
Biceps
Pectoralis major
Spine
Transversus abdominis

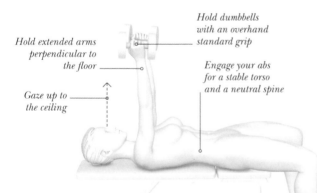

Hold extended arms perpendicular to the floor

Hold dumbbells with an overhand standard grip

Engage your abs for a stable torso and a neutral spine

Gaze up to the ceiling

PREPARATORY STAGE
Lie flat on the bench with your buttocks and head fully on it and place your feet flat on the floor, wider than hip-width apart; if working on the floor, bend your knees to improve stability. Hold the dumbbells above your knees, then lift them directly above your shoulders.

Spread weight evenly through your feet

Upper **body** and **arms**
This exercise places tension in the **triceps**. The **muscles of the shoulder** and **torso** help provide stability at the shoulder joint and the entire upper body, while those of the **forearm** aid in holding the weight in the hand. Think about flexing and extending at the elbow while maintaining a consistent shoulder position.

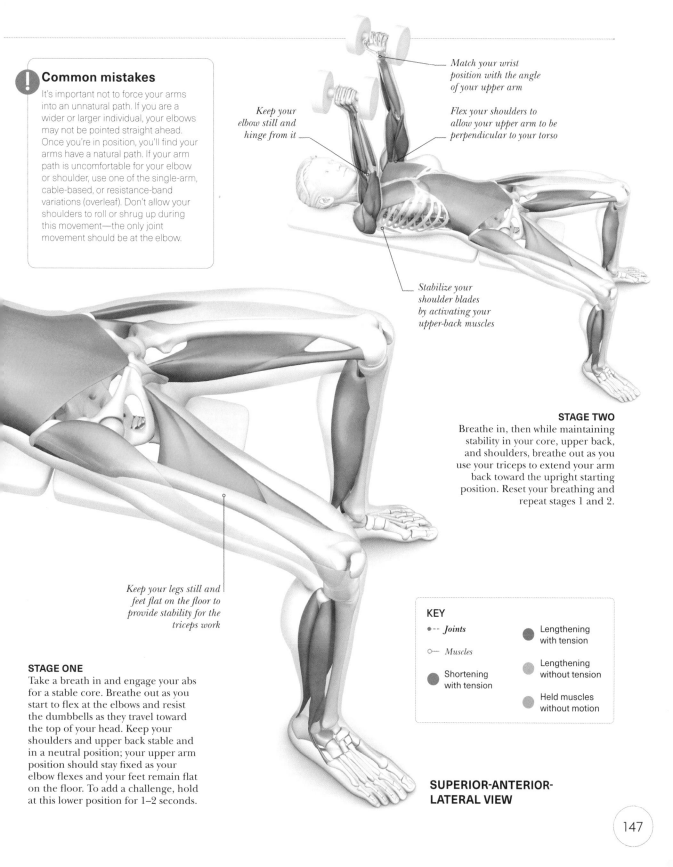

Match your wrist position with the angle of your upper arm

Keep your elbow still and hinge from it

Flex your shoulders to allow your upper arm to be perpendicular to your torso

Stabilize your shoulder blades by activating your upper-back muscles

STAGE TWO

Breathe in, then while maintaining stability in your core, upper back, and shoulders, breathe out as you use your triceps to extend your arm back toward the upright starting position. Reset your breathing and repeat stages 1 and 2.

Keep your legs still and feet flat on the floor to provide stability for the triceps work

KEY

- •-- *Joints*
- ○— *Muscles*
- ● Shortening with tension
- ● Lengthening with tension
- ● Lengthening without tension
- ● Held muscles without motion

STAGE ONE

Take a breath in and engage your abs for a stable core. Breathe out as you start to flex at the elbows and resist the dumbbells as they travel toward the top of your head. Keep your shoulders and upper back stable and in a neutral position; your upper arm position should stay fixed as your elbow flexes and your feet remain flat on the floor. To add a challenge, hold at this lower position for 1–2 seconds.

SUPERIOR-ANTERIOR-LATERAL VIEW

147

» VARIATIONS

These variations can be useful if you are new to the triceps extension. While ostensibly quite different, these exercises all target the triceps brachii. When working unilaterally, remember to perform the same number of reps on each arm.

KEY

● Primary target muscle

● Secondary target muscle

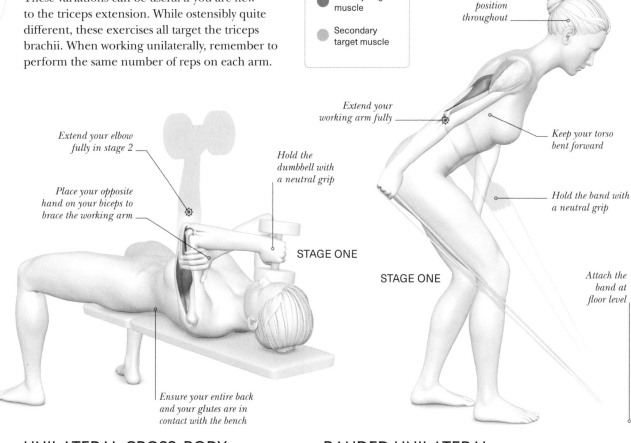

Extend your elbow fully in stage 2

Place your opposite hand on your biceps to brace the working arm

Hold the dumbbell with a neutral grip

STAGE ONE

Ensure your entire back and your glutes are in contact with the bench

Maintain a neutral head position throughout

Extend your working arm fully

Keep your torso bent forward

Hold the band with a neutral grip

STAGE ONE

Attach the band at floor level

UNILATERAL CROSS-BODY
TRICEPS EXTENSION

If you experience elbow discomfort, you may find it easier to perform a lying triceps extension unilaterally. This version also works well for those with wider frames.

PREPARATORY STAGE
Lie on the bench with your legs abducted, feet flat on the floor. Hold a dumbbell in your working arm, elbow extended, and support with your other arm.

STAGE ONE
Breathe in to brace your core. Then, while breathing out, flex your extended arm at the elbow to bring the dumbbell to your opposite cheek.

STAGE TWO
Breathe in to return your arm to the starting position. Repeat stages 1 and 2, then perform the exercise on the other side of your body.

BANDED UNILATERAL
TRICEPS EXTENSION

This exercise, performed on one side at a time, is often referred to as a "triceps kickback." Fix your shoulder into position first, then focus on extending your arm backward.

PREPARATORY STAGE
Stand with your feet hip-width apart in a staggered stance, knees soft, and bend forward at the hips to around 135°. Hold the band with your elbow flexed.

STAGE ONE
Breathe in and engage your core. Breathe out as you extend your arm fully. Keep some tension in your upper back to avoid rounding your shoulders.

STAGE TWO
Breathe in to return your arm to its starting position, with control. Repeat stages 1 and 2, then switch sides (remembering to reverse your stance, too).

TRICEPS **PUSH-UP**

This push-up variation with a modified hand position and arm path trains the chest, triceps, and shoulders. It is a useful bodyweight alternative to the lying triceps extension, challenging the body in a similar way.

PREPARATORY STAGE
Position yourself prone with your arms out in front of you, hands at or just inside shoulder-width. Flex your elbows slightly.

STAGE ONE
Engage your core, then breathe in as you lower your body toward the ground, flexing your elbows and squeezing your arms against your ribcage.

STAGE TWO
Breathe out as you drive up, extending your elbows almost fully to come back to the starting position. Repeat stages 1 and 2.

*Improving your knowledge of **triceps anatomy** helps you better understand whether an exercise works **one, two, or three triceps heads**.*

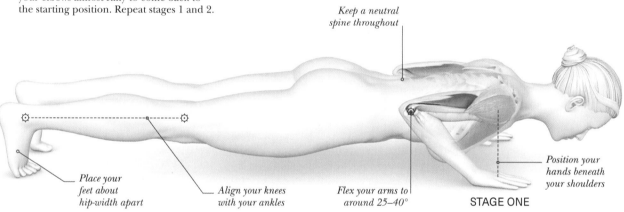

Keep a neutral spine throughout

Place your feet about hip-width apart

Align your knees with your ankles

Flex your arms to around 25–40°

STAGE ONE

Position your hands beneath your shoulders

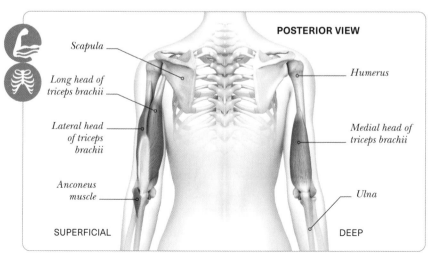

POSTERIOR VIEW

Scapula

Long head of triceps brachii

Lateral head of triceps brachii

Anconeus muscle

Humerus

Medial head of triceps brachii

Ulna

SUPERFICIAL

DEEP

A look at **the triceps**

The triceps brachii is unique in having three heads or divisions: the lateral and medial heads attach at the humerus and in the elbow, while the long head attaches at the scapula or shoulder blade. Some movements train all three heads at the same time, while others train just one or two. If you alter your shoulder position, you can potentially put more load on the long head without affecting the other two. Knowing more about the anatomy and where each head attaches and how it lines up with the resistance helps you make sense of why one exercise is better than another. The best example of an exercise that works all three triceps heads is the cross-cable pressdown (see p.153).

ROPE TRICEPS PUSHDOWN

This pushdown exercise targets the triceps, the large muscle at the back of the upper arm. Here, a cable machine with a rope attachment is used rather than a barbell or fixed attachment; this makes it easier to adapt the move to your individual mechanics and mobility limitations.

Upper **body** and **arms**
While the **triceps** are the focus of this exercise, **muscles of the shoulder, upper back,** and **torso** also help stabilize the shoulder joint, as well as the entire upper body. The rope attachment helps create the desired arm path without the restriction of a straight or fixed bar. Think about flexing and extending at the elbow while maintaining a consistent shoulder position. A bigger and stronger triceps can benefit other strength training exercises.

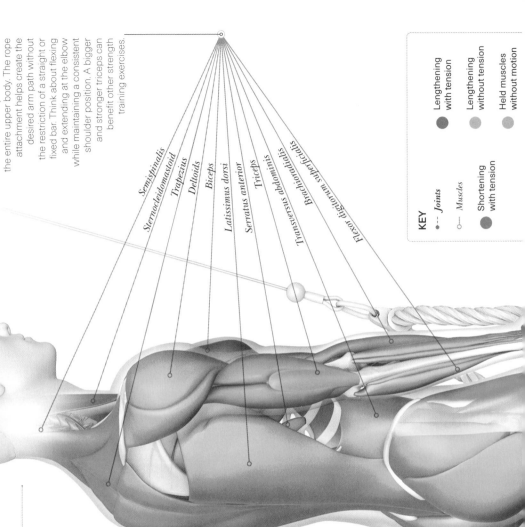

Semispinalis

Sternocleidomastoid

Trapezius

Deltoids

Biceps

Latissimus dorsi

Serratus anterior

Triceps

Transversus abdominis

Brachioradialis

Flexor digitorum superficialis

KEY

•--- *Joints*

o— *Muscles*

Shortening with tension

Lengthening with tension

Lengthening without tension

Held muscles without motion

THE BIG PICTURE

Holding the right posture and moving your arms only from the elbows are both essential for the success of this vertical pushing-down movement. Set the weights and fix a rope attachment (with two parts) to the cable pulley machine; adjust the cable pulley to its top position. If you experience any joint discomfort, try switching to other variations, including an alternative cable version and one using resistance bands (overleaf).

Beginners can start with 4 sets of 8–10 reps; discover other variations on pp.152–153 and other targeted sets in the training programs (see pp.201–214).

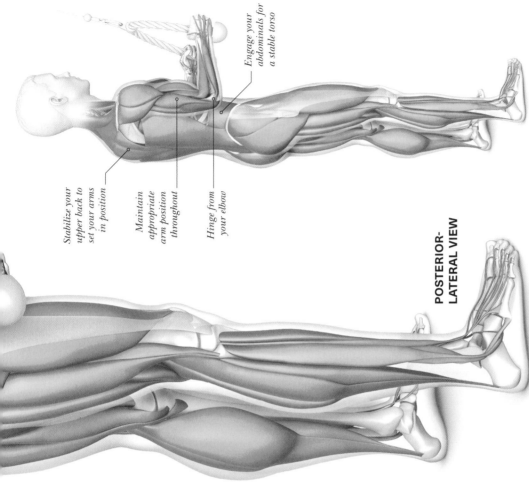

Engage your abdominals for a stable torso

Stabilize your upper back to set your arms in position

Maintain appropriate arm position throughout

Hinge from your elbow

POSTERIOR-LATERAL VIEW

STAGE TWO

Maintaining stability in your core, upper back, and shoulders, breathe in and resist the rope with your triceps as you return it to its starting position. Reset your breathing and repeat stages 1 and 2.

STAGE ONE

Inhale and engage your abs. Breathe out as you extend your elbows, using your triceps to push the rope down. Do not round your shoulders at the bottom of the range. To add a challenge, hold for 1–2 seconds in this position.

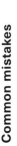

Common mistakes

Leaning your body forward past the cable's vertical hanging line is bad form and doesn't isolate the triceps for the work. Stand tall, not too close to the cable; the rope attachment should simply move up and down in the same vertical line without any forward or backward motion.

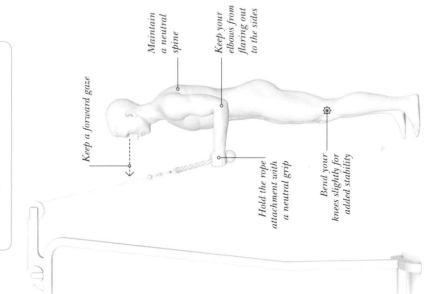

Keep a forward gaze

Maintain a neutral spine

Keep your elbows from flaring out to the sides

Hold the rope attachment with a neutral grip

Bend your knees slightly for added stability

PREPARATORY STAGE

Set up the machine and grasp the bottom of the rope attachment. Take 1–2 steps back and stand tall, feet shoulder-width apart. Place tension in the muscles of your upper back for stability and allow your elbows to flex to around 65–75°.

» VARIATIONS

It is important to position your shoulders correctly and avoid rounding them during each of these movements. These variations target the triceps brachii but are a great alternative if you experience any discomfort performing the rope pulldown.

BANDED TRICEPS EXTENSION

This resistance-band-based variation is useful for when you don't have access to machines. Bringing the bands over your shoulders also ensures the lines of resistance are properly lined up with your arm paths.

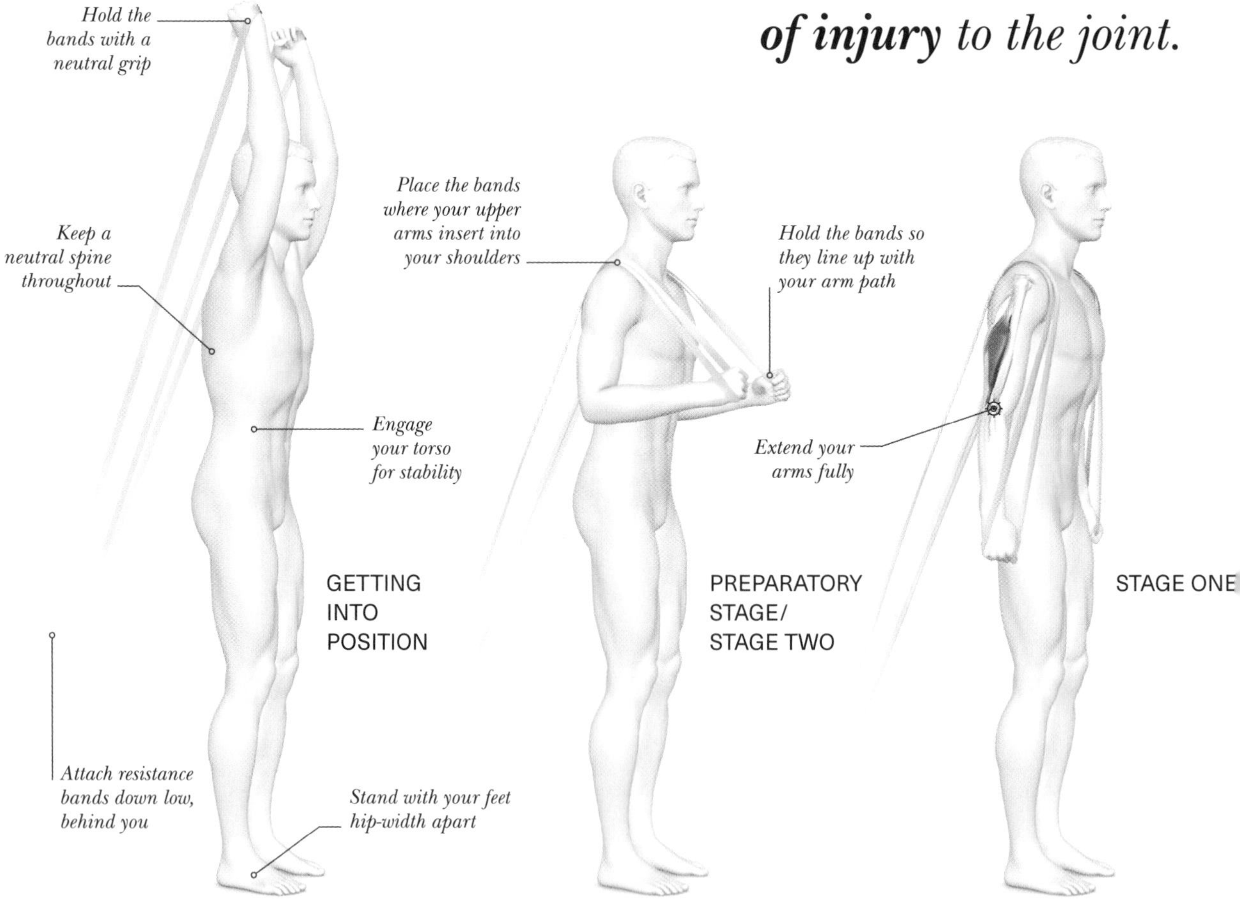

*Lining up **the path of resistance** (cable or band) with **the arm path** used in the exercise can **limit risk of injury** to the joint.*

Hold the bands with a neutral grip

Keep a neutral spine throughout

Place the bands where your upper arms insert into your shoulders

Hold the bands so they line up with your arm path

Engage your torso for stability

Extend your arms fully

GETTING INTO POSITION

PREPARATORY STAGE/ STAGE TWO

STAGE ONE

Attach resistance bands down low, behind you

Stand with your feet hip-width apart

GETTING INTO POSITION
Secure the resistance bands at a low level and stand facing away from them with a soft bend in your knees. Hold a band in each hand. Raise your arms high.

PREPARATORY STAGE
Extend your arms out to bring the resistance bands over your shoulders. Hold the ends of the bands in front of you, with your elbows flexed.

STAGE ONE
Inhale to engage your abs, then breathe out as you extend your elbows fully, shoulders pulled back, and upper arms remaining in line with your torso.

STAGE TWO
Breathe in to return your arms to the starting position, flexing at the elbows and moving the bands with control. Repeat stages 1 and 2.

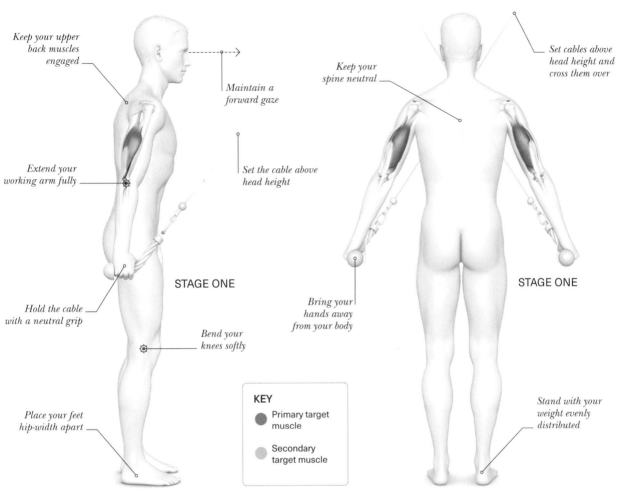

Keep your upper
back muscles
engaged

Maintain a
forward gaze

Extend your
working arm fully

Set the cable above
head height

Hold the cable
with a neutral grip

Bend your
knees softly

STAGE ONE

Place your feet
hip-width apart

Keep your
spine neutral

Set cables above
head height and
cross them over

Bring your
hands away
from your body

STAGE ONE

Stand with your
weight evenly
distributed

KEY

● Primary target
muscle

● Secondary
target muscle

CABLE UNILATERAL
TRICEPS **PRESSDOWN**

This variation requires only a single cable to train one
arm at a time. Focus on achieving the correct shoulder
position before extending your arm back.

PREPARATORY STAGE
Stand tall with your hips flexed slightly to bring your
upper body closer to the line of resistance. Hold the
cable with a neutral grip, arm flexed.

STAGE ONE
Breathe in to engage your core, then breathe out as
you extend your working arm fully. Your arm path
should follow the line of resistance of the cable.

STAGE TWO
Breathe out as you return your arm to the starting
position, keeping the movement controlled. Repeat
stages 1 and 2, then work your other side.

CROSS-CABLE
TRICEPS **PRESSDOWN**

Another option is to use two cables to train the triceps
on both sides simultaneously. Place tension in your upper
back to help prevent your shoulders from rounding.

PREPARATORY STAGE
Stand tall with your feet hip-width apart and hips
flexed slightly. Hold a cable in each hand with a
neutral grip and your elbows flexed.

STAGE ONE
Breathe in to brace your core. Breathe out to
extend your arms down, following the lines of
resistance formed by the cables.

STAGE TWO
Breathe out to flex your elbows, bringing your
arms back up to the starting position in a smooth,
even movement. Repeat stages 1 and 2.

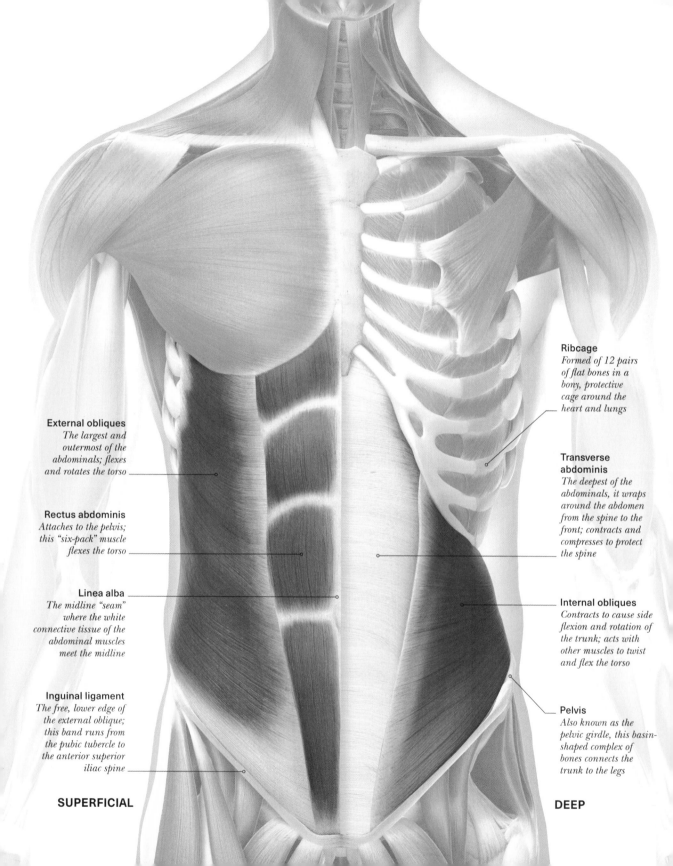

Ribcage
Formed of 12 pairs of flat bones in a bony, protective cage around the heart and lungs

External obliques
The largest and outermost of the abdominals; flexes and rotates the torso

Transverse abdominis
The deepest of the abdominals, it wraps around the abdomen from the spine to the front; contracts and compresses to protect the spine

Rectus abdominis
Attaches to the pelvis; this "six-pack" muscle flexes the torso

Linea alba
The midline "seam" where the white connective tissue of the abdominal muscles meet the midline

Internal obliques
Contracts to cause side flexion and rotation of the trunk; acts with other muscles to twist and flex the torso

Inguinal ligament
The free, lower edge of the external oblique; this band runs from the pubic tubercle to the anterior superior iliac spine

Pelvis
Also known as the pelvic girdle, this basin-shaped complex of bones connects the trunk to the legs

SUPERFICIAL

DEEP

ABDOMINAL EXERCISES

The main muscles responsible for movement in the abdominals are: the rectus abdominis (the "six pack" muscle); the external obliques and the internal obliques, both positioned at the sides of the torso; and the transverse abdominis, the deepest abdominal muscle.

The rectus abdominis (or RA) attaches to the sternum and the connective tissue of the ribs and pelvis. Both the external and the internal obliques attach to the ribs, pelvis, and linea alba—an area of connective tissue at the midline of the abdominal wall. The transverse abdominis (or TVA) attaches to the pelvis and the ribs, linea alba, and connective tissue of the lower back.

- **When flexing the trunk forward**, the RA creates this movement but also contributes structural support to other abdominals. It can be trained using bodyweight or load with exercises such as crunches or hanging knee raises.

- **When flexing the trunk to the side** (lateral flexion), your body uses the obliques, which also help in forward flexion and rotation. The obliques also act as antirotation and antiextension contributors for the trunk—keeping the spine safe and protected while adding stability to the torso.

The TVA functions as your internal "lifting belt," adding compression or cinching forces to stabilize the torso and protect the spine.

All of these muscles also support respiration and provide general strength and structure to the torso.

> *Strong abs lead to **a healthy core, a protected spine,** and **reduced lower-back injury**.*

FRONT PLANK
WITH ROTATION

Known by many as the "mountain climber," this exercise works multiple muscles—of the legs, core, and arms—at the same time while also giving you a cardio workout if you up the tempo. The twisting movement strengthens the muscles of the core, especially the oblique muscles.

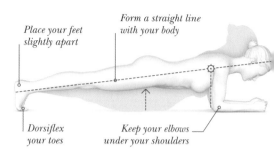

Place your feet slightly apart

Form a straight line with your body

Dorsiflex your toes

Keep your elbows under your shoulders

PREPARATORY STAGE

Lie on the floor in a prone position with your upper body supported by your forearms. To get into the starting position, raise your hips up to form a straight line from your head down to the ankle.

THE **BIG PICTURE**

For this exercise, you'll need to raise your hips into the plank position and hold your body in this straight line throughout as you twist to each side. By keeping tension through your arms, upper back, torso, and lower body, you help stabilize your lower back and protect it from injury.

Beginners can start with 4 sets of 8–10 reps; discover other targeted sets in the training programs (see pp.201–214). If you find this exercise too difficult, try holding the starting plank position without rotating.

KEY

- --- *Joints*
- o--- *Muscles*
- ● Shortening under tension
- ● Lengthening under tension
- ● Lengthening without tension (stretching)
- ● Held muscles without motion

Leg

The **quads** of the supporting leg remain engaged to help stabilize the body so that you can initiate the knee drive from the hips. Engaging the **hip flexors** powers the knee across the body to the opposite side.

Gastrocnemius

Knee

Vastus lateralis

Rectus femoris

Vastus medialis

Tensor fascia latae

! Common mistakes

Don't let your neck jut forward; keep your eyes fixed on the floor and a neutral head position. Be sure to keep your shoulders over your elbows.

ANTERIOR-LATERAL VIEW

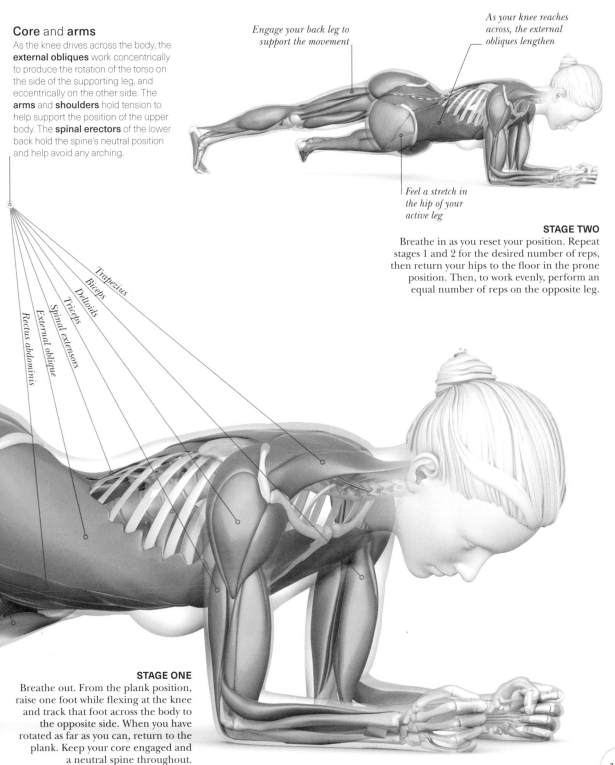

Core and arms

As the knee drives across the body, the **external obliques** work concentrically to produce the rotation of the torso on the side of the supporting leg, and eccentrically on the other side. The **arms** and **shoulders** hold tension to help support the position of the upper body. The **spinal erectors** of the lower back hold the spine's neutral position and help avoid any arching.

Engage your back leg to support the movement

As your knee reaches across, the external obliques lengthen

Feel a stretch in the hip of your active leg

Trapezius

Biceps

Deltoids

Triceps

Spinal extensors

External oblique

Rectus abdominis

STAGE TWO

Breathe in as you reset your position. Repeat stages 1 and 2 for the desired number of reps, then return your hips to the floor in the prone position. Then, to work evenly, perform an equal number of reps on the opposite leg.

STAGE ONE

Breathe out. From the plank position, raise one foot while flexing at the knee and track that foot across the body to the opposite side. When you have rotated as far as you can, return to the plank. Keep your core engaged and a neutral spine throughout.

SIDE PLANK
WITH ROTATION

⚠ Common mistakes

Incorrect body set-up (alignment is crucial) and sagging hips won't help you achieve tension from head to toe. Work to keep your hips off the floor.

This easy-to-do-at-home exercise strengthens the core and tones the waistline by working the muscles at the sides of the torso: the obliques. Be sure to breathe slowly throughout and to exercise one side, then the other.

Hips

The **hip flexors**, **hip adductors**, and **hip abductors** work to maintain the position of your lower body and help keep a neutral spine throughout the range of this movement.

THE **BIG PICTURE**

As with the front plank (see pp.156–157), your body is held in a straight line with abdominal muscles engaged throughout, but this time you're positioned on alternating sides. Keep your knees and chest facing forward throughout; rotate only from your hips.

Beginners can start with 4 sets of 8–10 reps; discover other targeted sets in the training programs (see pp.201–214).

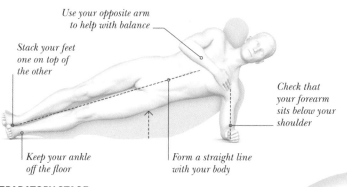

Use your opposite arm to help with balance

Stack your feet one on top of the other

Check that your forearm sits below your shoulder

Keep your ankle off the floor

Form a straight line with your body

PREPARATORY STAGE
Lie on one side with your feet stacked together and your upper body supported on your lower forearm. Fold your other arm across your chest. Lift your hips off the floor, holding a straight line from your head to your ankle.

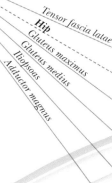

Tensor fascia latae
Hip
Gluteus maximus
Gluteus medius
Iliopsoas
Adductor magnus

ANTERIOR VIEW

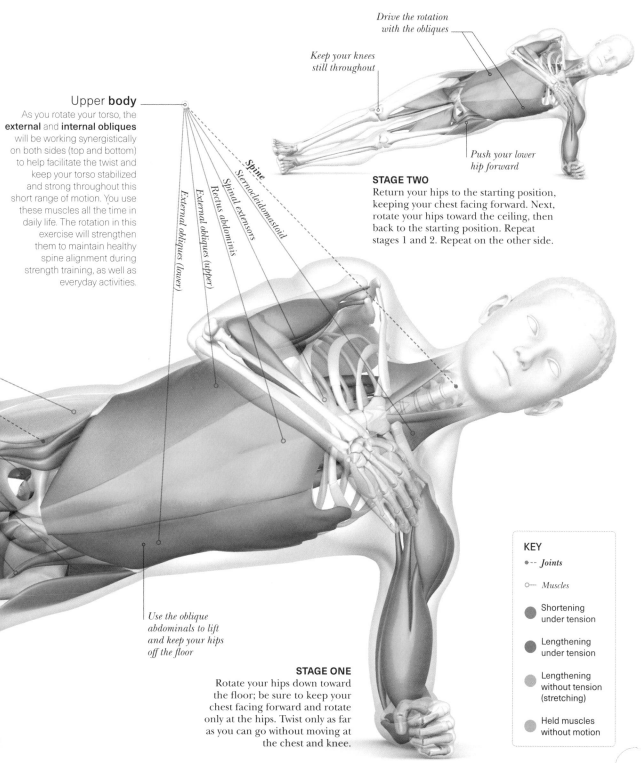

Upper **body**

As you rotate your torso, the **external** and **internal obliques** will be working synergistically on both sides (top and bottom) to help facilitate the twist and keep your torso stabilized and strong throughout this short range of motion. You use these muscles all the time in daily life. The rotation in this exercise will strengthen them to maintain healthy spine alignment during strength training, as well as everyday activities.

Drive the rotation with the obliques

Keep your knees still throughout

Push your lower hip forward

STAGE TWO
Return your hips to the starting position, keeping your chest facing forward. Next, rotate your hips toward the ceiling, then back to the starting position. Repeat stages 1 and 2. Repeat on the other side.

Spine

Sternocleidomastoid

Spinal extensors

Rectus abdominis

External obliques (upper)

External obliques (lower)

Use the oblique abdominals to lift and keep your hips off the floor

STAGE ONE
Rotate your hips down toward the floor; be sure to keep your chest facing forward and rotate only at the hips. Twist only as far as you can go without moving at the chest and knee.

KEY

●-- *Joints*

○— *Muscles*

● Shortening under tension

● Lengthening under tension

● Lengthening without tension (stretching)

● Held muscles without motion

TRANSVERSE ABDOMINAL BALL CRUNCH

This exercise safely trains the core, targeting the transverse and rectus abdominal muscles. The transversus abdominis (often shortened to TVA) is a deep muscle, whereas the rectus abdominis is the "six-pack" muscle nearer the surface.

THE BIG PICTURE

You'll need an exercise ball with a diameter of at least 21½–26 in (55–65 cm) for this abdominal crunch—a movement that involves lifting and lowering the upper body using the muscles of the core. You will feel your abdominal muscles compress and flex beneath your hands as you perform the movement.

Beginners can start with 4 sets of 8–10 reps; discover other variations on pp.162–163 and other targeted sets in the training programs (see pp.201–214).

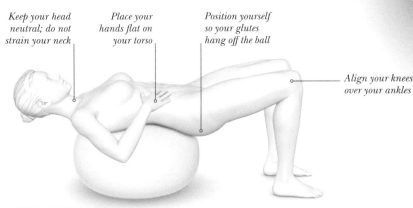

Keep your head neutral; do not strain your neck

Place your hands flat on your torso

Position yourself so your glutes hang off the ball

Align your knees over your ankles

PREPARATORY STAGE
Sit on top of the ball, with your feet shoulder-width apart and flat on the floor. Walk your feet out so that only the lower part of your back is in contact with the ball, then lower your upper body so that you adopt a supine position.

STAGE ONE
Take a breath in and engage your abdominals to help stabilize your core. Start the crunching motion by using your abs to flex at the spine as you breathe out; imagine "cinching in" your waist as you crunch. Once the abs are fully flexed and you've exhaled, that is the end of the range of motion. Do not flex further at the hips to bring the torso upward. To add a challenge, hold at the top position for 1 second.

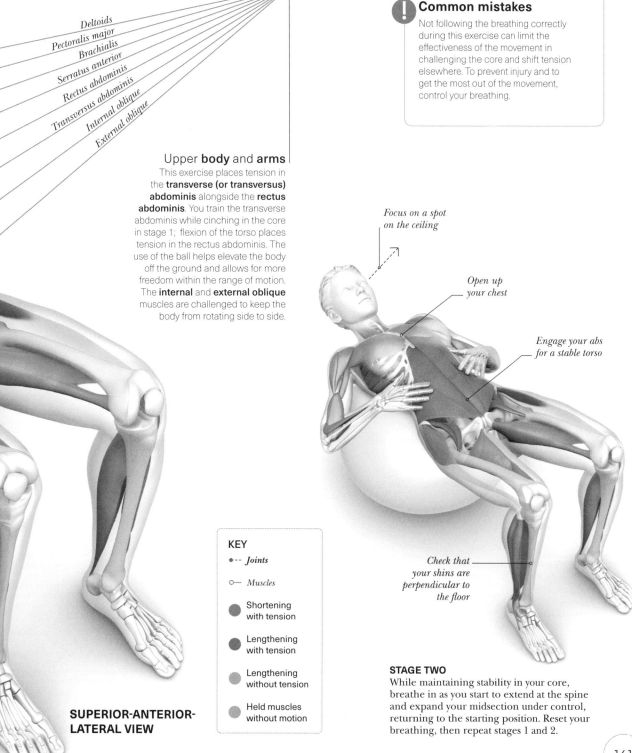

Deltoids
Pectoralis major
Brachialis
Serratus anterior
Rectus abdominis
Transversus abdominis
Internal oblique
External oblique

Upper **body** and **arms**

This exercise places tension in the **transverse (or transversus) abdominis** alongside the **rectus abdominis**. You train the transverse abdominis while cinching in the core in stage 1; flexion of the torso places tension in the rectus abdominis. The use of the ball helps elevate the body off the ground and allows for more freedom within the range of motion. The **internal** and **external oblique** muscles are challenged to keep the body from rotating side to side.

Focus on a spot on the ceiling

Open up your chest

Engage your abs for a stable torso

Check that your shins are perpendicular to the floor

KEY

●-- *Joints*

○— *Muscles*

● Shortening with tension

● Lengthening with tension

● Lengthening without tension

● Held muscles without motion

SUPERIOR-ANTERIOR-LATERAL VIEW

STAGE TWO

While maintaining stability in your core, breathe in as you start to extend at the spine and expand your midsection under control, returning to the starting position. Reset your breathing, then repeat stages 1 and 2.

» VARIATIONS

These exercises all target the abdominal muscles, including the transverse abdominis (TVA) and rectus abdominis (RA). Focus on core engagement and breathing control rather than speed.

CAT–COW KNEELING CRUNCH

Commonly referred to as "cat-cow," this yoga-inspired exercise targets muscles of the upper body—including those in the arms, shoulders, and back—as well as training the abdominals.

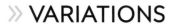

Alternate between arching your back up and down

Extend your neck and look forward in stage 2 (cow)

PREPARATORY STAGE/STAGE TWO

Engage your glutes for stability

Align your hips over your knees; your thighs should be perpendicular to the floor

STAGE ONE

Place the tops of your feet against the floor

Place your hands flat on the floor

Flex your neck forward in stage 1 (cat)

PREPARATORY STAGE (COW)
Kneel with your knees and feet aligned, hip-width apart. Your shins should be in contact with the floor. Place your hands on the floor beneath your shoulders.

STAGE ONE (CAT)
Breathe in to brace your core. As you breathe out, engage your TVA to lift your waist and flex at your spine using your rectus abdominis, so your back arches.

STAGE TWO (COW)
Breathe in to lower your back; contract your spinal erectors and upper-back muscles to open up your chest and lengthen your abs. Repeat stages 1 and 2.

STIR-THE-POT SWISS BALL

This exercise—so called because it emulates the motion of stirring a cooking pot—builds a connection between your core, hips, and lower back while strengthening and increasing the endurance of your core and lower back.

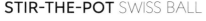

Keep your spine neutral without rounding your upper back

Maintain a neutral head position

Elbow position

Start on the smaller circle

Progress to the larger circle

SUPERIOR VIEW

Distribute your weight evenly through both feet

STAGE ONE

Engage your glutes throughout

Slowly does it
For this challenging exercise, start with small circles—as if you're drawing them slowly with your flexed elbows. As you become stronger, you'll be able to complete larger circles while, the entire time, holding the plank position.

PREPARATORY STAGE
Assume the plank position with your feet hip-width apart and your forearms supported securely on a stability ball; your elbows are in contact with the ball beneath your shoulders. Engage your abs and glutes and keep your knees extended.

STAGE ONE
Breathing in and out in a controlled manner, move your elbows in small circular motions, pressing down into the ball to guide it. Keep your hips still. Once you have mastered this exercise, you can make it harder by increasing the range of motion.

DEADBUG

This uniquely named abdominal exercise involves the transverse abdominis and rectus abdominis. It also challenges your ability to coordinate movements on both sides of your body while keeping your core engaged and your spine and pelvis neutral; the distance your arms and legs travel out will be determined, and limited, by this ability.

KEY

● Primary target muscle

● Secondary target muscle

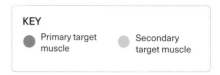

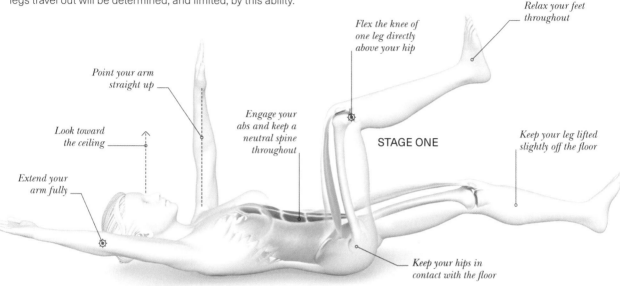

Point your arm straight up

Look toward the ceiling

Extend your arm fully

Engage your abs and keep a neutral spine throughout

Flex the knee of one leg directly above your hip

Relax your feet throughout

STAGE ONE

Keep your leg lifted slightly off the floor

Keep your hips in contact with the floor

PREPARATORY STAGE
Lie on your back with your arms flexed at the shoulders, legs flexed at the hips and knees, and head lifted off the ground in a neutral position.

STAGE ONE
Inhale to engage your abs. Exhale as you reach your right arm back and straighten your left leg simultaneously, keeping your hips in contact with the floor.

STAGE TWO
Breathe in to return to the starting position, then flex at the trunk to engage your rectus abdominis. Repeat on the other arm and leg.

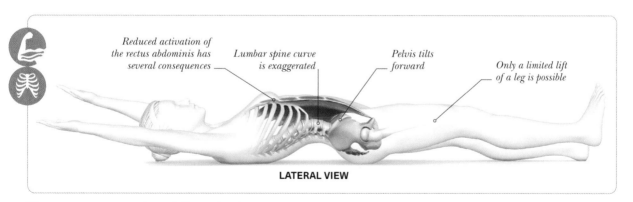

Reduced activation of the rectus abdominis has several consequences

Lumbar spine curve is exaggerated

Pelvis tilts forward

Only a limited lift of a leg is possible

LATERAL VIEW

The consequences of **not fully activating the abs**

Placing tension in the abs is crucial for creating stability in the pelvis and for protecting your spine during many other movements. In the illustration above, the exerciser struggles to lift a leg because she's not activating her abs and so can't transition to stage 1 of the deadbug exercise, above. Her pelvis starts to tilt forward, creating pelvic instability and increasing the risk of injury to her lower back.

HANGING
KNEE RAISE

Control and coordination of the hip and abdomen
are trained in this exercise, helping you better connect
with your body. The movement targets the hip flexors,
alongside the muscles of the rectus abdominis; just
lifting your bodyweight is enough to work against.

THE BIG PICTURE

It may look simple, but this exercise takes practice to achieve.
Hanging from a pull-up bar, you isolate muscles in your hip
and abdomen to flex your hips and your spine, lifting your
knees as high as you can. Tensing your abs before starting
neutralizes and stabilizes the spine. Arm straps can offer
additional support here so you can focus on working your abs.

Beginners can start with 4 sets of 8–10 reps; discover other
variations on pp.166–167 and other targeted sets in the
training programs (see pp.201–214).

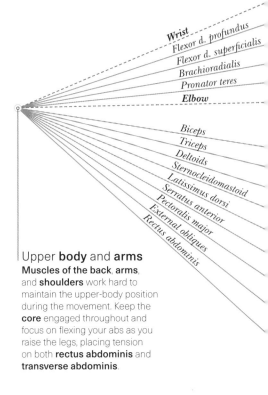

Upper **body** and **arms**
Muscles of the back, arms,
and **shoulders** work hard to
maintain the upper-body position
during the movement. Keep the
core engaged throughout and
focus on flexing your abs as you
raise the legs, placing tension
on both **rectus abdominis** and
transverse abdominis.

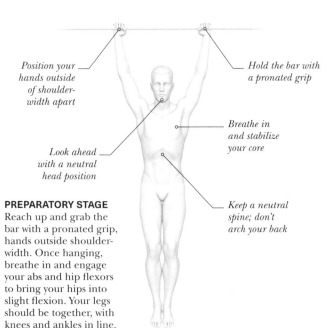

*Position your
hands outside
of shoulder-
width apart*

*Hold the bar with
a pronated grip*

*Look ahead
with a neutral
head position*

*Breathe in
and stabilize
your core*

*Keep a neutral
spine; don't
arch your back*

PREPARATORY STAGE
Reach up and grab the
bar with a pronated grip,
hands outside shoulder-
width. Once hanging,
breathe in and engage
your abs and hip flexors
to bring your hips into
slight flexion. Your legs
should be together, with
knees and ankles in line.

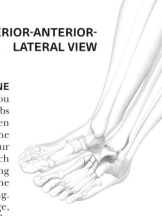

*Don't feel your knees
should touch your chest;
that is not the goal*

**SUPERIOR-ANTERIOR-
LATERAL VIEW**

STAGE ONE
Breathe out slowly as you
raise your knees. Your abs
will contract and shorten
as you raise and flex at the
hip—think to tuck your
pelvis under and crunch
your abs at the top to bring
your knees in. Control the
movement; do not swing.
For an added challenge,
hold for 1–2 seconds.

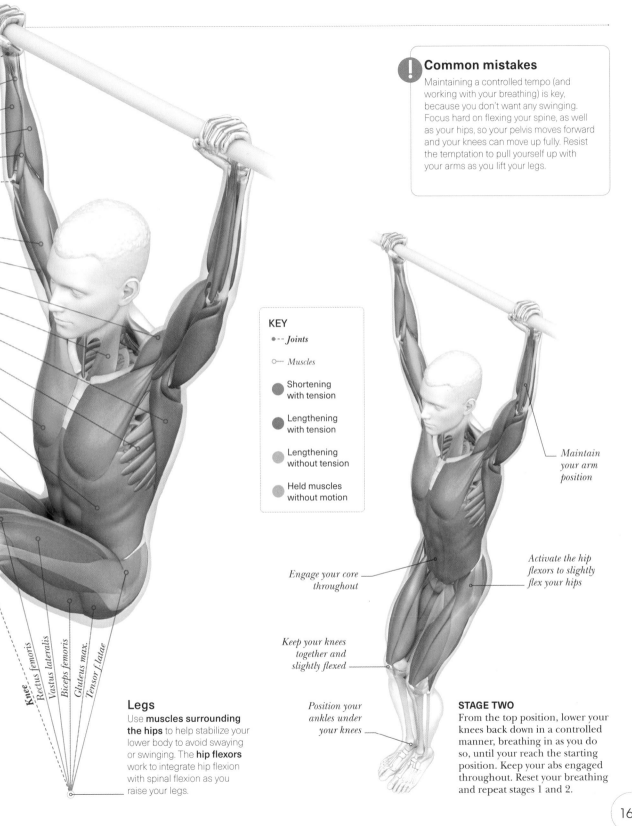

KEY

•--- *Joints*

○--- *Muscles*

● Shortening with tension

● Lengthening with tension

● Lengthening without tension

● Held muscles without motion

Maintain your arm position

Activate the hip flexors to slightly flex your hips

Engage your core throughout

Keep your knees together and slightly flexed

Position your ankles under your knees

Knee
Rectus femoris
Vastus lateralis
Biceps femoris
Gluteus max.
Tensor Fatae

Legs
Use **muscles surrounding the hips** to help stabilize your lower body to avoid swaying or swinging. The **hip flexors** work to integrate hip flexion with spinal flexion as you raise your legs.

STAGE TWO
From the top position, lower your knees back down in a controlled manner, breathing in as you do so, until your reach the starting position. Keep your abs engaged throughout. Reset your breathing and repeat stages 1 and 2.

›› VARIATIONS

These exercises are effective for training the visible ab muscles. A common mistake is to place too much importance on moving from preparatory stage to stage 1. Flex your trunk as you breathe out; once that is achieved, that is the end of your range of motion.

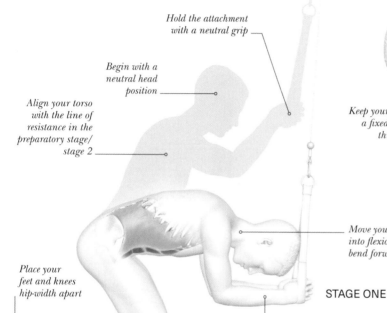

Stand tall in the preparatory stage/ stage 2

Hold the attachment on either side of your neck

Hold the attachment with a neutral grip

Begin with a neutral head position

Align your torso with the line of resistance in the preparatory stage/ stage 2

Keep your arms in a fixed position throughout

Point your elbows outward for stability

Move your neck into flexion as you bend forward

Stand with a soft bend in your knees

Place your feet and knees hip-width apart

STAGE ONE

STAGE ONE

Keep your arms in a fixed position throughout

Place your feet hip-width apart

CABLE ROPE CRUNCH

This exercise trains the abs in their most contracted range. Focus on bringing your sternum and pelvis toward each other—your hips will stay fixed while your abs do the work. For an added challenge, hold for 1–2 seconds after stage 1.

PREPARATORY STAGE
Facing the cable system with a rope, V-bar, or strap attachment in place, take hold of the attachment. Kneel down with your torso leaned forward.

STAGE ONE
Breathe in to brace your core. Breathe out as you flex at the trunk, engaging your rectus abdominis. Keep your arms in a fixed position.

STAGE TWO
Breathe in to rise back up; actively contract your spinal erectors to "pull" yourself up and lengthen your abdominals. Repeat stages 1 and 2.

FACING-AWAY STANDING CRUNCH

Use this variation to target the abs in their lengthened to midrange. Again, think about bringing your sternum and pelvis toward each other. To increase the challenge, hold for 1–2 seconds after stage 1.

PREPARATORY STAGE
Stand with your back toward the cable system, a rope, V-bar, or strap attachment in place. Hold the attachment with your hands on either side of your neck.

STAGE ONE
Breathe in to engage your core, then breathe out as you flex at the trunk, engaging the rectus abdominis and transverse abdominis muscles.

STAGE TWO
Breathe in as you return to the starting position, contracting your spinal erectors to "pull" yourself up and lengthening your abs. Repeat stages 1 and 2.

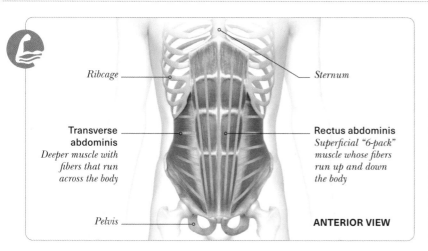

Ribcage — — *Sternum*

Transverse abdominis
Deeper muscle with fibers that run across the body

Rectus abdominis
Superficial "6-pack" muscle whose fibers run up and down the body

Pelvis

ANTERIOR VIEW

Muscles of the core

Your abdominal muscles help move, control, and support your spine and pelvis. The fibers in each layer of the abs (see also p.170) run in various directions, allowing the core to provide strength and power while withstanding the forces involved in movement in all planes of motion. Together, the core muscles provide stability and mobility for highly coordinated movements in strength training, sports, and everyday life.

DECLINE ABDOMINAL CRUNCH

This variation uses your bodyweight to train the core on a decline bench. Avoid the temptation to generate momentum at the start of the rep and allow that to carry you to the top position; this will take tension away from your abs.

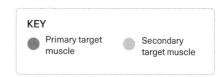

KEY

● Primary target muscle

● Secondary target muscle

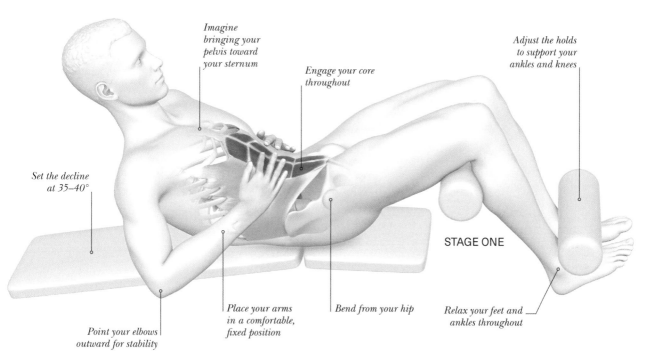

Imagine bringing your pelvis toward your sternum

Engage your core throughout

Adjust the holds to support your ankles and knees

Set the decline at 35–40°

Point your elbows outward for stability

Place your arms in a comfortable, fixed position

Bend from your hip

Relax your feet and ankles throughout

STAGE ONE

PREPARATORY STAGE
Position yourself on a decline bench with your feet and ankle secure in the foot holds and your hands either on your belly or at the sides of your head.

STAGE ONE
Breathe in to brace your core, then breathe out as you flex at the trunk, crunching upward. Be sure not to pull your head up with your hands.

STAGE TWO
Breathe in to return to the starting position, controlling the eccentric action and keeping tension on your abs. Repeat stages 1 and 2.

CABLE ROTATIONAL
OBLIQUE TWIST

This twisting exercise trains the internal and external oblique muscles at the sides of the torso. Building strength and endurance in these muscles helps protect the spine and aids bending and rotating. This movement goes from low to high, but you can go midlevel or high to low.

THE **BIG PICTURE**

The low-to-high rotational motion helps build strength in core muscles that, in turn, make everyday activities easier. This version has a more limited range of movement and, consequently, a lower risk of injury compared to others. Set the weights, adjust the height of the cable starting position, and set up a single handle attachment. If you are new to this exercise, use a lighter load and get used to the coordination of the movement across the body.

Beginners can start with 4 sets of 8–10 reps; discover other variations on pp.170–171 and other targeted sets in the training programs (see pp.201–214).

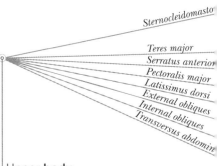

Sternocleidomasto
Teres major
Serratus anterior
Pectoralis major
Latissimus dorsi
External obliques
Internal obliques
Transversus abdomin

Upper **body**
Muscles of the back and **torso** help support a smooth and controlled movement from the low-to-high cable position. The **internal and external obliques** work in synchronicity to coordinate the passing off of tension from one side of the torso to the other. The **rectus abdominis** helps the oblique muscles manage the load as it comes across the body.

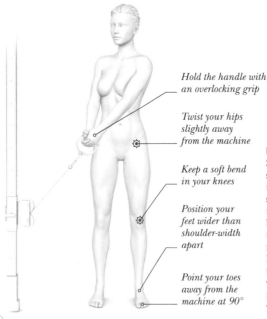

Hold the handle with an overlocking grip

Twist your hips slightly away from the machine

Keep a soft bend in your knees

Position your feet wider than shoulder-width apart

Point your toes away from the machine at 90°

PREPARATORY STAGE
Set up the machine and stand with your right side toward the cable pulley system. Take a wide step to your left and a step back to find a position that allows the cable to move freely. Grab the handle with both hands; the arm near the pulley will bend while the other reaches across your body, which will twist slightly.

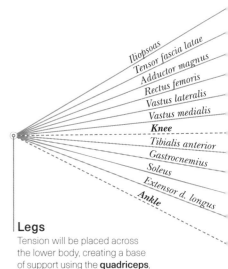

Iliopsoas
Tensor fascia latae
Adductor magnus
Rectus femoris
Vastus lateralis
Vastus medialis
Knee
Tibialis anterior
Gastrocnemius
Soleus
Extensor d. longus
Ankle

Legs
Tension will be placed across the lower body, creating a base of support using the **quadriceps**, **glutes**, **hamstrings**, and **calf muscles**. Stability comes from grounding your feet, thereby allowing more tension to be placed on the target muscles.

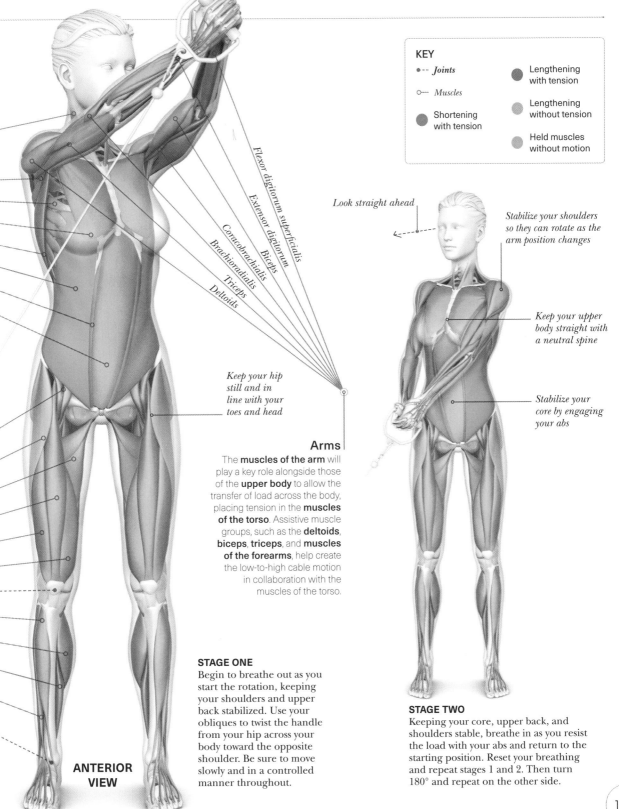

KEY

- •--- *Joints*
- o— *Muscles*
- ● Shortening with tension
- ● Lengthening with tension
- ● Lengthening without tension
- ● Held muscles without motion

Flexor digitorum superficialis

Extensor digitorum

Biceps

Coracobrachialis

Brachioradialis

Triceps

Deltoids

Look straight ahead

Stabilize your shoulders so they can rotate as the arm position changes

Keep your upper body straight with a neutral spine

Stabilize your core by engaging your abs

Keep your hip still and in line with your toes and head

Arms

The **muscles of the arm** will play a key role alongside those of the **upper body** to allow the transfer of load across the body, placing tension in the **muscles of the torso**. Assistive muscle groups, such as the **deltoids**, **biceps**, **triceps**, and **muscles of the forearms**, help create the low-to-high cable motion in collaboration with the muscles of the torso.

STAGE ONE
Begin to breathe out as you start the rotation, keeping your shoulders and upper back stabilized. Use your obliques to twist the handle from your hip across your body toward the opposite shoulder. Be sure to move slowly and in a controlled manner throughout.

ANTERIOR VIEW

STAGE TWO
Keeping your core, upper back, and shoulders stable, breathe in as you resist the load with your abs and return to the starting position. Reset your breathing and repeat stages 1 and 2. Then turn 180° and repeat on the other side.

169

» VARIATIONS

These rotational-crunch abdominal variations involve all the abs—transverse abdominis, rectus abdominis, and the internal and external obliques. When performing these variations, make sure to train both sides of your body evenly. Focus on your breathing and ensure both the lowering and rotation phases of each exercise are smooth and controlled.

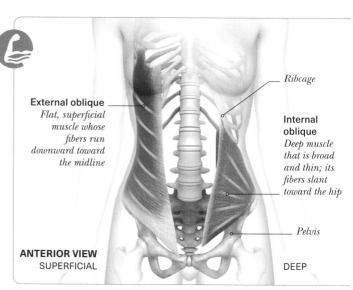

External oblique
Flat, superficial muscle whose fibers run downward toward the midline

Ribcage

Internal oblique
Deep muscle that is broad and thin; its fibers slant toward the hip

Pelvis

ANTERIOR VIEW
SUPERFICIAL

DEEP

Internal and **external** obliques
With their muscle fibers running perpendicular to one another, the internal and external obliques work synergistically across the torso to generate the rotational component of this movement.

OBLIQUE TWIST **WITH PLATE WEIGHT**

The internal and external obliques are the principal muscles used here, with the abdominals providing stability. You can increase the challenge of the exercise by keeping your legs lifted off the ground throughout the set.

KEY
● Primary target muscle
● Secondary target muscle

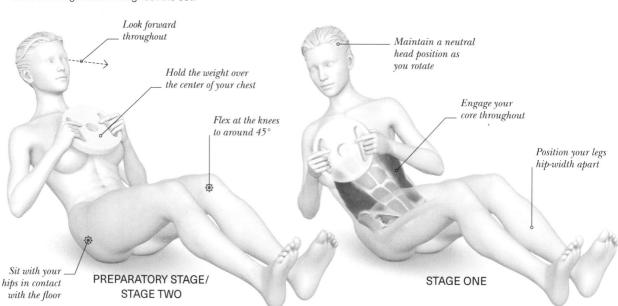

Look forward throughout

Hold the weight over the center of your chest

Flex at the knees to around 45°

Sit with your hips in contact with the floor

PREPARATORY STAGE/
STAGE TWO

Maintain a neutral head position as you rotate

Engage your core throughout

Position your legs hip-width apart

STAGE ONE

PREPARATORY STAGE
In a seated position, lean back and flex your legs at the hips and knees to form a V-shape between your torso and your thighs. Hold the weight over your chest.

STAGE ONE
Breathe in to engage your core, then breathe out as you rotate your upper body to one side, holding your legs still and maintaining tension in your core.

STAGE TWO
Breathe in to return to the starting position, with control. Repeat stages 1 and 2 rotating to the other side, then perform desired reps, alternating sides.

BICYCLE CRUNCH

This variation, which mimics the motions of a cyclist, is an accessible alternative to the more challenging alternating V-up crunch, below. To increase the difficulty, hold for 1 second at the top position and keep both legs raised throughout the set.

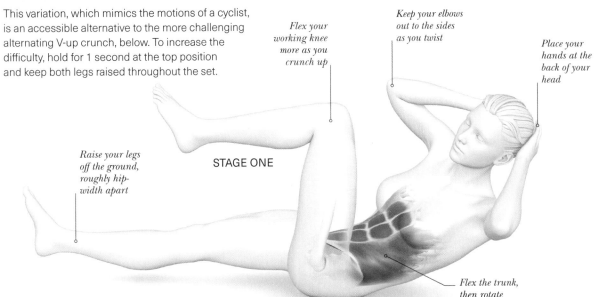

Flex your working knee more as you crunch up

Keep your elbows out to the sides as you twist

Place your hands at the back of your head

Raise your legs off the ground, roughly hip-width apart

STAGE ONE

Flex the trunk, then rotate

PREPARATORY STAGE
Lie flat on your back with your hands positioned behind your head and your legs slightly flexed at the hips and knees. Lift your head off the ground slightly.

STAGE ONE
Inhale to engage your core. Breathe out to lift your left knee and bring your opposite elbow toward it. Flex at the trunk and rotate your upper body toward your leg.

STAGE TWO
Breathe in as you return to the starting position, with control. Repeat, raising the opposite leg and elbow, then repeat an equal number of reps on both sides.

ALTERNATING V-UP CRUNCH

This exercise involves coordinating movements on opposite sides of the body while maintaining a neutral spine and pelvis. For more of a challenge, hold for 1 second at the top position and keep both legs raised throughout the set.

PREPARATORY STAGE
Lie flat on your back with your arms fully flexed at the shoulders, reaching behind you, and your legs straight. Lift your head off the ground slightly.

STAGE ONE
Breathe in to brace your core. Exhale as you lift your left leg up and bring your right arm toward it, then flex at the trunk to rotate your upper body toward your lifted leg.

STAGE TWO
Breathe in to return to the starting position, with control. Repeat, raising the opposite arm and leg, then repeat an equal number of reps on both sides.

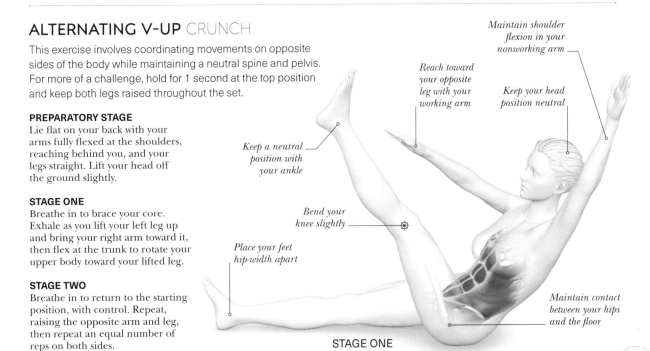

Maintain shoulder flexion in your nonworking arm

Reach toward your opposite leg with your working arm

Keep your head position neutral

Keep a neutral position with your ankle

Bend your knee slightly

Place your feet hip-width apart

Maintain contact between your hips and the floor

STAGE ONE

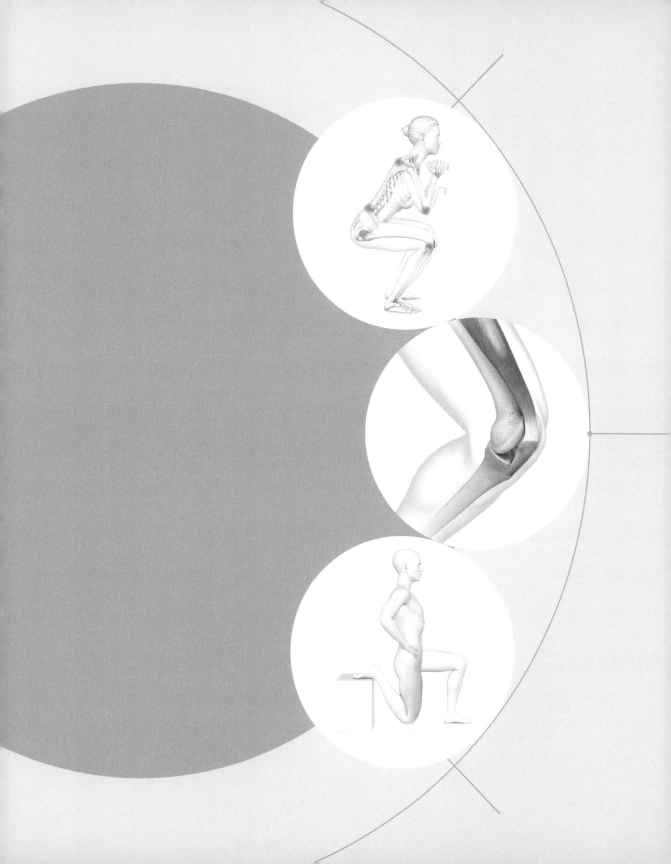

PREVENTING
INJURY

Strength training is among the safest of training modalities but is
not without risk of injury, so it pays to be aware of the common injuries
so that you can guard against them. Correct execution of any exercise
is the main way to avoid injury, but readying your body ahead of a
workout and letting it recover afterward are also key.

INJURY **RISK**

Strength training is a safe, effective way of improving your health, stimulating muscle growth, and improving body composition. That said, it does come with a risk of injury, but you can mitigate these risks by exercising regularly and focusing on the structure of your workout and on the execution of the exercises.

46%
OF INJURIES ARE
SPRAINS (DAMAGE
TO A LIGAMENT)
AND **STRAINS** (AN
OVERSTRETCH OR
TEAR IN A TENDON
OR MUSCLE).

A **CONSISTENT** APPROACH

Following a progressive training program gives your body time to adapt, get stronger, and build muscle mass. For this to happen, consistency is key. The benefits of strength training come only while you are consistently training. Set aside certain days of the week according to the split of your training program—how many times you want to train every week (see p.201). Long durations of time spent away from strength training reverses the good you've done, so sticking with the program is the route to success and the way to mitigate risk of injury. Track your progress to see your improvements that follow incrementally upward.

PREPARING THE BODY

Many injuries result from diving straight into a strength training session without warming up properly or mobilizing your joints ahead of the workout. Preparing your body is key to avoiding injury. With any program, it's more than just following the reps and sets and improving your execution of the exercises that are important. It's crucial to structure each and every workout in the same way (see below) and to stick to the routine, even as you make gains, to minimize the risk of injury while exercising regularly.

Routine safety

For optimum safety and for minimizing the risk of injuries in every training session, always tailor your workout routine to follow this structure.

Warm-up

Starting all training sessions with warm-up exercises (consisting of aerobic activities or dynamic stretches) is a must to prepare the body for the upcoming workout (see also p.186).

THE IMPORTANCE OF **EXECUTION**

Strength training's risk comes from performing exercises that place your body into unstable positions while under load. These positions will become more stable over time as you build flexibility and overall strength. A good exercise technique involves thought about a proper set-up, understanding what the exercise demands, concentration, proper breathing and bracing, and a controlled repetition tempo. Then it's a matter of repeating to improve.

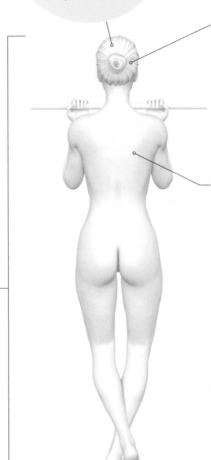

KNOWLEDGE

Find out exactly which muscles are involved in an exercise beforehand. The illustrated exercises (see pp.54–171) show both stages of a movement, as well as where to visualize tension in your muscles.

FOCUS

There is always a risk of injury if you don't concentrate on properly and safely executing an exercise. Here's where the mind–muscle connection comes into play (see p.39).

BREATHING AND BRACING

Breathing sets the rhythm of the reps—with breathing in and out tied to certain actions. Engaging the core stabilizes the torso so you can focus on target muscles.

PRACTICE DRIVES PROGRESSION

Strength training takes practice to improve its overall effectiveness and reduce the risk of injury. Proper exercise execution can lead to higher levels of mechanical tension in the target muscles and keeps the body within a safe and controlled movement pattern.

CONTROLLED TEMPO

The goal of each rep is to place tension from the loads on the muscles being trained. This takes focus but protects against injury. The last rep of a workout should be as controlled as the first.

Mobility exercises

See how your body responds to mobility exercises (and check for any areas of stiffness) once your body is warmed up. Mobilize the relevant parts ahead of the session's work (see also p.186).

Strength training exercises

Stick to your training program, ensuring you focus on the correct execution of the exercise (see above) and keep track of your progress (see also p.49).

Cool-down stretches

Stretch for at least 5–10 minutes (see also p.187). Short-hold (5–30 secs) static stretches improve flexibility and release tension in worked muscles. Plus, they provide an opportunity to wind down after exercise.

DELAYED-ONSET
MUSCLE SORENESS

Delayed-onset muscle soreness—DOMS—is when your muscles start to hurt and feel stiff in the days following a workout; your trained muscles won't generate as much force and your performance will decline during this time. While DOMS brings with it a host of detriments, it is a normal response to working your muscles harder.

IS SORENESS **NORMAL**?

Yes, and the soreness follows when you train at a higher intensity, frequency, duration, and resistance (see pp.198–199), such as when starting a new training program. Such workouts lead to mechanical tension, metabolic stress, and muscle damage (see pp.18–21)—all of which challenge your body, forcing it to adapt, build more muscle, and get stronger. Once your body adapts to the level of workout, you won't experience soreness until you introduce more of a challenge again.

What's a good level of soreness?

It's useful to register the level of soreness after a workout, as it can be a helpful indicator that target muscles were trained, but it's also important to tell when pain and/or restricted motion may indicate an injury. Use the table to help you assess if your soreness is DOMS or an injury.

DOMS VS. POTENTIAL INJURY

Muscle is tender to the touch.	Sharp, intense pains in muscle or near a joint.
Muscle fatigue reached much quicker than usual.	Continuous discomfort in daily activities, limiting your ability to perform simple tasks.
Loss of muscle strength or performance.	Loss of range of motion, strength, and performance within muscle or joint.
Discomfort subsides after 24–96 hours and improves as time goes on.	Discomfort persists past 48–96 hours and does not seem to improve.
DOMS A discomfort that limits muscles' range of motion or performance without long-term consequences. As the muscles recover, the discomfort will subside.	**INJURY** A discomfort or pain that persists and impacts structural abilities to perform exercises or activities of daily life. Seek medical guidance from a physiotherapist.

When DOMS strikes

Knowing what to expect when may help you deal with the muscle soreness after starting a new program or completing a particularly strenuous session. Time is the only healer for DOMS, so be sure to take the rest days in your training program.

TRAINING DAY

Undertaking a strenuous strength training workout stimulates the muscle damage and breakdown that ultimately leads to more muscle. Working at a higher-than-normal level forces your body to adapt and your fitness to improve.

SOME SORENESS

You'll feel the start of some muscle soreness when you wake the morning after your training session.

DAY 0

DAY 1

How best to limit DOMS?

To avoid working out when some muscles are already sore, it's crucial to follow a well-designed, progressive training program, as well as registering how you feel ahead of a workout. Large amounts of muscle damage will work against you and limit your ability to improve over time. So if you're looking to train several times a week, be sure to divide up your program so that it works different muscle groups each time (see p.201 to learn about the splits of training for working out 3x, 4x, or 5x a week).

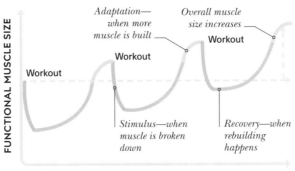

GOOD ROUTINE OF TRAINING AND REST

After a workout, there's a short period of muscle breakdown, which is followed by recovery and the rebuilding of those damaged muscle fibers. Afterward, a period of adaptation allows muscles to build new fibers as a response to being worked hard. This cycle builds muscle overall.

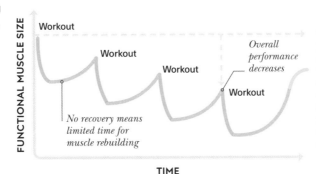

TRAINING TOO OFTEN

If recovery time is restricted or excluded altogether from training, the body has no opportunity to rebuild the damaged muscle, let alone adapt to build new muscle fibers. Such a cycle leads to diminishing overall muscle size and performance, despite the extra muscular work done.

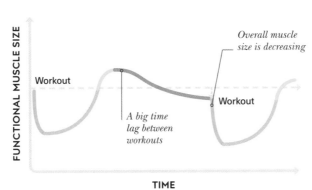

KEY
- Muscle breakdown
- Muscle rebuilding
- Building more muscle

TRAINING TOO INFREQUENTLY

If there are not enough training sessions across a certain time, the adaptation advantage is lost. Such a training cycle will not build muscle, and overall muscle size and training performance declines.

PEAK SORENESS

Beginners and advanced exercisers alike experience peak DOMS around day 2. Active rest is crucial for muscle recovery, so opt for light-intensity activity, such as walking or swimming, if you're eager to train again.

SORENESS SUBSIDES

Soreness starts to lessen around day 3. Being active is good for countering DOMS, but be sure to continue to take it easy. Active rest allows a period of recovery for rebuilding muscles.

SORENESS GONE

By day 4, the soreness in the muscle groups trained will be gone or almost gone.

DAY 2   DAY 3   DAY 4

COMMON INJURIES

An injury during a strength training workout—whether a muscular or an overuse injury—can happen to anyone, regardless of experience or fitness level. You can limit your risk of injury by learning how to spot the signs and symptoms of common injuries, as well as picking up tips on prevention and recovery after injury.

SELF-HELP MEASURES

Despite the relative safety of strength training, there is a risk of injury. If you do suffer from an injury, the word "POLICE" makes for a useful reminder of what to do: **P**rotection (protect the area injured); **O**ptimal **L**oading (do not overwork but keep moving); **I**ce (apply ice to relieve pain); **C**ompress (use a compression bandage); **E**levation (raise the injured site to reduce swelling).

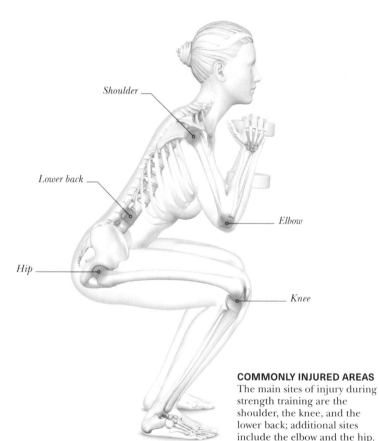

Shoulder

Lower back

Hip

Elbow

Knee

COMMONLY INJURED AREAS
The main sites of injury during strength training are the shoulder, the knee, and the lower back; additional sites include the elbow and the hip.

INJURY TYPES

The two most common types of injuries of strength training are overuse injuries and muscle strains. Injuries can be caused by: not properly warming up the body; overstretching a muscle beyond its range of motion; or demanding more than a muscle is capable of (overexertion).

Overuse injuries

Tendinitis is the inflammation of the tendon and the microtears resulting from overloading of the muscle–tendon unit with too much load or too sudden a movement. Tendinosis is the degeneration of the tendon in response to chronic overuse without proper time to heal.

Muscular injuries

A tension-based force exerted on a muscle can lead to excessive stretching of the muscle fibers and can potentially lead to a tear close to the myotendinous junction (see pp.12–13 and p.21).

IN THE **SHOULDER**

The shoulder is a complex ball-and-socket joint of muscles and supporting structures to create an integrated system of movement. Because the shoulders are involved with most actions performed at the gym, they are a common site of injury.

CAUSES AND SYMPTOMS

The shoulder's glenohumeral joint favors mobility at the expense of stability, relying on supporting structures, such as the rotator cuff. Repetitive use, explosive moves, and poor technique are common causes of injury.

- Tears—microtears to tendons or muscles or bigger tears in the muscle–tendon unit.
- Tendinitis—acute inflammation at the joint.
- Tendinosis—degeneration of the tendon from chronic overuse.
- Impingement—pinching of the tendons within the rotator cuff.

Symptoms include:
- Pain at and around the joint
- Inflammation

PREVENTION

Proper organization of your training sessions, as well as attention to correct exercise technique, can help prevent injury to the rotator cuff. A high rate of injury is from overuse, so limit your training frequency (see p.200) and ensure adequate rest to allow muscles and tendons to fully heal.

RETURNING TO TRAINING

After an injury, be sure to increase training volume and frequency (see also p.198) appropriately over the first 4–8 weeks. Too much too soon can set you back. Utilize mobility exercises that strengthen the shoulder and rotator cuff (see pp.189–191).

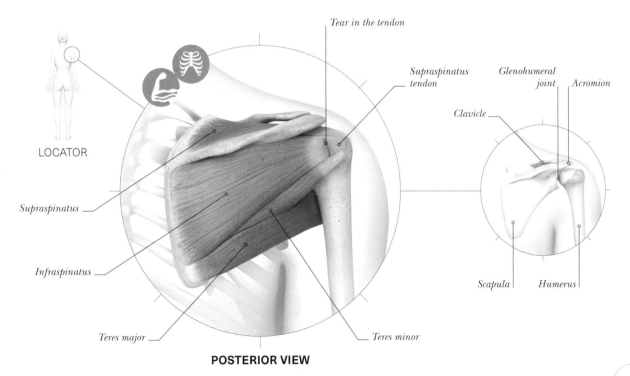

LOCATOR

Tear in the tendon

Supraspinatus tendon

Glenohumeral joint

Acromion

Clavicle

Supraspinatus

Infraspinatus

Teres major

Teres minor

Scapula

Humerus

POSTERIOR VIEW

IN THE **ELBOW**

The elbow is a hinge joint (similar to a door hinge) where there is movement happening in only one plane. The elbow is a common site of injury, because it helps most movements performed by the upper body.

CAUSES AND SYMPTOMS

The most common injury experienced in strength training at the elbow is "tennis elbow" (a.k.a. lateral epicondyle tendinopathy). Common causes include:

- Repetitive use or underuse of the extensor muscles of the forearm
- Poor exercise technique
- Repetitive use of barbells (can place large stress on the elbow)

Symptoms include:

- Pain at the lateral epicondyle (the bony bit of the elbow)
- Pain during loaded or resistive exercises involving the wrist or elbow joint

PREVENTION

Appropriate exercise selection and proper execution of exercises involving the elbow, alongside strengthening extensor forearm muscles, reduces the likelihood of injury. A high rate of injury is from overuse, so limit your training frequency (how many times you're training on this joint) and ensure adequate rest to allow muscles and tendons to fully heal.

RETURNING TO TRAINING

Be sure to increase training volume and frequency (see also p.198 and p.200) appropriately over the first 4–8 weeks. Too much too soon can set you back. Utilize mobility exercises that help add strength and stability to the extensor muscles of the forearm and elbow. Stretches of extensor muscles can also improve recovery time.

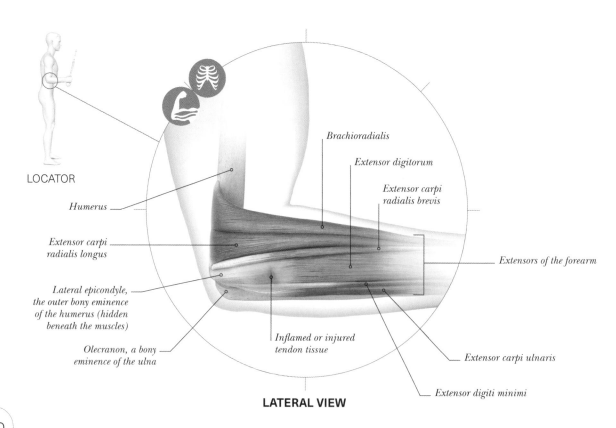

LOCATOR

Humerus

Extensor carpi radialis longus

Lateral epicondyle, the outer bony eminence of the humerus (hidden beneath the muscles)

Olecranon, a bony eminence of the ulna

Brachioradialis

Extensor digitorum

Extensor carpi radialis brevis

Extensors of the forearm

Inflamed or injured tendon tissue

Extensor carpi ulnaris

Extensor digiti minimi

LATERAL VIEW

IN THE **LOWER BACK**

Injuries of the lower back may be one of the most common strength training injuries, alongside the shoulder, due to the complexity of the hip and trunk muscles involved in generating and stabilizing movement of the lower body.

CAUSES AND SYMPTOMS

Lower-back muscle strain—one of the most common lower-back injuries—is most often due to a lack of pelvic control or lack of coordination with the abdominal muscles. Other causes include:

- Repetitive use
- Misalignment of the spine during an exercise
- Excessive loading without proper support or control

Symptoms include:
- Sharp pain
- Stiffness
- Inflammation
- Overall discomfort of the joint

PREVENTION

Proper exercise technique can help prevent lower-back muscle strain alongside building strength in your abdominals and core. It's a good idea to avoid excessive stresses or repetitive usage of movements that aggravate or worsen pain in your back.

RETURNING TO TRAINING

After an injury, be sure to increase training volume and frequency (see also p.198 and p.200) appropriately over the first 4–8 weeks. Too much too soon can set you back. Utilize mobility exercises (see pp.189 and 191) that will add strength and stability to the muscles of the lower back. Such exercises can offer relief alongside adjustments to your training to lessen the strain on this area.

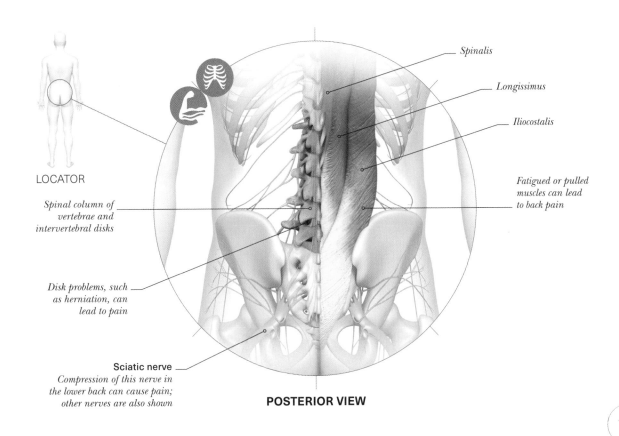

LOCATOR

Spinalis

Longissimus

Iliocostalis

Fatigued or pulled muscles can lead to back pain

Spinal column of vertebrae and intervertebral disks

Disk problems, such as herniation, can lead to pain

Sciatic nerve
Compression of this nerve in the lower back can cause pain; other nerves are also shown

POSTERIOR VIEW

IN THE **HIP**

Because the hip has a large range of motion in many planes (see p.50) and involves a complex system of supporting structures and muscles (attaching to the hip, knee, and torso), it can be injured from a variety of different actions.

CAUSES AND SYMPTOMS

One of the most common injuries experienced in strength training is gluteal tendinopathy (a.k.a. greater trochanteric pain syndrome or "rotator cuff syndrome of the hip"). Common causes include:

- Repetitive stress to the gluteal tendinous attachments of the gluteus medius and gluteus minimus muscles
- Bursitis of the hip—bursitis is the inflammation of small, fluid-filled sacs that cushion muscles, bones, and tendons near joints

Symptoms include:
- Pain at the site
- Discomfort when walking, trying to train, or even sitting or lying on the affected hip

PREVENTION

Appropriate exercise selection and proper execution of exercises can help prevent gluteal tendinopathy.

Avoiding excessive stress or repetitive use of movements such as hip abductions or "band walks" (with resistance bands around the legs). Overuse of mobility exercises can overload this area and lead to a higher risk of aggravation and injury.

RETURNING TO TRAINING

Be sure to increase training volume and frequency (see also p.198 and p.200) appropriately over the first 4–8 weeks. Too much too soon can set you back. Utilize mobility exercises (see pp.191–193) that help add strength and stability to the glutes and muscles of the hip.

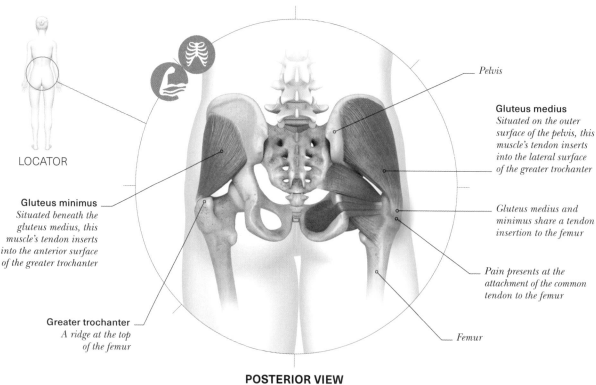

LOCATOR

Gluteus minimus
Situated beneath the gluteus medius, this muscle's tendon inserts into the anterior surface of the greater trochanter

Greater trochanter
A ridge at the top of the femur

Pelvis

Gluteus medius
Situated on the outer surface of the pelvis, this muscle's tendon inserts into the lateral surface of the greater trochanter

Gluteus medius and minimus share a tendon insertion to the femur

Pain presents at the attachment of the common tendon to the femur

Femur

POSTERIOR VIEW

IN THE **KNEE**

The knee is a common site of injury, as many strength training exercises load knee flexion and extension, such as back squats, lunges, and leg extension.

CAUSES AND SYMPTOMS

Pain around, behind, or below the patella (knee cap) is commonly known as "runner's knee" or, strictly, patellofemoral syndrome. It's the most common cause of anterior knee pain in exercisers. Common causes include:

- Overuse (the most common)
- Malalignment of the lower extremity and/or patella
- Muscular imbalances of the lower extremity
- Improper loading

Symptoms include:

- Pain around, behind, or below the anterior part of knee
- Pain that is exaggerated by loaded knee flexion exercises

PREVENTION

Proper execution technique can help prevent this condition alongside building up strength in your quadriceps, hamstrings, and muscles of the calves—all of which play a role in stabilization of the knee. Misalignment or poor tracking of the knee can exaggerate symptoms, so you'll need to rule this out as a direct cause. Avoid excessive stress or repeated movements that aggravate or worsen the condition.

RETURNING TO TRAINING

Be sure to increase training volume and frequency (see also p.198 and p.200) appropriately over the first 4–8 weeks. Utilize appropriate repetition tempo and exercises (limit those that stress the knee) to help alleviate any unnecessary stress on the joint.

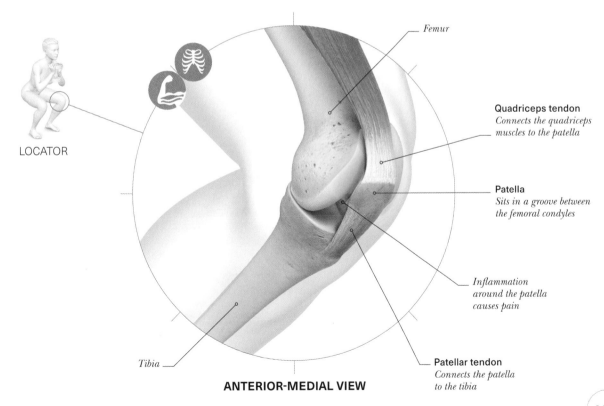

LOCATOR

Femur

Quadriceps tendon
Connects the quadriceps muscles to the patella

Patella
Sits in a groove between the femoral condyles

Inflammation around the patella causes pain

Tibia

Patellar tendon
Connects the patella to the tibia

ANTERIOR-MEDIAL VIEW

RETURNING TO TRAINING
AFTER INJURY

The return to regular exercise after an injury can be tough. You'll probably feel motivated to get back to full performance but may be limited by your ability to perform at first, which can bring frustration. Choose from the various strategies available to find those that work for you.

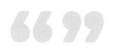

*Utilizing **several strategies** can **cut recovery time** and help you **regain your previous performance levels**.*

RECOVERY **STRATEGIES**

The ability to restore range of motion, function, and overall strength and performance will depend on your ability to remain patient, strategic, and listen to your body during the recovery process. One of the most common ways of reinjuring yourself or worsening a condition is doing too much too soon.

When returning to strength training, there are several strategies at your disposal to ensure you are able to start training and to rebuild your strength and performance safely.

MODIFY YOUR PROGRAM
You can make tweaks to your training program, such as by reducing training volume and training intensity on the affected or injured area. Ensure you adjust the potential variables—the training load, the amount of training volume, and the frequency of training the affected area—and are not making the condition or discomfort worse by overloading or overuse. If avoiding volume and intensity on a specific muscle

group or joint, you can continue to train as normal with other muscles and joints. For example, if dealing with a biceps injury, you could continue with lower-body strength training as long as it does not directly affect your recovery.

ADJUST YOUR POSITION
Implement variations of an exercise or positional adjustments to be able to work around any discomfort. Use cables or machines whenever possible to ensure that your training environment is safe and that your range of motion is limited. Altering the range of motion in a given exercise can help train a specific area while also working around an injury or any discomfort.

For example, if you still experience pain or discomfort in the knee through a full range of motion when performing a leg extension (see Altering range of motion, opposite), you can adjust the range of motion to train in a range where there is no discomfort, such as the upper two-thirds of a leg extension.

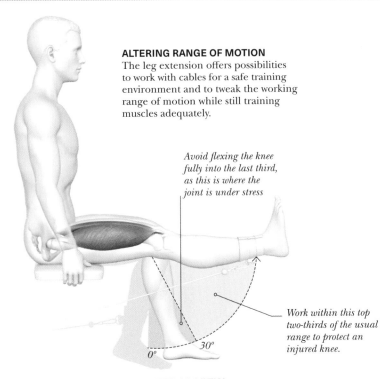

ALTERING RANGE OF MOTION
The leg extension offers possibilities to work with cables for a safe training environment and to tweak the working range of motion while still training muscles adequately.

Avoid flexing the knee fully into the last third, as this is where the joint is under stress

Work within this top two-thirds of the usual range to protect an injured knee.

0°   30°

LATERAL VIEW

TWEAK THE TEMPO

Altering the repetition tempo (the time spent in the eccentric and concentric phases of a movement; see also p.204) can allow you to work around an injured muscle or any tendon-related discomfort.

Expanding on the leg extension exercise above, if you cannot heavily load the exercise due to joint discomfort, you can alter your repetition tempo to increase the amount of time the quads are under tension and still enable adequate stimulus. For example, you could insert a pause at the top of the exercise—while continuously maintaining tension on and contracting the quads— for 2–4 seconds. Likewise, with the eccentric, you could up the time under tension by extending the time in the lowering portion.

FOCUS ON THE LOCAL

Choose an exercise that localizes a given muscle group or joint. If you have knee pain, for instance, you could continue to train the quads by performing leg extensions instead of barbell back squats and adjust the rep tempo.

Don't rush recovery

There is a psychological component to returning from an injury. Depending on the severity of the injury, it is worth building confidence in performing an exercise before returning to your previous training loads or performance levels. Do not rush your recovery—"no pain, no gain" does not apply to this process. If you are in any discomfort, utilize training adaptations or medication or seek qualified medical guidance to properly address the situation.

 Blood flow restriction training

KAATSU training—a patented training style developed in Japan in the 1970s by Dr. Yoshiaki Sato—uses engineered cuffs to shut off blood flow to a specific limb. Blood flow restriction (BFR) training is a variation of this method and has been shown to be an effective way to work around an injury and keep training. BFR training involves the application of a cuff on the training limb nearest its point of attachment to the body while exercising (see the cuff positions below). The application of the cuff partially restricts arterial blood flow (blood coming into the muscle) and significantly or completely restricts venous return (blood flowing out of the working muscle).

This method of training is shown to:
● Help work around injuries
● Help the rehabilitation process
● Minimize pain while doing exercises
● Act as a way to train more effectively with lower loads—as low as 20–30 percent of 1RM
Compared to high-load strength training, where 70–85 percent of 1RM is often recommended (you can work at lower levels), with BFR training, you can continue to work out effectively using lower loads. It can also boost muscle growth (hypertrophy), combat muscle loss (atrophy), and improve muscle strength and function.

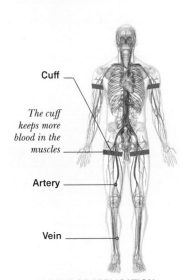

Cuff

The cuff keeps more blood in the muscles

Artery

Vein

PLACES OF APPLICATION

DESIGNING A ROUTINE

Exercising effectively but safely is key to avoiding injury. Following a routine of warming up and mobilizing your body before a strength training session sets you up for a great workout. Finishing off with a cool-down session allows your body to recover and your mind to transition back to everyday life.

5–30 SECS
STATIC STRETCHES
COULD HELP
REDUCE
MYOTENDINOUS-
RELATED INJURIES
(SEE P.178)

AN ACTIVE WARM-UP

A well-designed warm-up helps reduce the risk of injury and readies you for a training session without tiring you out.

A WARM-UP ALSO AIMS TO:

- Increase **heart rate** and **blood flow**
- Raise **body temperature**
- Activate the **nervous system**
- Prepare you for **physical work**
- Ready your mind for the **mental challenges** of focusing on exercise technique, skill acquisition, and overall coordination

MODES OF STRETCHING

Static stretching, where a pose is held for a time, is not an integral part of a warm-up; only short-duration stretches (<45 secs) don't impact strength and performance.

Dynamic stretching, where you actively move a limb from its neutral position to its end range of motion within the movement's normal plane of motion, is the most recommended type of stretching before strength training. The goal is to perform a series of smooth, controlled, and rhythmic moves for a given time or number of repetitions.

ELEMENTS OF A STRENGTH TRAINING ROUTINE

Get into good workout habits from the start. Following a structured approach to each and every workout will protect you against injury. Waking your body up and preparing it for the workout ahead is key, as is tuning in to how your body is moving during a series of mobility exercises. The length of your strength training routine will vary by the session and what your muscle priorities are that day, but always be sure to finish with a cool-down—whether passive, active, or a combination of the two.

Warm-up

Even just 5 minutes of intense physical activity can get you ready. You can choose whatever exercises you like to get your blood pumping and heart rate up combined with some dynamic stretching.

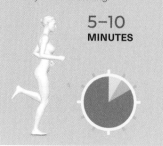

5–10
MINUTES

Mobility exercises

Now that you're warm, your body will move more easily. Maybe start with a simple neck flexion (see p.188), then work on the body areas you're targeting in your workout. Note any areas of stiffness.

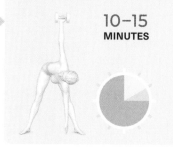

10–15
MINUTES

MOBILITY WORK

Mobility represents our body's ability to move through a particular range of motion actively before being restricted.

CHOOSING THE EXERCISES

Mobility work is a great addition to any warm-up; it allows you to see how your body moves and feels on any given day. Day to day, depending on previous workouts or stressors, your body can change in its ability to work through a given range of motion without restriction.

Mobility work is specific to getting your body ready for that day's demands. For example, if you are training your upper body, it is a good idea to perform mobility exercises that prepare your shoulders and upper body for the challenges of that day's workout. The same goes for the lower body on a lower body–focused day.

Foam rolling

You can do foam rolling before or after a workout. While bearing your weight, roll slowly on the roller until you find a tender area, then focus on that spot by rolling back and forth until you feel it soften or release. Such self-massage (or administered myofascial release) could produce short-term improvements in flexibility without decreasing muscular performance when done before a training session. Postworkout foam rolling could improve recovery by alleviating the perception of muscle pain. The physiological mechanisms are still unknown. However, there is thought to be a large placebo effect to its positive impacts, which is significant enough to give it merit.

THE COOL-DOWN

There are two types of common cool-down approaches; choose what works for you and limit it to less than 30 minutes. A passive cool-down may involve sitting rest, saunas, foam rolling, static stretching, massage, or controlled and slow rhythmic breathing. An active version comprises a series of low-intensity activities, such as swimming and walking.

A COOL-DOWN AIMS TO:

- Remove **accumulated lactate** from blood and muscle (see p.28)
- Help prevent the depression of **immune cell numbers**
- **Speed recovery** of respiratory and cardiovascular systems
- Reduce the **risk of injury**
- Improve **psychological mood**
- Help you **unwind** from the intensity of your workout

Strength training exercises

Whether you're training three, four, or five times a week, it's crucial to follow a plan for a workout to ensure you're reaping the biggest rewards possible. See the ready-made training programs (pp.201–213) if you'd like to start there; there are some suitable for beginners and other advanced versions for those who are already training.

| **LEGS** (See pp.52–53) | **CHEST** (See pp.90–91) | **BACK** (See pp.108–109) |
| **SHOULDERS** (See pp.122–123) | **ARMS** (See pp.140–141) | **ABDOMINALS** (See pp.154–155) |

Cool-down stretches

Be sure to give yourself adequate time for your heart rate to return to normal and for you to psychologically unwind from the training session. Enjoy this stretching time.

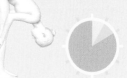

5–10 MINUTES

MOBILITY EXERCISES

As we've seen on p.187, mobility work allows you to see how your body moves and feels on any given day. The range of exercises given here start at the neck and work their way down the body through the shoulders, hips, and legs, but you can perform them in any order you like.

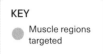
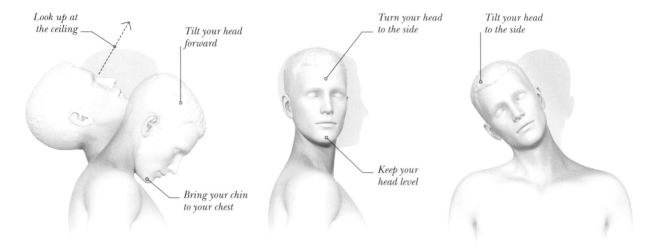

Look up at the ceiling

Tilt your head forward

Bring your chin to your chest

Turn your head to the side

Keep your head level

Tilt your head to the side

NECK **FLEXION/ EXTENSION**

Because much of our waking days are spent looking down at screens, it is important to take the neck through a guided range of motion to ensure muscles of the neck and upper back are ready for the exertion ahead.

PREPARATORY STAGE
Stand in a neutral position with your feet shoulder-width apart and your core muscles engaged.

STAGE ONE
Flex your neck to stretch the muscles of your upper back and the back of your neck—bring your chin toward your chest. Return your head to neutral.

STAGE TWO
Extend your head back to stretch the muscles of the front of the neck—look up at the ceiling. Do not force beyond comfort. Return your head to neutral. Perform 5–10 reps.

NECK **ROTATION**

Modern life limits our time spent naturally rotating our head throughout the day, with computer screens and phones as the culprits. This exercise ensures the muscles of the neck and upper back are prepared for a workout.

PREPARATORY STAGE
Stand in a neutral position with your feet shoulder-width apart and your core muscles engaged.

STAGE ONE
Rotate your head to the right, feeling a light stretch in the muscles of your neck to help work out any tightness or stiffness before training.

STAGE TWO
Return to neutral (facing front) and rotate your head to the left, feeling a light stretch in the muscles of your neck. Perform 5–10 reps on both sides.

NECK **SIDE FLEXION**

Another neck exercise completes the range of motion of the head on its axis. This easy exercise helps you avoid hurting neck and upper back muscles when you start to train (which can be common).

PREPARATORY STAGE
Stand in a neutral position with your feet shoulder-width apart and your core muscles engaged.

STAGE ONE
Flex your neck to one side, feeling a stretch in the muscles of the upper trap and neck—as if trying to put your ear on your shoulder, as far as is comfortable to do so.

STAGE TWO
Return to neutral, then flex your neck to the other side. Perform 5–10 reps on both sides.

DUMBBELL WINDMILLS

This exercise works on the mobility and stability of the shoulder, plus it's great for challenging thoracic extension and rotational mobility. Such shoulder mobility work helps prepare your upper body for the resistance it will be challenged with during a training session.

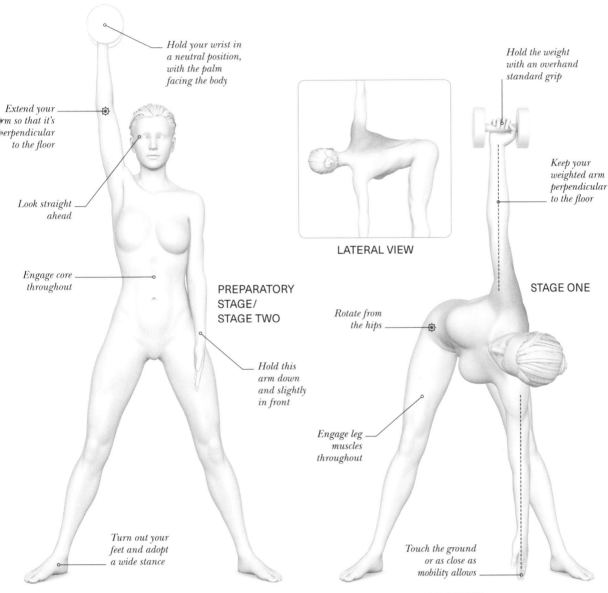

Hold your wrist in a neutral position, with the palm facing the body

Extend your arm so that it's perpendicular to the floor

Look straight ahead

Engage core throughout

PREPARATORY STAGE/ STAGE TWO

Hold this arm down and slightly in front

Turn out your feet and adopt a wide stance

LATERAL VIEW

Hold the weight with an overhand standard grip

Keep your weighted arm perpendicular to the floor

STAGE ONE

Rotate from the hips

Engage leg muscles throughout

Touch the ground or as close as mobility allows

PREPARATORY STAGE
Grab the dumbbell (or kettlebell) and raise it to shoulder height. Then raise the weight straight up above your shoulder, with your other arm straight in front.

STAGE ONE
Turn the palm of the hand holding the weight so it faces forward while simultaneously rotating your body and touching the ground with your free hand.

STAGE TWO
Rotate back to the starting position—with your working arm held upright—and repeat stages 1 and 2 for 5–10 reps. Then repeat on the other side.

DUMBBELL BOTTOMS-UP PRESS

This drill challenges the rotator cuff's role in stabilizing external resistive forces at the shoulder. Improving your overhead mobility and the amount of load you can push up from below (in a bottoms-up press) will help stabilize and strengthen muscles of the rotator cuff, and also help improve your shoulder's ability to stabilize heavy loads overhead. For the maximum challenge in this exercise, switch to a kettlebell, as the resistive forces differ from that of a dumbbell.

KEY

- Muscle regions targeted

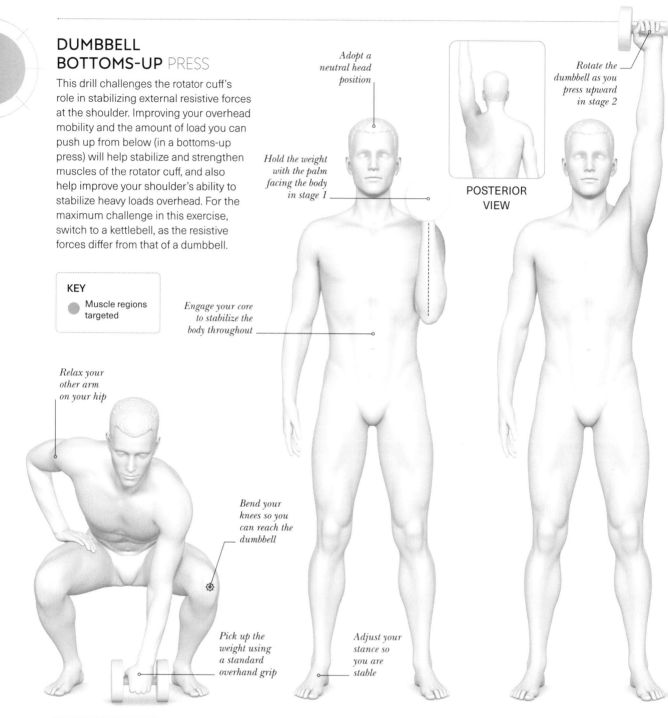

Adopt a neutral head position

Hold the weight with the palm facing the body in stage 1

Rotate the dumbbell as you press upward in stage 2

POSTERIOR VIEW

Engage your core to stabilize the body throughout

Relax your other arm on your hip

Bend your knees so you can reach the dumbbell

Pick up the weight using a standard overhand grip

Adjust your stance so you are stable

PREPARATORY STAGE
With the weight on the floor in front of you, adopt a hip-width or wider stance. Reach down and pick up the weight with one hand—you can adjust your stance once you are in the stage 1 position.

STAGE ONE
Drive up through the legs to help you raise the weight to shoulder height. Align the dumbbell with your wrist; hold your forearm perpendicular to the floor.

STAGE TWO
As you press the weight up, rotate your wrist so that your palm faces forward. Return to stage 1, then repeat stages 1 and 2 for 5–10 reps. Repeat with the other arm.

BANDED EXTERNAL ROTATION

Tasked with the role of stabilizing the shoulder, the rotator cuff is an important group of muscles in terms of maximizing mobility and stability. External rotation is a common deficit many people struggle with in their overhead pressing work. This drill helps challenge stability and strength within the external rotators of the shoulder.

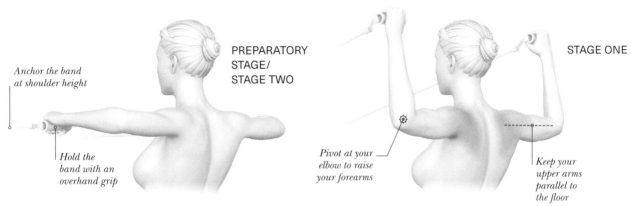

Anchor the band at shoulder height

PREPARATORY STAGE/ STAGE TWO

Hold the band with an overhand grip

STAGE ONE

Pivot at your elbow to raise your forearms

Keep your upper arms parallel to the floor

PREPARATORY STAGE
Fix a low-resistance band at shoulder height and stand with a neutral spine and shoulder-width stance. Face toward the band and flex the elbow so your upper arm is parallel to the floor.

STAGE ONE
Externally rotate at the elbow—move your forearm so that it's perpendicular to the floor, keeping your upper arm level. Keep your elbow in line with your shoulder throughout the movement.

STAGE TWO
Resist the band's tension as you allow the arm to rotate back toward a neutral position in a controlled manner. Repeat stages 1 and 2 for 5–10 reps.

INCHWORM

This mobility exercise offers a superb total body warm-up. It challenges muscle tissue crossing all major joints in the body as you walk your feet in, then walk your hands out, priming the body for your workout.

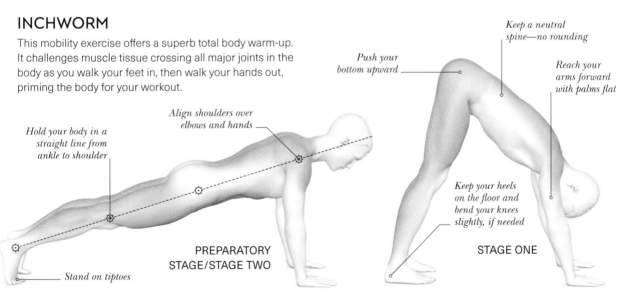

Keep a neutral spine—no rounding

Push your bottom upward

Reach your arms forward with palms flat

Align shoulders over elbows and hands

Hold your body in a straight line from ankle to shoulder

Stand on tiptoes

PREPARATORY STAGE/STAGE TWO

Keep your heels on the floor and bend your knees slightly, if needed

STAGE ONE

PREPARATORY STAGE
Start off in the push-up high plank position (see p.95). Engage your core, holding your body in a straight line, and maintain a neutral head position.

STAGE ONE
From here, inch your feet up toward your hands one foot at a time while maintaining a neutral spine and engaged core. Do not round at the back.

STAGE TWO
When you reach the final position, return to the starting position by inching your hands forward until your reach the push-up plank. Perform 5–10 reps.

SUPINE HIP **FLEXION WITH BAND**

The hip flexor muscles—most notably the psoas and rectus femoris—aid coordination of pelvic stability, alongside hip flexion. This exercise helps challenge the rectus femoris and psoas in a more contracted position, getting them activated and ready to be loaded on your lower body workouts.

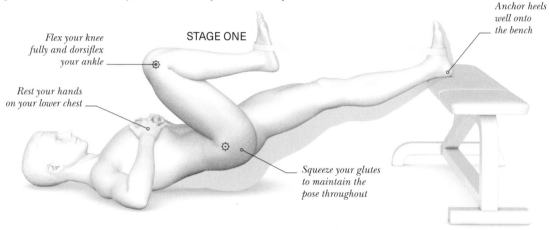

STAGE ONE

Flex your knee fully and dorsiflex your ankle

Rest your hands on your lower chest

Anchor heels well onto the bench

Squeeze your glutes to maintain the pose throughout

PREPARATORY STAGE
From a supine position with feet on the bench and a resistance band across your feet, raise your hips into a glute bridge (see p.78); keep your elbows on the floor.

STAGE ONE
While maintaining a glute bridge, flex at the hip and knee to bring the working knee up toward the body as far as it comfortably goes.

STAGE TWO
With control, extend the same leg and return your foot to the bench. Repeat on the other leg. Repeat stages 1 and 2 for 5–10 reps on each side.

90/90 **HIP STRETCH**

This exercise is effective at challenging overall hip mobility—external and internal—and acts as a "hip opener," helping combat tight or stiff hips. Having good internal and external rotation at the hip can help alleviate common pain in the hips and lower back.

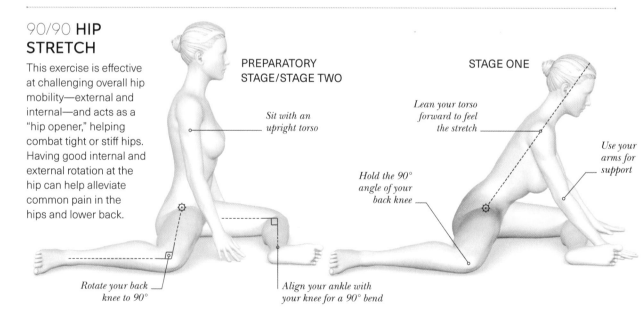

PREPARATORY STAGE/STAGE TWO

Sit with an upright torso

STAGE ONE

Lean your torso forward to feel the stretch

Use your arms for support

Hold the 90° angle of your back knee

Rotate your back knee to 90°

Align your ankle with your knee for a 90° bend

PREPARATORY STAGE
Start seated upright on the floor with both legs bent at 90°—one in front of you with knee internally rotated, the other behind you externally rotated.

STAGE ONE
Move your torso to align your belly button with your knee. Lean forward, keeping your chest high, and hold for 3–5 seconds to feel a stretch in the glutes of your lead leg.

STAGE TWO
Sit up tall to return to the starting position. Repeat stages 1 and 2 for 3–5 reps, then repeat on the other side.

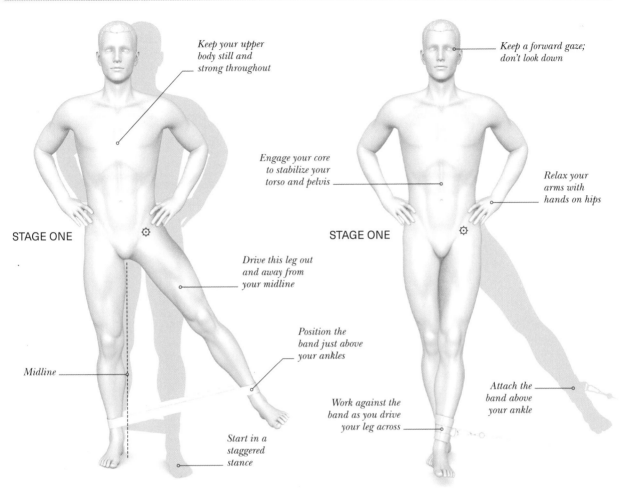

Keep your upper body still and strong throughout

Engage your core to stabilize your torso and pelvis

STAGE ONE

Drive this leg out and away from your midline

Position the band just above your ankles

Midline

Start in a staggered stance

Keep a forward gaze; don't look down

Relax your arms with hands on hips

STAGE ONE

Attach the band above your ankle

Work against the band as you drive your leg across

LEG ABDUCTION WITH BAND

This exercise helps warm up the external rotators and abductors of the hip. In a world where people sit for long periods throughout the day, it is important to maintain stability and strength within the hip abductors.

PREPARATORY STAGE
Stand within a resistance band in a staggered stance with your working leg slightly in front of the other. Stand tall with your hands resting on your hips.

STAGE ONE
Engage your core and maintain a neutral spine. Drive the working leg out and away from your midline while keeping your pelvis stable.

STAGE TWO
Return the working leg to the starting position by resisting the band tension in a controlled motion. Repeat stages 1 and 2 for 5–10 reps. You can touch the ground between reps to regain balance.

LEG ADDUCTION WITH BAND

This exercise focuses on warming up the internal rotators and adductors of the hip. The hip adductors get little use during a sedentary life, so this move complements the abduction (see left) for healthy hip stability.

PREPARATORY STAGE
Stand tall with a resistance band attached to your working leg, which is slightly in front of the other. Shift from the band's fitting to get enough resistance.

STAGE ONE
Engage your core and maintain a neutral spine. Drive the working leg in toward the midline of your body while keeping your pelvis stable.

STAGE TWO
Return the working leg to the starting position by resisting the band tension in a controlled motion. Repeat stages 1 and 2 for 5–10 reps. You can touch the ground between reps to regain balance.

COOL-DOWN STRETCHES

Cool-down stretching, also known as passive cool-down, can be part of a longer cool-down routine that includes other low-intensity dynamic activities such as swimming, cycling, and walking. The stretching component of your cool-down routine promotes relaxation and shifts your body into the "rest and digest" state, helping promote recovery and a sense of calm and well-being.

 Breathe to help recovery

Slow, controlled, rhythmic breathing helps stimulate the vagus nerve and promotes rest, relaxation, and recovery. Controlled rhythmic breathing paired with short static stretching can promote recovery and a higher sense of well-being, as well as elevating your mood. During your stretching session, aim to breathe slowly and rhythmically—around 6–10 breaths per minute—which will help you find a calm, relaxed state so that you can sink deeper into your stretches.

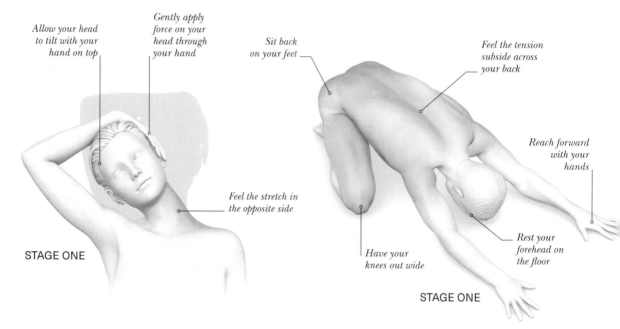

Allow your head to tilt with your hand on top

Gently apply force on your head through your hand

Feel the stretch in the opposite side

STAGE ONE

Sit back on your feet

Feel the tension subside across your back

Reach forward with your hands

Rest your forehead on the floor

Have your knees out wide

STAGE ONE

SCALENE STRETCH

During training, you can place lots of tension on the upper back (trapezius) and muscles of the neck (scalene), either directly or indirectly through stabilization. This stretch helps lengthen those muscles and reduce tension.

PREPARATORY STAGE
Stand tall. Maintain a neutral head position and reach one arm across the top of your head and place it over the top of your ear.

STAGE ONE
Gently apply force through your hand to stretch your neck, pulling on the opposite side of the head.

STAGE TWO
Return to neutral, then repeat stages 1 and 2 on the other side. On each side, hold for 5 seconds for a total of 3–5 reps.

CHILD'S POSE

This stretch, with origins in yoga, is performed as a seated pose (or asana). It is a safe way to release tension through the breath while stretching back muscles and also those surrounding joints of the hip, knee, and ankle.

PREPARATORY STAGE
Start in a table-top position (on all fours).

STAGE ONE
Shift your knees out slightly so you can sink your hips back while reaching your hands forward—stretching your back and shoulders. Focus on the breath and do your best to control your breathing as you transition into the seated back position.

STAGE TWO
Return to the starting position by raising your hips up and forward into the table-top position. Repeat for 3–5 controlled reps.

KEY

● Muscle regions targeted

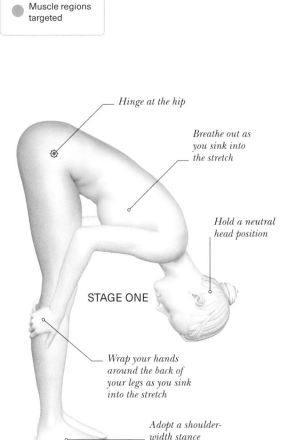

Hinge at the hip

Breathe out as you sink into the stretch

Hold a neutral head position

STAGE ONE

Wrap your hands around the back of your legs as you sink into the stretch

Adopt a shoulder-width stance

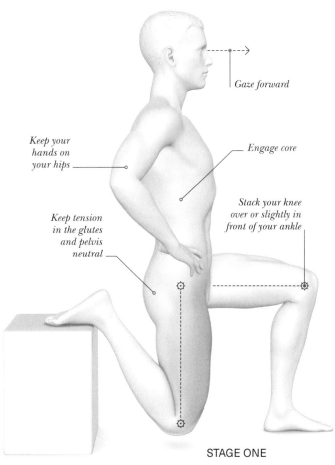

Gaze forward

Keep your hands on your hips

Engage core

Stack your knee over or slightly in front of your ankle

Keep tension in the glutes and pelvis neutral

STAGE ONE

FORWARD FOLD

Another yoga-inspired stretch, the forward fold is a standing pose (asana) that is easy to match to your own limitations or needs. This excellent stretch relieves tension in the lower back and hips.

PREPARATORY STAGE
Stand tall with your feet shoulder-width apart.

STAGE ONE
Flex at the hips, bending your torso over toward 45°. Keep your core engaged and spine neutral with maybe a slight rounding at the upper back. Feel a light to moderate stretch in the lower back, hamstrings, and glutes.

STAGE TWO
Control your breathing, exhaling on the way down and inhaling on the way up. Perform 3–5 reps, holding each stretch for 5–10 seconds.

QUAD STRETCH

Also known as the "couch stretch," this cool-down stretch helps relieve tension and works on a limited range of motion in the hip flexors. This stretch helps mobilize and stabilize the muscles surrounding the pelvis.

PREPARATORY STAGE
Stand tall with a block about 24 in (60 cm) high positioned behind one leg. Place your foot on top of the block.

STAGE ONE
Drop your elevated back knee toward the floor, keeping the same leg's thigh perpendicular to the floor. As you descend, feel the stretch down the quadriceps muscle of the working leg.

STAGE TWO
Return to the upright pose, then complete 3–5 controlled reps. Repeat on the other leg.

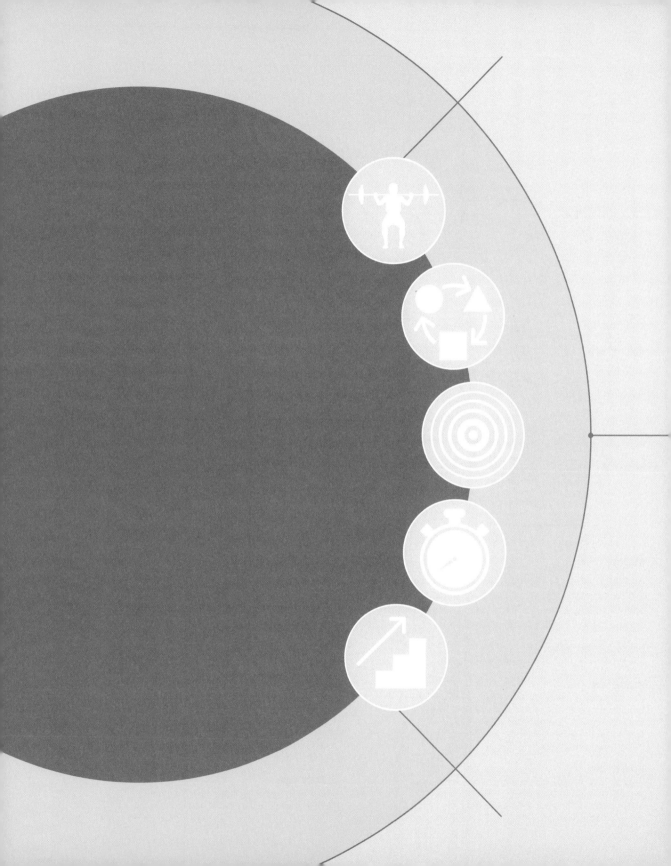

HOW TO TRAIN

One of the most challenging parts of strength training is understanding how to take a grouping of exercises and turn them into a well-structured program to achieve your goals. This section dives right into the most important training principles—how to implement and progress them—with examples of putting it all together to build muscle, strength, and endurance.

VARIABLES WITHIN STRENGTH TRAINING

The training programs in this book are built around the following key variables: training volume, training intensity, exercise selection, and fatigue management. In addition, the programs are organized by difficulty and by frequency, so you can choose a session based on your experience level and how much time out of your week you can dedicate to training.

TRAINING **VOLUME**

Volume refers to the amount of exercise performed over a given period of time, usually a training session or week of training. It is often represented by the number of reps for a given number of sets at a given load (weight).

As you gain experience, you can further adjust volume by altering the specific exercises you select, their range of motion and resistance profile (at what point in the rep the movement is hardest), and the tempo and rest periods used.

Total weekly volume

Each training week will be measured by the amount of training volume performed per muscle group.

EXAMPLE

If you perform 4 sets of chest exercises per workout and you work out 3 times per week, then you will perform 12 total sets of chest exercises. This is your total weekly volume for chest workouts.

4x sets x @ 3x per week
= **12x sets** per week for specific body part

Training volume by training program

Training can be geared toward building muscle, increasing strength endurance, or increasing strength; training volume will vary depending on which of these three is the end goal of training. Volume can be progressed by adding reps or load or by adding a set.

Muscle building	Strength	Strength endurance
Focus on gradually increasing total training volume by load, reps, or sets (see above). The goal is to increase the total volume week-on-week for the target muscle group.	Focus on volume of intensity per training session or training week. The goal is to work up to higher relative intensities (% of 1RM; see right) to train the nervous system.	Focus on the density of work—the amount of work performed in a given amount of time. The goal is to increase the total density per session so you do more work in the same time.

TRAINING INTENSITY

Intensity of load is expressed as a percentage of the maximum weight you can support in one rep of an exercise (known as 1 rep maximum or 1RM).

Training load will dictate how many reps you can do in a set. Higher intensity most often correlates with lower reps (6 or fewer), moderate loads with moderate reps (6–12), and lower loads with higher reps (12–20 or more). When your goal is to build strength, lower rep ranges are best to maximize intensity. For muscle building, use moderate intensity, and for strength endurance, lighter intensity.

Low reps	Moderate reps	High reps
1–6	6–12	12+
Best for building strength	Best for building muscle	Best for building endurance

← **STRENGTH–ENDURANCE CONTINUUM** →

EXERCISE **SELECTION**

Each exercise trains a muscle at a specific part of its range of motion. Different exercises can also challenge a muscle more eccentrically or concentrically (see pp.12–13).

For example, a back squat challenges the lengthened range of the quadriceps, whereas a leg extension targets their mid-shortened range, even with the same load and rep number. Different machines also challenge muscles differently. It's important to find exercises that work for your skill level, structure, and mechanics.

RANGE OF MOTION

The contribution of muscles changes depending on joint angle and exercise. At each point along the range of motion, different parts of a muscle will be under demand; this is why it is important to use the full range of motion possible within your exercise technique, keeping in mind your individual limitations.

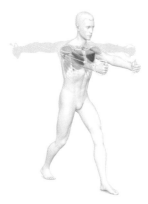

TRAINING TARGET MUSCLES
Consider your abilities when choosing exercises; for instance, adjusting the cable height in a chest fly may allow you to better rotate your shoulders.

FATIGUE MANAGEMENT

Managing fatigue is crucial for maximizing muscle growth and strength, as well as lowering your risk of injury.

PROXIMITY TO FAILURE

This research-based approach to managing fatigue uses a number, often given on a 1–10 scale (see right), to represent "reps in reserve" (RIR): how many reps you have "left in the tank" on a given set. It correlates with your rate of perceived exertion (RPE).

AUTOREGULATION

This refers to the concept of adjusting your training based on the feel of the load on any given day, such as by making a session easier if you feel particularly fatigued. An individualized approach will keep you motivated and prevent injury.

DELOAD

A deload is a light week or back-off week during which you train at the minimum volume needed to maintain muscle or strength to facilitate recovery and muscle repair. The harder you have trained, the longer the deload you will need before you can return to or build on that level. Every fifth week is an ideal time in a training schedule for a deload. Beginners should reduce loads by around 10–20 percent for this week, while those at a more advanced level should reduce set volume by around 30–50 percent of where it peaked over the previous weeks of training, as well as reducing RIR by 2 points.

RIR-based RPE scale

SCORE	DESCRIPTION
10	Maximal effort
9.5	No RIR, but could increase load
9	1 RIR
8.5	Definitely 1, maybe 2 RIR
8	2 RIR
7.5	Definitely 2, maybe 3 RIR
7	3 RIR
5-6	4-6 RIR
3-4	Light effort
1-2	Little to no effort

The importance of rest

Rest is time between sets of an exercise, which is crucial for recovery. In advanced training programs, the amount of rest taken should vary from 15 seconds up to 5 minutes, depending on your training goal (see right) and according to intensity, set duration, and training experience. Beginners to strength training may want to use the higher end of the range to ensure training response is appropriately managed.

00:15–1:00
strength endurance

00:30–3:00
muscle building

2:00–5:00
strength

» TRAINING **FREQUENCY**

Training frequency represents how many times in a training week you are training a given muscle group (see the example on p.198).

As you need to reach a determined training volume per muscle group per week to gain muscle or strength, training more days per week allows you to vary the work.

TRAINING MORE OFTEN
You can train each muscle group more frequently and with fewer sets per day.

TRAINING LESS OFTEN
You can have more days of recovery between sessions for a specific muscle group but more sets for that muscle group per session.

As well as manipulating training frequency, you can also simply manipulate training volume per session by adding reps, load, or sets (see also below) to your current program. Understand that everything you add increases the total stress of that training session.

TRAINING **PROGRESSION**

Progressive overload is defined as the proactive addition of stress or stimulus (in the form of sets, reps, or load) over time (see also graphs, opposite) used to help your training progress.

Being able to do more reps of a given weight or lift heavier loads confirms that overload has occurred. There are several factors you can change in order to ensure your training progresses over time.

ADDING REPS AND LOAD
A repetition, or rep, is one complete motion, eccentric and concentric, of an exercise. Adding reps or extra weight are good ways to progress your training, by increasing the amount of tension placed on the

target muscle(s). The more tension, the more muscle tissue is active, both from a contractile and a metabolic perspective.

ADDING SETS
A popular way to progress your training volume or intensity is to add whole sets into the workout. A higher volume provides an increased ability to boost muscle growth, but only to a point; if you exceed your maximum recoverable threshold, you will only see diminishing returns.

PROGRESSIVE REPS IN RESERVE (RIR)
Monitoring your RIR focuses on increasing the overall fatigue in a program by raising the total

work intensity. Keeping a number of RIR helps manage fatigue and ensures consistency in performance (see also Fatigue management, p.199).

RECOVERY
Recovery is one of the most important variables of training. Because strength training breaks down muscle fibers (see pp.18–21), maximizing recovery time helps your body repair itself to build muscle, strength, and endurance. Without adequate recovery, your training performance will suffer and you will not be able to properly adapt to your training. This is why rest days are so important, alongside good-quality sleep, nutrition, and stress management.

Progressive overload

ADDING REPS AND LOAD	ADDING SETS	PROGRESSIVE RIR	RECOVERY
If you reach a plateau adding weight or reps to your sets, boost volume by adding entire extra sets.	The productive volume range is somewhere between 10 and 18 sets per week for most people.	Beginners should stay 2–4 reps shy of failure; advanced trainees can reduce RIR by 1 point per week.	Schedule rest days into your program to avoid your training performance suffering.

THE **TRAINING PROGRAMS**

Training sessions are governed by training split—how you choose to organize your training week and sessions. There are three programs aimed at a beginner and three at an advanced level, with options to train more or less often.

TRAINING **SPLIT**

Based on your experience level, training goal, and available training time, you can choose from workouts 3x, 4x, or 5x a week, varying between beginner and advanced programs. Find the program that matches your goal—muscle building, strength endurance, or strength.

- **3x per week**—this is a **full body training split**, best distributing the volume between muscle groups throughout the training week. It focuses on major muscle groups and multijoint, integrated exercises to place tension on smaller muscle groups, such as the shoulders.

- **4x per week**—this is a **half body training split**. With the added training day, you can split the training volume up per muscle group, allowing for more volume per muscle group in each session.

- **5x per week**—this will be a **one-third body training split**. Each day trains about one-third of the body, placing more volume per muscle group per workout with less weekly training frequency per muscle group.

ADJUSTING TRAINING VOLUME WITHIN PROGRAMS

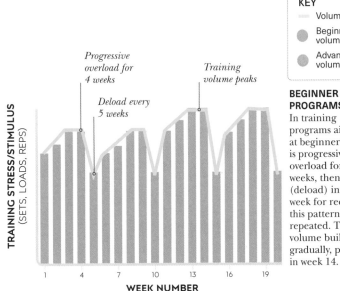

KEY
- Volume trend
- Beginner volume
- Advanced volume

BEGINNER PROGRAMS

In training programs aimed at beginners, there is progressive overload for four weeks, then a drop (deload) in the fifth week for recovery; this pattern is then repeated. Training volume builds gradually, peaking in week 14.

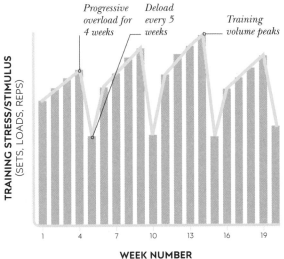

ADVANCED PROGRAMS

Advanced training follows the same pattern as above, but with higher training volume throughout; increase in volume week-on-week is also greater, allowing for more progressive overload. In weeks 16–19, the amount of stress dips back down to facilitate recovery.

MUSCLE BUILDING BEGINNER

Training to build muscle via the process of hypertrophy (see p.18) is rooted in performing high-quality repetitions for a certain amount of volume at a certain level of intensity or proximity to failure (see p.199).

Training all the way to failure on every set is not productive long term. Instead, aim to train to near failure on each set, using the rate of perceived exertion (RPE) scale on p.199 to gauge your reps in reserve (RIR). Training within 4–5 reps of failure has been shown to contribute enough stimulus to promote muscle growth.

Begin each workout by warming up (see p.186). Where indicated, you can choose a variation of the given exercise according to your preference and situation.

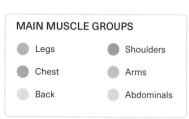

MAIN MUSCLE GROUPS

- Legs
- Chest
- Back
- Shoulders
- Arms
- Abdominals

For all workouts

Any beginner muscle-building workout uses the following reps, sets, rest between sets, RIR, and tempo guidance however often you're training:

8–10 REPS
4 SETS
60–90 SECONDS REST
3–4 RIR
CONTROLLED TEMPO

Guidance on tempo

Tempo is the rhythm with which you perform each rep. "Controlled" tempo means the pace should be monitored with each rep: complete the eccentric phase with a controlled 2–3-second count and the concentric with a 1-second count to maintain proper technique and tension on the muscle.

MUSCLE BUILDING—3x PER WEEK

	EXERCISE
WORKOUT 1	Barbell back squat or variation (pp.54–57)
	Leg curl (seated or lying) (pp.68–70)
	Dumbbell bench press (p.96) or Push-up (p.95)
	Wide-grip vertical pulldown (p.110) or Pull-up (p.113)
	Dumbbell shoulder press (p.127)
	Front plank with rotation (p.156)
WORKOUT 2	Barbell bench press or variation (pp.92–95)
	Romanian deadlift (p.89)
	Neutral-grip horizontal row (p.114)
	Machine or dumbbell shoulder press (pp.126–127)
	Leg extension or variation (pp.74–77)
	TVA ball crunch (p.160) or Cat–cow kneeling crunch (p.162)
WORKOUT 3	Traditional deadlift (p.86) or Step up with dumbbells (p.66)
	Neutral-grip vertical pulldown (p.112) or Chin-up (p.113)
	Mid-cable chest fly (p.103) or Machine chest fly (p.104)
	Leg curl (seated or lying) (pp.68–70)
	Machine or dumbbell shoulder press (pp.126–127)
	Cable rotational oblique twist (p.168)

MUSCLE BUILDING—5x PER WEEK

	EXERCISE
WORKOUT 1	Incline barbell bench press or variation (pp.94–95)
	Neutral-grip vertical pulldown (p.112)
	Prone bench rear deltoid raise (p.138)
	Dumbbell biceps curl (p.142)
	Rope triceps pushdown (p.150) or Close-grip barbell bench press (p.94)
	Cable rope crunch (p.166)
WORKOUT 2	Romanian deadlift (p.89)
	Hack squat (p.60)
	Dumbbell glute bridge or variation (pp.80–81)
	Leg extension (p.74)
	Calf raise (p.82)
WORKOUT 3	Dumbbell shoulder press or variation (pp.126–127)
	Dumbbell lateral raise or variation (pp.128–131)
	Banded biceps curl (p.144)
	Cross-cable triceps pressdown (p.153)
	Cable rotational oblique twist (p.168)
	Decline abdominal crunch (p.167)
WORKOUT 4	Neutral-grip horizontal row (p.114)
	Wide-grip vertical pulldown (p.110)
	Dumbbell bench press (p.96) or Push-up (p.95)
	Dumbbell bent-over row (p.116)
	Chest or back exercise of choice
WORKOUT 5	Leg press (p.58) or Dumbbell squat (p.56)
	Leg extension or variation (pp.74–77)
	Leg curl (seated or lying) (pp.68–70)
	Dumbbell glute bridge or variation (pp.80–81)
	Prone bench rear deltoid raise (p.138)
	Dumbbell lateral raise or variation (pp.128–131)

MUSCLE BUILDING—4x PER WEEK

	EXERCISE
WORKOUT 1	Barbell bench press or variation (pp.92–95)
	Leg press (p.58)
	Rope triceps pushdown or variation (p.150–153)
	Dumbbell lateral raise or variation (pp.128–131)
	Cable rope crunch (p.166)
WORKOUT 2	Neutral-grip vertical pulldown or Chin-up (pp.112–113)
	Leg curl or variation (pp.68–71)
	Dumbbell glute bridge or variation (pp.80–81)
	Dumbbell biceps curl or variation (pp.142–145)
	Leg extension or variation (pp.74–77)
WORKOUT 3	Calf raise (p.82)
	High–low cable chest fly or variation (pp.100–103)
	Dumbbell triceps extension or variation (pp.146–149)
	Dumbbell shoulder press or variation (pp.126–127)
	Cable rotational oblique twist (p.168)
WORKOUT 4	Neutral-grip horizontal row (p.114)
	Romanian deadlift (p.89)
	Dumbbell glute bridge or variation (pp.80–81)
	Banded biceps curl (p.144)
	Seated calf raise (p.84)

203

MUSCLE BUILDING ADVANCED

In these advanced muscle-building programs, the progression is mostly achieved through increasing training volume and expanding exercise selection.

A wider variety of exercises appear in these advanced training programs compared to the beginner workouts,

and volume is upped to increase the metabolic stress and tension placed on muscles. As with beginner programs, you should aim to train to near failure on each set by gauging your RIR or RPE (see p.199). Pay attention to the tempo, or rhythm, required for each exercise (see below left).

MAIN MUSCLE GROUPS

- Legs
- Shoulders
- Chest
- Arms
- Back
- Abdominals

For all workouts

Any advanced muscle-building workout uses the following rest between sets and RIR however often you're training:

60–90 SECONDS REST
2–3 RIR

Guidance on tempo

In more advanced programs, tempo is expressed as a ratio of four numbers that correspond to the duration, in seconds, of each stage in a rep: eccentric contraction, rest at the bottom of the rep, concentric contraction, and rest at the top of the rep. A tempo of 3011, for instance, requires a controlled 3-second count during eccentric contraction (such as descending in a squat), 0 seconds of rest at the bottom of the rep, a controlled 1-second count of concentric contraction (such as rising explosively from a squat), and 1 second of hold at the top of the rep, where you contract the target muscle. Other common tempos used in the training programs in this book are 3010 and 3110.

FOR GUIDANCE ON SUPERSETS SEE P.212

Superset pairings are indicated by blue and between bold lines

MUSCLE BUILDING—3x PER WEEK

	EXERCISE	SETS	REPS	TEMPO
WORKOUT 1	Barbell back squat (p.54) or Leg press (p.58)	4	6–8	3010
	Leg curl (seated or lying) (pp.68–70)	4	6–8	3010
	DB bench press (p.96) or Barbell bench press (p.92)	4	6–8	3010
	Wide-grip vertical pulldown (p.110) or Pull-up (p.113)	4	6–8	3010
	DB shoulder press (p.127)	4	6–8	3010
	Front plank with rotation (p.156)	4	6–8	Controlled
WORKOUT 2	Barbell bench press (p.92) or DB bench press (p.96)	4	6–8	3010
	Romanian deadlift (p.89)	4	6–8	3010
	Neutral-grip horizontal row (p.114)	4	6–8	3010
	Machine or DB shoulder press (pp.126–127)	4	6–8	3010
	Leg extension (p.74)	4	6–8	3010
	TVA ball crunch or variation (pp.160–163)	4	6–8	Controlled
WORKOUT 3	Traditional deadlift or variation (pp.86–89)	4	8–10	2010
	Neutral-grip vertical pulldown or Chin-up (pp.112–113)	4	8–10	3010
	Mid-cable chest fly (p.103) or Machine chest fly (p.104)	4	8–10	3010
	Leg curl (seated or lying) (pp.68–70)	4	8–10	3010
	Machine shoulder press (p.126) or Front delt shoulder press (p.135)	4	8–10	3010
	Cable rotational oblique twist (p.168)	4	8–10	Controlled

MUSCLE BUILDING—4x PER WEEK

	EXERCISE	SETS	REPS	TEMPO
WORKOUT 1	DB bench press or var. (pp.96–99)	4	6–8	3110
	Barbell back squat (p.54) or Leg press (p.58)	5	6–8	3010
	Cross-cable triceps pressdown (p.153)	4	8–10	3011
	High–low cable chest fly (p.100)	4	8–10	3011
	DB lateral raise or var. (pp.128–131)	4	8–10	3010
	DB triceps extension or variation (pp.146–149)	4	8–10	3010
	Cable rope crunch (p.166)	5	8–10	Controlled
WORKOUT 2	Neutral-grip vertical pulldown or Chin-up (pp.112–113)	4	6–8	3010
	Lying leg curl or var. (pp.68–71)	5	6–8	3011
	Barbell glute bridge or variation (pp.78–81)	4	6–8	3011
	Machine biceps curl (p.144)	4	6–8	3011
	DB biceps curl or var. (pp.142–145)	4	8–10	3011
	DB bent-over row (p.116)	4	8–10	3010
	Calf raise or variation (p.82–85)	5	8–10	Controlled
WORKOUT 3	Leg extension or var. (pp.74–77)	5	8–10	3011
	Mid-cable chest fly (p.103)	4	8–10	3010
	DB triceps extension or variation (pp.146–149)	4	8–10	3110
	Barbell overhead shoulder press or variation (pp.124–127)	4	8–10	3010
	DB lateral raise or var. (pp.128–131)	4	8–10	3010
	Cable rotational oblique twist (p.168)	5	6–8	Controlled
WORKOUT 4	Neutral-grip horizontal row (p.114)	4	6–8	3010
	Romanian deadlift (p.89)	5	6–8	3010
	Barbell glute bridge or variation (pp.78–81)	4	6–8	3011
	Banded biceps curl (p.144)	4	8–10	3011
	Seated calf raise (p.84)	5	8–10	3011

MUSCLE BUILDING—5x PER WEEK

	EXERCISE	SETS	REPS	TEMPO
WORKOUT 1	Incline DB bench press or var. (p.98)	4	6–8	3110
	Neutral-grip vertical pulldown (p.112)	4	6–8	3010
	DB rear delt fly (p.136)	4	8–10	3011
	DB chest fly (p.106)	4	8–10	3010
	DB biceps curl (p.142)	4	8–10	3011
	Rope triceps pushdown (p.150)	4	8–10	3011
	Face-away standing crunch (p.166)	4	8–10	Controlled
WORKOUT 2	Romanian deadlift (p.89)	4	6–8	3010
	Hack squat (p.60)	3	8–10	3110
	Barbell glute bridge or variation (pp.78–81)	4	8–10	3011
	Leg curl (p.68)	4	8–10	3011
	Leg extension (p.74)	3	8–10	3011
	Calf raise (p.82) or Leg press calf raise (p.85)	4	8–10	3011
WORKOUT 3	Machine or DB shoulder press (p.126–127)	4	6–8	3110
	DB lateral raise or var. (pp.128–129)	4	8–10	3010
	DB front raise or var. (pp.132–135)	4	8–10	3011
	Banded biceps curl (p.144)	4	8–10	3011
	DB rear delt fly or var. (pp.136–139)	4	8–10	3011
	Cross-cable triceps pressdown (p.153)	4	8–10	3011
	Side plank with rotation (p.158)	4	8–10	Controlled
	Stir-the-pot Swiss ball (p.162)	4	8–10	Controlled
WORKOUT 4	Neutral-grip horizontal row (p.114)	4	6–8	3010
	Vertical pulldown (p.110)	4	8–10	3011
	DB bench press (p.96) or Push-up (p.95)	3	8–10	3110
	Low–high cable chest fly (p.103)	3	8–10	3011
	DB trap shrug (p.118)	4	8–10	3010
	Chest or back exercise of choice	4	8–10	Controlled
WORKOUT 5	Barbell back squat (p.54) or Hack squat (p.60)	4	8–10	3110
	Leg extension or var. (pp.74–77)	4	8–10	3011
	Leg curl (seated or lying) (pp.68–70)	4	8–10	3010
	DB glute bridge or var. (pp.80–81)	4	8–10	3011
	Prone bench rear delt raise (p.138)	4	8–10	3011
	DB lateral raise or var. (pp.128–131)	4	10–12	3010
	Cable rope crunch (p.166) or Hanging knee raise (p.164)	4	8–10	Controlled

STRENGTH BEGINNER

Training with the goal of building muscular strength requires high-intensity (high-load) training paired with lower rep ranges and longer rest periods.

In strength-specific programs, the intent is to use the muscle mass you have to generate contractile force and to train your nervous system, allowing it to recruit and activate muscles to generate force more intensively

and efficiently (see p.38). Training for strength is also an expression of skill and coordination.

In these programs, you should complete the main exercise with the goal of increasing the load used with each set. Use warm-up sets on main exercises as needed to ready your body for heavier loads. Where indicated, you can choose a variation of the given exercise according to your preference and situation.

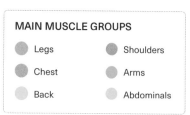

MAIN MUSCLE GROUPS

- Legs
- Chest
- Back
- Shoulders
- Arms
- Abdominals

For all workouts

Any beginner strength workout uses the following reps, sets, rest between sets, RIR, and tempo guidance however often you're training:

CONTROLLED TEMPO

1 MINUTE REST for exercises with
2 SETS and **2–3** MINUTES REST
for others, except for those
marked *, which should have
2–5 MINUTES REST

STRENGTH—3x PER WEEK

EXERCISE	SETS	REPS	RIR
WORKOUT 1			
Machine horizontal row (p.116)	2	6–8	3–4
Machine shoulder press (p.126)	2	6–8	3–4
Barbell bench press (p.92) or DB bench press (p.96) *	5	5	2–3
Barbell overhead shoulder press (p.124) or DB shoulder press (p.127)	3	6	2–3
Cross-cable triceps pressdown or variation (pp.152–153)	3	6	2–3
WORKOUT 2			
Calf raise (p.82)	2	6–8	3–4
DB glute bridge (p.80)	2	6–8	3–4
Barbell back squat (p.54) or Hack squat (p.60) *	5	5	2–3
Leg press (p.58)	3	6	2–3
Seated calf raise (p.84)	3	6	2–3
WORKOUT 3			
Calf raise (p.82)	2	6–8	3–4
DB glute bridge (p.80)	2	6–8	3–4
Barbell bent-over row (p.117) or Machine horizontal row (p.116) *	5	5	2–3
Neutral-grip vertical pulldown (p.112)	3	6	2–3
DB biceps curl (p.142) or Machine biceps curl (p.144)	3	6	2–3

STRENGTH—4x PER WEEK

	EXERCISE	SETS	REPS	RIR
WORKOUT 1	Calf raise (p.82)	2	6–8	3–4
	DB glute bridge (p.80)	2	6–8	3–4
	Barbell back squat (p.54) or Hack squat (p.60) *	5	5	2–3
	Leg press (p.58)	3	6	2–3
	Leg extension (p.74)	3	6	2–3
	Seated calf raise (p.84)	3	6	2–3
WORKOUT 2	Machine horizontal row (p.116)	2	6–8	3–4
	Machine shoulder press (p.126)	2	6–8	3–4
	Barbell bench press (p.92) or DB bench press (p.96) *	5	5	2–3
	Barbell overhead shoulder press (p.124) or DB shoulder press (p.127)	3	6	2–3
	Mid-cable chest fly (p.103) or DB lateral raise (p.128)	3	6	2–3
	Cross-cable triceps pressdown or variation (pp.152–153)	3	6	2–3
WORKOUT 3	Calf raise (p.82)	2	6–8	3–4
	Walking lunge with DBs (p.65)	2	6–8	3–4
	Romanian deadlift (p.89) *	5	5	2–3
	Leg curl (seated or lying) (pp.68–70)	3	6	2–3
	Barbell glute bridge or variation (pp.78–81)	3	6	2–3
	Calf raise (p.82)	3	6	2–3
WORKOUT 4	Banded biceps curl (p.144)	2	6–8	3–4
	Wide-grip vertical pulldown (p.110)	2	6–8	3–4
	Barbell bent-over row (p.117) or Machine horizontal row (p.116) *	5	5	2–3
	Neutral-grip vertical pulldown (p.112)	3	6	2–3
	Prone bench rear delt raise (p.138)	3	6	2–3
	DB biceps curl (p.142) or Machine biceps curl (p.144)	3	6	2–3

STRENGTH—5x PER WEEK

	EXERCISE	SETS	REPS	RIR
WORKOUT 1	Calf raise (p.82)	2	6–8	3–4
	DB glute bridge (p.80)	2	6–8	3–4
	Barbell back squat (p.54) or Hack squat (p.60) *	5	5	2–3
	Leg press (p.58)	3	6	2–3
	Leg extension (p.74)	3	6	2–3
	Seated calf raise (p.84)	3	6	2–3
WORKOUT 2	Machine horizontal row (p.116)	2	6–8	3–4
	Machine shoulder press (p.126)	2	6–8	3–4
	Barbell bench press (p.92) or DB bench press (p.96)	5	5	2–3
	Barbell overhead shoulder press (p.124) or DB shoulder press (p.127)	3	6	2–3
	Mid-cable chest fly (p.103) or DB lateral raise (p.128)	3	6	2–3
	Cross-cable triceps pressdown or variation (pp.152–153)	3	6	2–3
WORKOUT 3	Calf raise (p.82)	2	6–8	3–4
	Walking lunge with DBs (p.65)	2	6–8	3–4
	Romanian deadlift (p.89) *	5	5	2–3
	Leg curl (seated or lying) (pp.68–70)	3	6	2–3
	Barbell glute bridge or var. (pp.78–81)	3	6	2–3
	Calf raise (p.82)	3	6	2–3
WORKOUT 4	Banded biceps curl (p.144)	2	6–8	3–4
	Wide-grip vertical pulldown (p.110)	2	6–8	3–4
	Barbell bent-over row (p.117) or Machine horizontal row (p.116) *	5	5	2–3
	Neutral-grip vertical pulldown (p.112)	3	6	2–3
	Prone bench rear delt raise (p.138)	3	6	2–3
	DB biceps curl (p.142) or Machine biceps curl (p.144)	3	6	2–3
WORKOUT 5	Machine horizontal row (p.116)	2	6–8	3–4
	Machine shoulder press (p.126)	2	6–8	3–4
	Incline DB bench press (p.98) or Mid-cable chest fly (p.103) *	3	6–8	2–5
	DB or Machine shoulder press (pp.126–127)	3	6–8	2–3
	DB lateral raise (p.128)	3	6–8	2–3
	Rope triceps pushdown or variation (pp.150–153)	3	6–8	2–3

STRENGTH ADVANCED

These advanced strength-focused programs achieve progression through increasing training volume and expanding exercise selection.

Building strength at a more advanced level is achieved primarily through upping the load used—as with the beginner programs, you should aim to ascend load with each set working up to peak intensity on the last set of each exercise within each workout. Again, use warm-up sets as needed on main exercises to acclimatize to heavier loads.

MAIN MUSCLE GROUPS

- Legs
- Chest
- Back
- Shoulders
- Arms
- Abdominals

For all workouts

Any advanced muscle-building workout uses the following rest between sets and RIR however often you're training:

60 SECONDS Rest for exercises with 2 sets, **2–3 MINUTES REST** for those with 4 sets, and **2–5 MINUTES** for those with **5 SETS**

FOR GUIDANCE ON TEMPO SEE P.202 AND P.204

 Biasing muscle groups

Many of us have particular muscle groups that we wish to improve. Once you have built a solid foundational base of muscle and strength, you can start to bias training volume toward your target muscle groups by increasing the number of sets you dedicate to them in each training week. Watch out that you don't overshoot your limits: if you add something for your goal muscle group(s), reduce volume on another body part to compensate.

STRENGTH—3x PER WEEK

	EXERCISE	SETS	REPS	RIR	TEMPO
WORKOUT 1	Machine horizontal row (p.116)	2	6–8	3–4	Controlled
	Machine shoulder press (p.126)	2	6–8	3–4	Controlled
	Barbell bench press (p.92) or DB bench press (p.96)	5	5	2	3110
	Barbell overhead shoulder press or DB shoulder press (pp.124–127)	4	6	2	3110
	Cross-cable triceps pressdown (p.153)	4	6	2	3110
WORKOUT 2	Calf raise (p.82)	2	6–8	3–4	Controlled
	DB glute bridge (p.80)	2	6–8	3–4	Controlled
	Barbell back squat (p.54) or Hack squat (p.60)	5	5	2	3110
	Leg press (p.58)	4	6	2	3110
	Seated calf raise (p.84)	4	6	2	3110
WORKOUT 3	Banded biceps curl (p.144)	2	6–8	3–4	Controlled
	Wide-grip vertical pulldown (p.110)	2	6–8	3–4	Controlled
	Barbell bent-over row or Machine horizontal row (pp.116–117)	5	5	2	3110
	Neutral-grip vertical pulldown (p.112)	4	6	2	3110
	DB biceps curl or Machine biceps curl (pp.142–144)	4	6	2	3010

STRENGTH

ADVANCED

STRENGTH BUILDING—4x PER WEEK

	EXERCISE	SETS	REPS	RIR	TEMPO
WORKOUT 1	Calf raise (p.82)	2	6–8	3–4	Controlled
	DB glute bridge (p.80)	2	6–8	3–4	Controlled
	Barbell back squat (p.54) or Hack squat (p.60)	5	5	2	3110
	Leg press (p.58) or Trap bar deadlift (p.88)	4	6	2	3110
	Leg extension (p.74)	4	6	2	3010
	Seated calf raise (p.84)	4	6	2	3110
WORKOUT 2	Machine horizontal row (p.116)	2	6–8	3–4	Controlled
	Machine shoulder press (p.126)	2	6–8	3–4	Controlled
	Barbell (p.92) or DB bench press (p.96)	5	5	2	3110
	Barbell overhead press or DB shoulder press (pp.124–127)	4	6	2	3110
	Mid-cable chest fly (p.103) or DB lateral raise (p.128)	4	6	2	3010
	Cross-cable triceps pressdown (p.153)	4	6	2	3110
WORKOUT 3	Calf raise (p.82)	2	6–8	3–4	Controlled
	Walking lunge with DBs (p.65)	2	6–8	3–4	Controlled
	Romanian deadlift (p.89)	5	5	2	3110
	Leg curl (seated or lying) (pp.68–70)	4	6	2	3110
	Barbell glute bridge or variation (pp.78–81)	4	6	2	3010
	Calf raise (p.82)	4	6	2	3110
WORKOUT 4	Banded biceps curl (p.144)	2	6–8	3–4	Controlled
	Wide-grip vertical pulldown (p.110)	2	6–8	3–4	Controlled
	Barbell bent-over or Machine horizontal row (pp.116–117)	5	5	2	3110
	Neutral-grip vertical pulldown (p.112)	4	6	2	3110
	Prone bench rear delt raise (p.138)	4	6	2	3010
	DB biceps curl or Machine biceps curl (pp.142–144)	4	6	2	3110

STRENGTH—5x PER WEEK

	EXERCISE	SETS	REPS	RIR	TEMPO
WORKOUT 1	Calf raise (p.82)	2	6–8	3–4	Controlled
	DB glute bridge (p.80)	2	6–8	3–4	Controlled
	Barbell back squat (p.54) or Hack squat (p.60)	5	5	2	3110
	Leg press (p.58) or Trap bar deadlift (p.88)	4	6	2	3110
	Leg extension (p.74)	4	6	2	3010
	Seated calf raise (p.84)	4	6	2	3110
WORKOUT 2	Machine horizontal row (p.116)	2	6–8	3–4	Controlled
	Machine shoulder press (p.126)	2	6–8	3–4	Controlled
	Barbell bench press (p.92) or DB bench press (p.96)	5	5	2	3110
	Barbell overhead press or DB shoulder press (pp.124–127)	4	6	2	3110
	Mid-cable chest fly (p.103) or DB lateral raise (p.128)	4	6	2	3010
	Cross-cable triceps press-down or var. (pp.152–153)	4	6	2	3110
WORKOUT 3	Calf raise (p.82)	2	6–8	3–4	Controlled
	Walking lunge with DBs (p.65)	2	6–8	3–4	Controlled
	Romanian deadlift (p.89)	5	5	2	3110
	Leg curl (seated or lying) (pp.68–70)	4	6	2	3110
	Barbell glute bridge or variation (pp.78–81)	4	6	2	3010
	Calf raise (p.82)	4	6	2	3110
WORKOUT 4	Banded biceps curl (p.144)	2	6–8	3–4	Controlled
	Wide-grip vertical pulldown (p.110)	2	6–8	3–4	Controlled
	Barbell bent-over row or variation (pp.116–117)	5	5	2	3110
	Neutral-grip vertical pulldown (p.112)	4	6	2	3110
	Prone bench rear delt raise (p.138)	4	6	2	3010
	DB biceps curl or Machine biceps curl (pp.142–144)	4	6	2	3110
WORKOUT 5	Machine horizontal row (p.116)	2	6–8	3–4	Controlled
	Machine shoulder press (p.126)	2	6–8	3–4	Controlled
	Incline DB bench press (p.98) or Cable chest fly (p.100)	4	6–8	2–3	3010
	DB or Machine shoulder press (pp.126–127)	4	6–8	2–3	3010
	DB lateral raise (p.128)	4	6–8	2–3	3010
	Rope triceps pushdown or variation (pp.150–153)	4	6–8	2–3	3010

STRENGTH ENDURANCE BEGINNER

Also known as muscular-endurance training, this training focuses on using low to moderate loads with shorter rest periods to challenge local muscular endurance.

During these programs, you increase the total work capacity, or the total density of work per session. This style of training can also aid in the development of

muscle and strength and is effective when used in combination with other forms of training or sports. Exercise combinations—known as supersets or giant sets—will help challenge the body to sustain work capacity deeper into fatigue.

Begin each workout by warming up. Where indicated, you can choose a variation of the given exercise.

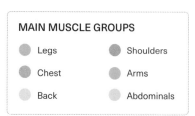

MAIN MUSCLE GROUPS

- Legs
- Chest
- Back
- Shoulders
- Arms
- Abdominals

For all workouts

Any beginner strength-endurance workout uses the following reps, sets, rest between sets, RIR, and tempo guidance however often you're training:

12–15 REPS
3 SETS
(**4** SETS when training **4x** or **5x** a week)
45–60 SECONDS REST
3–4 RIR
CONTROLLED TEMPO

STRENGTH ENDURANCE—3x PER WEEK

	EXERCISE
WORKOUT 1	Leg press (p.58) or DB squat (p.56)
	Leg curl (seated or lying) (pp.68–70)
	DB bench press (p.96) or Push-up (p.95)
	Wide-grip vertical pulldown (p.110) or Pull-up (p.113)
	DB shoulder press (p.127) or DB lateral raise (p.128)
	Alternating V-up crunch (p.171)
WORKOUT 2	Mid-cable chest fly (p.103) or Push-up (p.95)
	Seated leg curl or variation (pp.70–71)
	Neutral-grip horizontal row (p.114)
	Machine shoulder press (p.126) or DB lateral raise (p.128)
	Leg extension or variation (pp.74–77)
	Transverse abdominal ball crunch (p.160)
WORKOUT 3	Leg extension or variation (pp.74–77)
	Neutral-grip vertical pulldown or Chin-up (pp.112–113)
	DB bench press (p.96) or Machine chest fly (p.104)
	Hamstring ball curl (p.72)
	Machine shoulder press (p.126) or Front delt shoulder press (p.135)
	Bicycle crunch (p.171)

STRENGTH ENDURANCE—4x PER WEEK

EXERCISE
WORKOUT 1
Mid-cable chest fly (p.103) or Push-up (p.95)
Leg press (p.58) or DB squat (p.56)
Rope triceps pushdown or variation (pp.150–153)
DB shoulder press (p.127) or DB lateral raise (p.128)
Cable rope crunch (p.166)
WORKOUT 2
Neutral-grip vertical pulldown or Chin-up (pp.112–113)
Seated leg curl or variation (pp.70–71)
DB glute bridge or variation (pp.80–81)
DB biceps curl or variation (pp.142–145)
Calf raise (p.82)
WORKOUT 3
Leg extension or variation (pp.74–77)
DB bench press (p.96) or Push-up (p.95)
DB triceps extension or variation (pp.146–149)
Machine or DB shoulder press (pp.126–127)
Cable rotational oblique twist (p.168)
WORKOUT 4
Neutral-grip horizontal row (p.114)
Seated leg curl or variation (pp.70–71)
DB glute bridge or variation (pp.80–81)
Banded biceps curl (p.144)
Seated calf raise (p.84)

STRENGTH ENDURANCE—5x PER WEEK

EXERCISE
WORKOUT 1
Mid-cable chest fly or variation (pp.102–103)
Wide-grip vertical pulldown (p.110)
DB rear delt fly or variation (pp.136–139)
DB biceps curl or variation (pp.142–145)
Cross-cable triceps pressdown or variation (pp.152–153)
Cable rope crunch or variation (pp.166–167)
WORKOUT 2
Romanian deadlift or variation (pp.88–89)
Leg press (p.58)
DB glute bridge or variation (pp.80–81)
Leg extension (p.74)
Calf raise (p.82)
WORKOUT 3
DB shoulder press (p.127)
DB lateral raise (p.128)
Hammer curl (p.145)
Cross-cable triceps pressdown (p.153)
Cable rotational oblique twist (p.168)
Decline ab crunch (p.167) or Deadbug (p.163)
WORKOUT 4
Horizontal row (p.114) or Barbell bent-over row (p.117)
Wide-grip or Machine vertical pulldown (pp.110–112)
DB bench press (p.96) or Push-up (p.95)
DB bent-over row (p.116)
Chest or back exercise of choice
WORKOUT 5
Leg press (p.58) or DB squat (p.56)
Leg extension or variation (pp.74–77)
Leg curl (seated or lying) (pp.68–70)
DB glute bridge or variation (pp.80–81)
Machine rear delt fly (p.138)
DB lateral raise or variation (pp.128–131)

STRENGTH ENDURANCE ADVANCED

These advanced strength-endurance programs achieve progression mostly through increasing training volume and expanding exercise selection.

These programs build on the beginner strength-endurance training by including a greater number and variety of exercises in each workout. The shorter rest periods used in these workouts, paired as in beginner-level programs with low to moderate loads, further increase the density of work, training your muscles to last longer under stress before you become fatigued.

MAIN MUSCLE GROUPS

- Legs
- Chest
- Back
- Shoulders
- Arms
- Abdominals

For all workouts

Any advanced muscle-building workout uses the following rest between sets and RIR however often you're training:

12–15 REPS

2–3 RIR

**FOR GUIDANCE ON TEMPO
SEE P.202 AND P.204**

Supersets

A superset is a combination of exercises performed one after another. For instance, in a chest press superset with a pulldown, you would perform the chest press reps, rest for the prescribed time, then perform the pulldown reps. This example is an agonist–antagonist superset: it trains opposing muscle groups, saving you time without impacting performance. Other pairings include exercises that work the same body part, upper body–lower body, and agonist–synergist. You do not have to do supersets, but doing so is an effective way to work out.

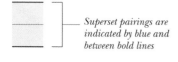

Superset pairings are indicated by blue and between bold lines

STRENGTH ENDURANCE—3x PER WEEK

	EXERCISE	SETS	REST	TEMPO
WORKOUT 1	Hack squat (p.60) or Leg press (p.58)	4	45s	Controlled
	Leg curl (seated or lying) (pp.68–70)	4	45s	Controlled
	DB bench press (p.96) or Mid-cable chest fly (p.103)	4	45s	Controlled
	Vertical pulldown (p.110) or Pull-up (p.113)	4	45s	Controlled
	DB shoulder press (p.127) or DB lateral raise (p.128)	4	45s	Controlled
	Cable rope crunch (p.166)	4	45s	Controlled
WORKOUT 2	Mid-cable chest fly (p.103) or Push-up (p.95)	4	45s	Controlled
	Leg curl or variation (pp.68–71)	4	45s	Controlled
	Neutral-grip horizontal row (p.114)	4	45s	Controlled
	Machine shoulder press (p.126) or DB lateral raise (p.128)	4	45s	Controlled
	Leg extension or variation (p.74–77)	4	45s	Controlled
	TVA ball crunch (p.160)	4	45s	Controlled
WORKOUT 3	Leg extension or variation (pp.74–77)	4	45s	Controlled
	Machine vertical pulldown (p.112) or Chin-up (p.113)	4	45s	Controlled
	DB bench press (p.96) or Machine chest fly (p.104)	4	45s	Controlled
	Seated leg curl (p.70)	4	45s	Controlled
	Machine shoulder press (p.126) or Front delt shoulder press (p.135)	4	45s	Controlled
	Cable rotational oblique twist (p.168)	4	45s	Controlled

STRENGTH ENDURANCE—4x PER WEEK

WORKOUT 1 / WORKOUT 2

EXERCISE	SETS	REST	TEMPO
Mid-cable or Machine chest fly (pp.103–104)	3	30s	3010
Leg press (p.58) or DB squat (p.56)	3	45–60s	3010
DB bench press (p.96) or Push-up (p.95)	3	30s	3010
Leg extension (p.74)	3	45–60s	3010
Rope triceps pushdown or variation (pp.150–153)	3	30s	3010
DB shoulder press (p.127)	3	45–60s	3010
DB triceps extension (p.146)	3	30s	3010
DB lateral raise (p.128)	3	45–60s	3010
Cable rope crunch (p.166)	4	30–45s	Controlled
Neutral-grip vertical pulldown or Chin-up (pp.112–113)	3	30s	3010
Seated leg curl or variation (pp.70–71)	3	45–60s	3010
Neutral-grip horizontal row (p.114)	3	30s	3010
Romanian deadlift (p.89)	3	45–60s	3010
DB glute bridge or variation (pp.80–81)	3	30s	3010
DB biceps curl (p.142) or Banded biceps curl (p.144)	3	45–60s	3010
Standing cable glute kickback (p.80)	3	30s	3010
Hammer curl (p.145)	3	45–60s	3010
Calf raise (p.82)	4	30–45s	Controlled

WORKOUT 3 / WORKOUT 4

EXERCISE	SETS	REST	TEMPO
Leg extension or variation (pp.74–77)	3	30s	3010
DB bench press (p.96) or Push-up (p.95)	3	45–60s	3010
DB goblet squat (p.56) or Stationary lunge with DBs (p.62)	3	30s	3010
Mid-cable chest fly or variation (pp.102–103)	3	45–60s	3010
DB triceps extension or variation (pp.146–149)	3	30s	3010
Machine shoulder press or DB shoulder press (pp.126–127)	3	45–60s	3010
Cross-cable triceps pressdown (p.153)	3	30s	3010
DB lateral raise or variation (pp.128–131)	3	45–60s	3010
Side plank with rotation (p.158)	4	30–45s	Controlled
Neutral-grip horizontal row (p.114)	3	30s	3010
Romanian deadlift (p.89)	3	45–60s	3010
Wide-grip vertical pulldown (p.110) or Pull-up (p.113)	3	30s	3010
Seated leg curl or variation (pp.70–71)	3	45–60s	3010
Standing cable glute kickback (p.80)	3	30s	3010
Hammer curl (p.145)	3	45–60s	3010
DB glute bridge or variation (pp.80–81)	3	30s	3010
DB biceps curl (p.142) or Banded biceps curl (p.144)	3	45–60s	3010
Seated calf raise (p.84)	4	30–45s	Controlled

» STRENGTH ENDURANCE ADVANCED

STRENGTH ENDURANCE—5x PER WEEK

	EXERCISE	SETS	REST	TEMPO
WORKOUT 1	Mid-cable chest fly or variation (pp.102–103)	3	30s	3010
	Wide-grip vertical pulldown (p.110)	3	45–60s	3010
	DB bench press or variation (pp.96–99)	3	30s	3010
	DB bent-over row or variation (pp.116–117)	3	45–60s	3010
	Machine rear delt fly or variation (pp.138–139)	4	30s	3010
	DB biceps curl or variation (pp.142–145)	4	45–60s	3010
	Cross-cable triceps pressdown (p.153)	4	30s	3010
	Cable rope crunch or variation (pp.166–167)	4	45–60s	3010
WORKOUT 2	Romanian deadlift (p.89)	3	30s	3010
	Leg press (p.58)	3	45–60s	3010
	Leg curl or variation (pp.68–71)	3	30s	3010
	Leg extension or variation (pp.74–77)	3	45–60s	3010
	DB glute bridge or variation (pp.80–81)	3	30s	3010
	Back foot elevated split squat (p.64)	3	45–60s	3010
	Calf raise (p.82)	4	30–45s	Controlled
WORKOUT 3	DB shoulder press or variation (pp.126–127)	3	30s	3010
	DB lateral raise (p.128)	3	45–60s	3010
	Hammer curl (p.145)	3	30s	3010
	Cross-cable triceps pressdown (p.153)	3	45–60s	3010
	Cable upright row (p.121)	3	30s	3010
	Decline ab crunch (p.167)	3	45–60s	3010
	Cable or Banded front raise (pp.134–135)	3	30s	3010
	Cable rotational oblique twist or variation (pp.168–171)	3	45–60s	3010

MAIN MUSCLE GROUPS

- Legs
- Chest
- Back
- Shoulders
- Arms
- Abdominals

	EXERCISE	SETS	REST	TEMPO
WORKOUT 4	Barbell bent-over row (p.117)	3	30s	3010
	Machine vertical pulldown (p.112)	3	45–60s	3010
	DB bench press (p.96) or Push-up (p.95)	3	30s	3010
	Neutral-grip horizontal row (p.114)	3	45–60s	3010
	High–low cable chest fly or variation (pp.100–103)	3	30s	3010
	Dumbbell bent-over row (p.116)	3	45–60s	3010
	Chest or back variation of choice	4	30–45s	Controlled
WORKOUT 5	Leg press (p.58)	3	30s	3010
	Walking lunge with DBs (p.65)	3	45–60s	3010
	Leg curl (p.68)	3	30s	3010
	DB glute bridge or variation (pp.80–81)	3	45–60s	3010
	Prone bench rear delt raise (p.138)	3	30s	3010
	DB lateral raise or variation (pp.128–131)	3	45–60s	3010
	TVA ball crunch (p.160)	3	30s	3010
	Cable rope crunch (p.166)	3	45–60s	3010

GLOSSARY

1 rep maximum (1RM) The maximum amount of weight a person can lift during one repetition of an exercise; training intensity is measured by expressing the load used as a percentage of this amount.

Abdominals (abs) A group of muscles in the torso consisting of the rectus abdominis, the external abdominal obliques, the internal abdominal obliques, and the transverse abdominis.

Abduction The action of moving a limb away from the midline of the body.

Actin A protein that interacts with myosin to cause muscle contraction.

Adduction The action of moving a limb toward the midline of the body.

Adductors A group of muscles that are used to draw the thighs toward the midline, consisting of the adductor longus, the adductor brevis, the adductor magnus, the pectineus, and the gracilis.

Agonist A muscle that, opposing another muscle, causes a movement to happen.

Amino acids Organic compounds that combine to form proteins; they are necessary for a number of processes in the body.

Antagonist A muscle that acts as the opposing force in muscle contraction or relaxation.

Anterior Positioned at the front.

ATP Adenosine triphosphate; a molecule that is the energy currency of a cell.

Barbell A piece of exercise equipment consisting of a long bar with weights at either end.

Bilateral On both sides of the body simultaneously.

Cable pulley An exercise machine consisting of an adjustable pulley system and a cable with a handle.

Carbohydrates Naturally occurring chemical substances that contain carbon, hydrogen, and oxygen; they are the primary source of energy when stored in the body.

Cluster set A set that is broken up into subsets with additional short rest periods in between them; the reps within a cluster set can be performed at greater intensity thanks to the additional rest intervals.

Coactivation When multiple muscles activate simultaneously.

Concentric contraction Muscle shortening in response to a load, as in lifting a weight in a biceps curl.

Deadlift An exercise that involves extending at the knees and/or hips to lift a weight from the ground.

Deep (of muscles) Further in from the skin.

Deltoid (delts) A muscle of the shoulder.

Dropsets Sets performed consecutively with incremental reductions in load.

Dumbbell A type of exercise equipment consisting of a short bar with weights at either end; usually used in a pair.

Eccentric contraction Muscle lengthening in response to a load, as in lowering a weight in a biceps curl.

Elbow flexors A group of muscles that are used to flex the arm at the elbow, consisting of the biceps brachii, the brachialis, and the brachioradialis.

Extension A movement that increases the angle of a joint.

EZ bar A type of barbell with a waved bar.

Fascicle A bundle of muscle fibers.

Fat A nutrient with several necessary functions in the body, including protecting internal organs and nerves and assisting the absorption of vitamins.

Fatigue management The process of keeping track of and adjusting the amount of fatigue experienced during training.

Flexion A movement that decreases the angle of a joint.

Form The manner in which an exercise is performed; good form maximizes the safety and benefits of the exercise.

Glucose A simple sugar that is the body's preferred energy source.

Glutes A group of muscles in the buttocks consisting of the gluteus maximus, the gluteus medius, and the gluteus minimus.

Glycogen A carbohydrate formed of connected glucose molecules that is used by the body to store glucose primarily in skeletal muscles and the liver.

Hip extensors A group of muscles that are used to extend the hips and draw the thighs back, consisting of the glutes, the adductor magnus, and the hamstrings (the biceps femoris, the semitendinosus, and the semimembranosus).

Hypertrophy Muscle growth due to an increase in the size of cells.

Isometric contraction When a muscle is activated, but instead of lengthening or shortening, it is held at a constant length.

Isotonic contraction Muscle engagement where the muscle changes length; can be either eccentric or concentric.

Lateral Positioned at the side(s).

Latissimus dorsi (lats) A muscle of the back.

Load The amount of weight used in an exercise.

Metabolic stress The accumulation of metabolites (such as lactate) in muscles due to exercise.

Muscle building Training to promote muscle growth.

Myosin A protein that interacts with actin to cause muscle contraction.

Neutral grip Holding a weight, cable, and so on with the wrists not rotated so the palms face each other.

Neutral spine Position of optimal load distribution for the spine; maintains the natural curves of the spine.

Pectorals (pecs) A group of muscles in the chest, consisting of the pectoralis major and the pectoralis minor.

Posterior Positioned at the back.

Pronated grip Holding a weight, cable, and so on with the wrists rotated so the palms face downward or away from you.

Prone Lying on your front.

Protein A molecule made up of amino acids; dietary protein is necessary for life and bodily maintenance.

Quadriceps (quads) A group of muscles in the thigh, consisting of the rectus femoris, the vastus medialis, the vastus lateralis, and the vastus intermedius.

Range of motion The extent of possible movement of a joint.

Repetition (rep) An instance of performing the complete motion of an exercise.

Resistance An external force against which muscles contract, such as weight.

Rhomboids A group of muscles in the upper back, consisting of the rhomboid minor and the rhomboid major.

RIR Reps in reserve; a measure of the difficulty of a set that refers to the number of further reps that the person could have performed before giving way to fatigue.

Sarcomere The basic functional unit of contraction of a muscle fiber.

Semisupinated grip Holding a weight, cable, and so on with the wrists partly rotated so the palms face diagonally upward and inward; halfway between a neutral and a supinated grip.

Set A combined group of consecutive repetitions of an exercise performed for a desired or prescribed number of repetitions.

Skeletal muscle Striated muscle tissue connected to the skeletal system that allows for movement.

Strength The amount of force a muscle or muscle group can produce.

Strength endurance Also known as muscular endurance; the ability of muscles to support load continuously over time.

Stress Mechanical, metabolic, or psychological demands placed on the body.

Superficial (of muscles) Closer to the skin.

Superset A combination of sets of different exercises performed sequentially.

Supinated grip Holding a weight, cable, and so on with the wrists rotated so the palms face upward or toward you.

Supine Lying on your back.

Synergist A muscle that acts around a joint to support the action of an agonist muscle.

Tempo The rhythm with which exercises are performed during sets.

Tendon A fibrous cord made up of collagen that attaches muscle to bone.

Training intensity The amount of load used during an exercise, normally expressed as a percentage of 1 rep maximum.

Training volume The amount of exercise or work performed over a given period of time.

Trapezius A muscle of the upper back.

Unilateral On one side of the body.

INDEX

BIBLIOGRAPHY

6–7 G. Ashdown-Franks et al., "The evidence for physical activity in the management of major mental illnesses", *Curr Opin Psychiatry* 32, no. 5 (2019), 375–380. K. I. Erickson et al., "Exercise training increases size of hippocampus and improves memory", *Proc Natl Acad Sci USA* 108, no. 7 (2011), 3017–3022. F. Herold et al., "Functional and/or structural brain changes in response to resistance exercises and resistance training lead to cognitive improvements", *Eur Rev Aging Phys Act* 16, no. 10 (2019). J. Mcleod et al., "Resistance Exercise Training as a Primary Countermeasure to Age-Related Chronic Disease", *Front Physiol* 10 (2019), 645. D. Tavoian et al., "Perspective: Pragmatic Exercise Recommendations for Older Adults", *Front Physiol* 11 (2020), 799. J. M. Northey et al., "Exercise interventions for cognitive function in adults older than 50", *Br J Sports Med* 52, no. 3 (2018), 154–160. F. J. Penedo and J. R. Dahn, "Exercise and well-being: a review of mental and physical health benefits associated with physical activity", *Curr Opin Psychiatry* 18, no. 2 (2005), 189–193. S. Walker, "Neural Adaptations to Strength Training", in M. Schumann and B. Rønnestad (eds), *Concurrent Aerobic and Strength Training*, Cham, Springer, 2019. J. Xiao (ed), *Physical Exercise for Human Health*, Singapore, Springer Singapore, 2020. **8–9** A. D. Faigenbaum et al., "Youth resistance training: updated position statement paper from the national strength and conditioning association", *J Strength Cond Res* 23, no. 5 (2009), S60–S79. J. Mcleod et al., "Resistance Exercise Training as a Primary Countermeasure to Age-Related Chronic Disease" (2019). G. Nuckols, "The Effects of Biological Sex on Fatigue During and Recovery from Resistance Exercise" (2019). J. M. Northey et al., "Exercise interventions for cognitive function in adults older than 50" (2018). F. J. Penedo and J. R. Dahn, "Exercise and well-being" (2005). B. Schoenfeld, *Science and Development of Muscle Hypertrophy*, 2nd ed., Champaign, IL, Human Kinetics, 2020. D. Tavoian et al., "Perspective: Pragmatic Exercise Recommendations for Older Adults: The Case for Emphasizing Resistance Training" (2020). J. Xiao (ed), *Physical Exercise for Human Health*, Springer Singapore, 2020. **12–13** T. W. Nesser (ed), *The Professional's Guide to Strength & Conditioning: Safe and Effective Principles for Maximizing Athletic Performance*, Provo, UT, BYU Academic Publishing, 2019. **14–15** G. Haff and N. T. Triplett (eds), *Essentials of Strength Training and Conditioning*, 4th ed., Champaign, IL, Human Kinetics, 2016. M. L. Latash, "Muscle coactivation: definitions, mechanisms, and functions", *J Neurophysiol* 120, no. 1 (2018), 88–104. J. G. Betts et al., *Anatomy and Physiology*, Houston, TX, OpenStax, 2013. B. Schoenfeld, *Science and Development of Muscle Hypertrophy*, 2020. **16–17** B. R. MacIntosh et al., *Skeletal Muscle: Form and Function*, Champaign, IL, Human Kinetics, 2006. T. W. Nesser (ed), *The Professional's Guide to Strength & Conditioning*, 2019. **18–19** R. Csapo et al., "Skeletal Muscle Extracellular Matrix – What Do We Know About Its Composition, Regulation, and Physiological Roles?", *Front Physiol* 11 (2020). C. T. Haun et al., "A Critical Evaluation of the Biological Construct Skeletal Muscle Hypertrophy", *Front Physiol* 10 (2019). E. Helms, A Progression Framework for Hypertrophy, MASS Research Review, July 2020. S. K. Powers et al., "Disease-Induced Skeletal Muscle Atrophy and Fatigue", *Med Sci Sport Exer* 48, no. 11 (2016), 2307–2319. R. A. Saxton and D. M. Sabatini, "mTOR Signaling in Growth, Metabolism, and Disease", *Cell* 169, no. 2 (2017), 361–371. B. Schoenfeld, *Science and Development of Muscle Hypertrophy*, 2020. T. Snijders et al., "Satellite cells in human skeletal muscle plasticity", *Front Physiol* 6 (2015). J. Xiao (ed), *Physical Exercise for Human Health*, Springer Singapore, 2020. **20–23**

R. J. Bloch and H. Gonzalez-Serratos, "Lateral force transmission across costameres in skeletal muscle", *Exerc Sport Sci Rev* 31, no. 2 (2003), 73–78. C. A. Goodman, "The Role of mTORC1 in Regulating Protein Synthesis and Skeletal Muscle Mass in Response to Various Mechanical Stimuli", *Rev Physiol Bioch P* 166 (2013), 43–95. T. A. Hornberger, "Mechanotransduction and the regulation of mTORC1 signaling in skeletal muscle", *Int J Biochem Cell B* 43, no. 9 (2011), 1267–1276. T. W. Nesser (ed), *The Professional's Guide to Strength & Conditioning*, 2019. B. Schoenfeld, *Science and Development of Muscle Hypertrophy*, 2020. **24–25** N. H. Hart et al., "Mechanical basis of bone strength", *J Musculoskeletal Neuronal Interactions* 17, no. 3 (2017), 114–139. H. P. Hirschfeld et al., "Osteosarcopenia: where bone, muscle, and fat collide", *Osteoporosis Int* 28, no. 10 (2017), 2781–2790. S. K. Powers and E. T. Howley, *Exercise Physiology: Theory and Application to Fitness and Performance*, 10th ed., New York, NY, McGraw Hill Education, 2018. R. Nikander et al., "Targeted exercise against osteoporosis", *BMC Medicine* 8, no. 1 (2010). **26–27** R.S. Behnke, Kinetic Anatomy, 3rd ed., Champaign, IL, Human Kinetics, 2016. T. W. Nesser (ed), *The Professional's Guide to Strength & Conditioning*, 2019. D. A. Neumann et al., *Kinesiology of the Musculoskeletal System: Foundations for Rehabilitation*, 3rd ed., Amsterdam, Elsevier, 2016. **28–29** O. K. Berg et al., "Maximal strength training increases muscle force generating capacity and the anaerobic ATP synthesis flux without altering the cost of contraction in elderly", *Exp Gerontol* 111 (2018), 154–161. G. Haff and N. T. Triplett (eds), *Essentials of Strength Training and Conditioning*, 2016. T. W. Nesser (ed), *The Professional's Guide to Strength & Conditioning*, 2019. **30–31** B. M. Roberts et al., "Nutritional Recommendations for Physique Athletes", *J Hum Kinet* 7, no. 1 (2020), 79–108. B. Pramuková et al., "Current knowledge about sports nutrition", *Australas Med J* 4, no. 3 (2011), 107–110. T. W. Nesser (ed), *The Professional's Guide to Strength & Conditioning*, 2019. B. Schoenfeld, *Science and Development of Muscle Hypertrophy*, 2020. **32–33** E. Derbyshire, "Micronutrient Intakes of British Adults Across Mid-Life", *Front Nutrition* 5 (2018). B. Misner, "Food Alone May Not Provide Sufficient Micronutrients for Preventing Deficiency", *J Int Soc Sport Nutr* 3, no. 1 (2006), 51–55. B. M. Roberts et al., "Nutritional Recommendations for Physique Athletes" (2020). R. Jäger et al., "International Society of Sports Nutrition Position Stand: protein and exercise", *J Int Soc Sport Nutr* 14, no. 20 (2017). J. Iraki et al., "Nutrition Recommendations for Bodybuilders in the Off-Season", *Sports (Basel)* 7, no. 7 (2019), 154. T. W. Nesser (ed), *The Professional's Guide to Strength & Conditioning*, 2019. B. Schoenfeld, *Science and Development of Muscle Hypertrophy*, 2020. E. T. Trexler et al., "Metabolic adaptation to weight loss", *J Int Soc Sport Nutr* 11, no. 1 (2014), 7. **34–35** M. J. Arnaud and T. D. Noakes, "Should humans be encouraged to drink water to excess?", *Eur J Clin Nutr* 65, no. 7 (2011), 875–876. S. M. Arent et al., "Nutrient Timing: A Garage Door of Opportunity?" *Nutrients* 12, no. 7 (2020), 1948. J. Berardi et al., *The Essentials of Sport and Exercise Nutrition: Certification Manual*, 3rd ed., Toronto, Precision Nutrition Inc., 2017. "Calcium: Fact Sheet for Health Professionals", NIH Office of Dietary Supplements [web article], 26 March 2020, ods.od.nih.gov/factsheets/Calcium-HealthProfessional/. D. Liska et al., "Narrative Review of Hydration and Selected Health Outcomes in the General Population", *Nutrients* 11, no. 1 (2019), 70. E. Jéquier and F. Constant, "Water as an essential nutrient: the physiological basis of hydration", *Eur J Clin Nutr* 64, no. 2 (2010), 115–123.

P. R. Harris et al., "Fluid type influences acute hydration and muscle performance recovery in human subjects", *J Int Soc Sport Nutr* 16, no. 15 (2019). J. McKendry et al., "Nutritional Supplements to Support Resistance Exercise in Countering the Sarcopenia of Aging", *Nutrients* 12, no. 7 (2020), 2057. B. J. Schoenfeld and A. A. Aragon, "How much protein can the body use in a single meal for muscle-building?", *J Int Soc Sport Nutr* 15, no. 10 (2018). T. Snijders et al., "The Impact of Pre-sleep Protein Ingestion on the Skeletal Muscle Adaptive Response to Exercise in Humans", *Front Nutrition* 6, no. 17 (2019). J. Trommelen and L.J. van Loon, "Pre-Sleep Protein Ingestion to Improve the Skeletal Muscle Adaptive Response to Exercise Training", *Nutrients* 8, no. 12 (2016), 763. B. Schoenfeld, *Science and Development of Muscle Hypertrophy*, 2020. **36–37** A. Banaszek et al., "The Effects of Whey vs. Pea Protein on Physical Adaptations Following 8 Weeks of High-Intensity Functional Training (HIFT)", *Sports (Basel)* 7, no. 1 (2019), 12. I. Berrazaga et al., "The Role of the Anabolic Properties of Plant- versus Animal-Based Protein Sources in Supporting Muscle Mass Maintenance", *Nutrients* 11, no. 8 (2019), 1825. D. Rogerson, "Vegan diets: practical advice for athletes and exercisers", *J Int Soc Sport Nutr* 14, no. 36 (2017). F. Mariotti and C.D. Gardner, "Dietary Protein and Amino Acids in Vegetarian Diets", *Nutrients* 11, no. 11 (2019), 2661. B. Schoenfeld, *Science and Development of Muscle Hypertrophy*, 2020. S. H. M. Gorissen et al., "Protein content and amino acid composition of commercially available plant-based protein isolates", *Amino Acids* 50, no. 12 (2018), 1685–1695. **38–39** B. K. Barry and R. G. Carson, "The consequences of resistance training for movement control in older adults", *J Gerontol A Biol Sci Med Sci* 59, no. 7 (2004), 730–754. K. I. Erickson et al., "Exercise training increases size of hippocampus and improves memory" (2011). J. M. Northey et al., "Exercise interventions for cognitive function in adults older than 50" (2018). F. Herold et al., "Functional and/or structural brain changes in response to resistance exercises and resistance training" (2019). Y. Netz, "Is There a Preferred Mode of Exercise for Cognition Enhancement in Older Age?", *Front Med (Lausanne)* 6, no. 57 (2019). N. J. Gates et al., "Study of Mental Activity and Regular Training (SMART) in at-risk individuals", *BMC Geriatrics* 11, no. 1 (2011). A. Törpel et al., "Strengthening the Brain – Is Resistance Training with Blood Flow Restriction an Effective Strategy for Cognitive Improvement?", *J Clin Med* 7, no. 10 (2018), 337. S. Walker, "Neural Adaptations to Strength Training", in *Concurrent Aerobic and Strength Training*, 2019. **40–41** G. Ashdown-Franks et al., "The evidence for physical activity in the management of major mental illnesses" (2019). U. Arnautovska et al., "Applying the Integrated Behavior Change Model to Understanding Physical Activity Among Older Adults", *J Sport Exer Psychol* 39, no. 1 (2017), 43–55. R. Brand and B. Cheval, "Theories to Explain Exercise Motivation and Physical Inactivity", *Front Psychol* 10 (2019), 1147. T. J. H. Bovend'Eerdt et al., "Writing SMART rehabilitation goals and achieving goal attainment scaling", *Clin Rehabil* 23, no. 4 (2009), 352–361. J. Clear, *Atomic Habits: an Easy & Proven Way to Build Good Habits & Break Bad Ones*, New York, NY, Penguin Random House LLC, 2018. K. I. Erickson et al., "Exercise training increases size of hippocampus and improves memory" (2011). K. Geller et al., "Intrinsic and Extrinsic Motives Support Adults' Regular Physical Activity Maintenance", *Sports Med Int Open* 2, no. 3 (2018), E62–E66. A. W. Kruglanski and E. Szumowska, "Habitual Behavior Is Goal-Driven", *Perspect Psychol Sci* 15, no. 5 (2020), 1256–1271. H. H. Lee et al., "The Exercise–affect–adherence pathway: An evolutionary perspective", *Front Psychol* 7, no. 1285 (2016). E. K. Olander et al., "What are the most effective techniques in changing obese individuals' physical activity self-efficacy and behaviour", *Int J Behav Nutr Phys Act* 10, no. 29 (2013). F. J. Penedo and J. R. Dahn, "Exercise and well-being" (2005). B. S. McEwen, "Physiology and neurobiology of stress and adaptation", *Physiol Rev* 87, no. 3 (2007), 873–904. J. M. Northey et al., "Exercise interventions for cognitive function in adults older than 50" (2018).

N. Ntoumanis et al., "A meta-analysis of self-determination theory-informed intervention studies in the health domain", *Health Psychol Rev* (2020), 1–31. H. Raison et al., "A systematic review of interventions using cue-automaticity to improve the uptake of preventive healthcare in adults", *Community Dent Health* 35, no. 1 (2018), 37–46. **68–69** D. Landin et al., "Actions of Two Bi-Articular Muscles of the Lower Extremity", *J Clin Med Res* 8, no. 7 (2016), 489–494. **80–81** D. A. Neumann et al., *Kinesiology of the Musculoskeletal System*, 2017. **98–99** R. Paine and M. L. Voight, "The role of the scapula", *Int J Sports Phys Ther* 8, no. 5 (2013), 617–629. **112–113** J. A. Dickie et al., "Electromyographic analysis of muscle activation during pull-up variations", *J Electromyogr Kinesiol* 32 (2017), 30–36. **172–173** R. Aicale et al., "Overuse injuries in sport", *J Orthop Surg Res* 13, no. 1 (2018). J. W. Keogh and P. W. Winwood, "The Epidemiology of Injuries Across the Weight-Training Sports", *Sports Med* 47, no. 3 (2017), 479–501. **176–177** P. M. Clarkson et al., "Muscle function after exercise-induced muscle damage and rapid adaptation", *Med Sci Sports Exerc* 24, no. 5 (1992), 512–520. K. Cheung et al., "Delayed onset muscle soreness: treatment strategies and performance factors", *Sports Med* 33, no. 2 (2003), 145–164. D. Chapman et al., "Greater muscle damage induced by fast versus slow velocity eccentric exercise", *Int J Sports Med* 27, no. 8 (2006), 591–598. D. A. Connolly et al., "Treatment and prevention of delayed onset muscle soreness", *J Strength Cond Res* 17, no. 1 (2003), 197–208. T. Mori et al., "Stretch speed-dependent myofiber damage and functional deficits in rat skeletal muscle induced by lengthening contraction", *Physiol Rep* 2, no. 11 (2014), E12213. **178–183** E. Bass, "Tendinopathy: Why the Difference Between Tendinitis and Tendinosis Matters", *Int J Ther Massage Bodywork* 5, no. 1 (2012), 14–17. C. M. Bleakley et al., "PRICE needs updating, should we call the POLICE?", *Br J Sports Med* 46, no. 4 (2011), 220–221. J. M. Bump and L. Lewis, "Patellofemoral Syndrome", in *StatPearls*, Treasure Island, FL, StatPearls Publishing, 2020. J. Charnoff and U. Naqvi, "Tendinosis (Tendinitis)", in *StatPearls*, Treasure Island, FL, StatPearls Publishing, 2020. T. L. Fernandes et al., "Muscle Injury – Physiopathology, Diagnosis, Treatment and Clinical Presentation", *Rev Bras Ortop* 46, no. 3 (2015), 247–255. M. Gupton et al., "Anatomy, Hinge Joints", in *StatPearls*, Treasure Island, FL, StatPearls Publishing, 2020. "Tennis elbow: Strengthening and stretching exercises", InformedHealth.org [web article], Cologne, Institute for Quality and Efficiency in Health Care (IQWiG), 30 May 2018, https://www.ncbi.nlm.nih.gov/books/NBK506995/. D. A. Neumann et al., *Kinesiology of the Musculoskeletal System*, 2017. **184–185** B. S. Baker et al., "Does Blood Flow Restriction Therapy in Patients Older Than Age 50 Result in Muscle Hypertrophy, Increased Strength, or Greater Physical Function?", *Clin Orthop Relat Res* 478, no. 3 (2010), 593–606. Q. Henoch, *ClinicalAthlete*, www.clinicalathlete.com, 2020. L. Hughes et al., "Blood flow restriction training in clinical musculoskeletal rehabilitation", *Br J Sports Med* 51, no. 13 (2017), 1003–1011. W. Kraemer et al., "Recovery from injury in sport", *Sports Health* 1, no. 5 (2009), 392–395. S. D. Patterson et al., "Blood Flow Restriction Exercise", *Front Physiol* 10 (2019), 533. **186–187** H. Chaabene et al., "Acute Effects of Static Stretching on Muscle Strength and Power", *Front Physiol* 10 (2019), 1468. T. W. Nesser (ed), *The Professional's Guide to Strength & Conditioning*, 2019. J. L. Nuzzo, "The Case for Retiring Flexibility as a Major Component of Physical Fitness", *Sports Med* 50, no. 5 (2020), 853–870. B. Van Hooren and J. M. Peake, "Do We Need a Cool-Down After Exercise?", *Sports Med* 48, no. 7 (2018), 1575–1595. T. Wiewelhove et al., "A Meta-Analysis of the Effects of Foam Rolling on Performance and Recovery", *Front Physiol* 10 (2019), 376. **198–201** G. Haff and N. T. Triplett (eds), *Essentials of Strength Training and Conditioning*, 2016. E. Helms, *A Progression Framework for Hypertrophy*, MASS Research Review, July 2020. E. Helms et al., *The Muscle and Strength Pyramid: Training*, 2nd ed., 2019. T. W. Nesser (ed), *The Professional's Guide to Strength & Conditioning*, 2019. B. Schoenfeld, *Science and Development* of Muscle Hypertrophy, 2020. M. C. Zourdos et al., "Novel Resistance Training-Specific Rating of Perceived Exertion Scale Measuring Repetitions in Reserve", *J Strength Cond Res* 30, no. 1 (2016), 267–275. **206–207** G. Haff and N. T. Triplett (eds), *Essentials of Strength Training and Conditioning*, 2016. E. Helms et al., *The Muscle and Strength Pyramid: Training*, 2019. **210–211** G. Haff and N. T. Triplett (eds), *Essentials of Strength Training and Conditioning*, 2016. J. A. Mettler and L. Griffin, "Muscular endurance training and motor unit firing patterns during fatigue", *Exp Brain Res* 234, no. 1 (2016), 267–276.

ABOUT THE AUTHOR

Austin Current, BSc, CSCS, CISSN, is a fitness coach and educator. He holds a Bachelor's Degree in Exercise Science and is a National Strength and Conditioning Association Certified Strength Coach Specialist (NSCA-CSCS) as well as a Certified Sports Nutritionist from the International Society of Sports Nutrition (CISSN). He is the co-owner of Physique Development Consulting, LLC (physiquedevelopment.com), and coaches clients in person and online from all over the world. Austin has helped run seminars around North America and Europe since early 2018, teaching anatomy, exercise execution, biomechanics, nutrition, and program design. He has also had a successful competitive career as a natural physique bodybuilder, earning his professional status in the International Federation of Bodybuilding (IFBB) in 2014 at age 20, as the second-youngest male in the organization's history. In his work with clients and personal trainers around the globe, he has been recognized for his ability to break down complex topics into digestible information, and for merging results with the learning experience in a way that educates and empowers.

For more about Austin, head to **www.CoachAustinCurrent.com**, or find **@austincurrent_** on Instagram.

ACKNOWLEDGMENTS

Author acknowledgments

Writing this book has been one of the most challenging and rewarding experiences of my professional life. Every coach and educator owes immense credit and thanks for those who have come before us, paving the way to the information we get to research, assimilate, make our own, and eventually share.

I first want to thank my amazing wife, KaSandra, for her patience, understanding, and encouragement. Thank you and I love you. I want to thank my wonderful and supportive parents, Kelly, Frank, Keith, and Michele, without whom much of what I've accomplished would not have been possible. Your commitment to giving me every opportunity will never be forgotten. Thanks to my loving and supportive grandparents, Ted and Maureen. You have been a guiding light in my life and I have so much to thank you for. And to my brother, Zach: you have always had my back and I love you for that.

Thanks to my colleagues, Alex and Sue, for their patience during this lengthy and demanding process. I owe my good friend, Miguel Blacutt, for his time and effort during the writing of this book. His feedback was invaluable.

I want to thank Miranda Card for her help in the psychology section. Thank you to N1 Education for years of education on program design, specifically Adam Miller for his help in the training program section of this book. Thank you to Jarrad Griffin and the team at PRIME Fitness for their hospitality while I captured reference images for Chapter 2; they made the process of getting the 1,000+ images so much easier! Thank you to Dr. Cody Haun and Dr. Brandon Roberts for help with reference materials and information.

Lastly, thank you to the entire DK team: Nikki, Alastair, Arran, Clare, Megan, Karen, and more. Without you, this book would never have been possible. I am so grateful that you gave me this opportunity.

Publisher acknowledgments

DK would like to thank Kiron Gill for editorial assistance, Constance Novis for proofreading, and Marie Lorimer for providing the index.

Picture credits